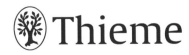

The Nose—Revision & Reconstruction

A Manual and Casebook

Hans Behrbohm, MD, PhD
Professor
Department of Otorhinolaryngology
  and Facial Plastic Surgery
Park-Klinik Weissensee
Academic Teaching Hospital of the Charité University Hospital
Berlin, Germany

With contributions by
Johanna Brehm, MD, PhD
Walter Briedigkeit, MD, PhD†
Jacqueline Eichhorn-Sens, MD, PhD
Holger Gassner, MD, PhD, FACS
Wolfgang Gubisch, MD, PhD
Thomas Hildebrandt, MD, PhD
Joachim Quetz, MD, PhD

Forewords by
M. Eugene Tardy, MD, FACS
Claus Walter, MD, PhD

1052 illustrations

Thieme
Stuttgart • New York • Delhi • Rio de Janeiro

Library of Congress Cataloging-in-Publication Data

Behrbohm, Hans, author.
The nose—revision & reconstruction / Hans Behrbohm.
    p. ; cm.
Includes bibliographical references and index.
ISBN 978-3-13-143591-0 — ISBN 978-3-13-150511-8 (eISBN)
I. Title.
[DNLM: 1. Rhinoplasty—methods. 2. Nose—surgery. WV 312]
RD119.5.N67
617.5′230592—dc23   2014036178

Important note: Medicine is an ever-changing science undergoing continual development. Research and clinical experience are continually expanding our knowledge, in particular our knowledge of proper treatment and drug therapy. Insofar as this book mentions any dosage or application, readers may rest assured that the authors, editors, and publishers have made every effort to ensure that such references are in accordance with the state of knowledge at the time of production of the book.

Nevertheless, this does not involve, imply, or express any guarantee or responsibility on the part of the publishers in respect to any dosage instructions and forms of applications stated in the book. Every user is requested to examine carefully the manufacturers' leaflets accompanying each drug and to check, if necessary in consultation with a physician or specialist, whether the dosage sche- dules mentioned therein or the contraindications stated by the manufacturers differ from the statements made in the present book. Such examination is particularly important with drugs that are either rarely used or have been newly released on the market. Every dosage schedule or every form of application used is entirely at the user's own risk and responsibility. The authors and publishers request every user to report to the publishers any discrepancies or inaccuracies noticed. If errors in this work are found after publication, errata will be posted at www.thieme.com on the product description page.

Some of the product names, patents, and registered designs referred to in this book are in fact registered trademarks or proprietary names even though specific reference to this fact is not always made in the text. Therefore, the appearance of a name without designation as proprietary is not to be construed as a representation by the publisher that it is in the public domain.

© 2016 by Georg Thieme Verlag KG

Thieme Publishers Stuttgart
Rüdigerstrasse 14, 70469 Stuttgart, Germany
+49 [0]711 8931 421, customerservice@thieme.de

Thieme Publishers New York
333 Seventh Avenue, New York, NY 10001 USA
+1 800 782 3488, customerservice@thieme.com

Thieme Publishers Delhi
A-12, Second Floor, Sector-2, Noida-201301
Uttar Pradesh, India
+91 120 45 566 00, customerservice@thieme.in

Thieme Publishers Rio, Thieme Publicações Ltda.
Edifício Rodolpho de Paoli, 25º andar
Av. Nilo Peçanha, 50 – Sala 2508
Rio de Janeiro 20020-906 Brasil
+55 21 3172 2297 / +55 21 3172 1896

Cover design: Thieme Publishing Group
Typesetting by Prairie Papers

Printed in China by Everbest Printing Ltd   5 4 3 2 1

ISBN 978-3-13-143591-0

Also available as an e-book:
eISBN 978-3-13-150511-8

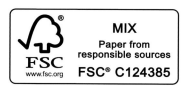

Contents

Foreword

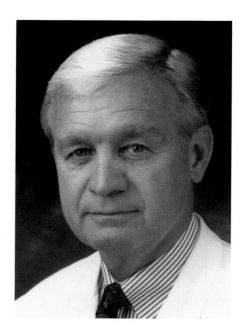

Every primary rhinoplasty is an adventure. Revision rhinoplasty, in contrast, constitutes an exploration into an unknown anatomic landscape, scarred and significantly altered by previous surgical procedures. Multiple pathways exist in the quest to correct previously altered anatomic components. As difficult as this surgical effort often is, more difficult still is the struggle to satisfy patients quite naturally unfulfilled by earlier operations on their nose.

Before undertaking revision rhinoplasty, four fundamental questions must be posed:

1. Can definitive improvement be reasonably predicted?

2. Will the potential improvements realized result in patient satisfaction?

3. Will the approach and techniques employed result in improvement without great risk of further adverse healing outcomes?

4. Is the surgeon sufficiently experienced and confident of an improved outcome?

Absolutely essential to the undertaking of a rhinoplasty revision is painstaking and detailed analysis of the disturbed anatomy. Tissues scarred and rendered less vascular by previous surgery, devastating natural tissue dissection planes, lend themselves less well to preoperative analysis. A judgment must be made about whether the abnormalities encountered may be safely repaired. It is axiomatic that *functional* nasal problems must be initially addressed.

At the outset, a fundamental and critical decision must be made about whether it may be more appropriate and safe to engage in a major tissue dissection and exploration created by the *external (open) approach*, or whether more limited incisions and dissection available through *endonasal approaches* place the damaged tissues—and therefore the patient surgical outcome—at less risk.

In this beautifully illustrated and written volume designed to highlight patient-centered clinical problems, Professor Behrbohm reveals the surgical principles underlying common and unique cases encountered in a busy clinical practice. Following an erudite analysis and evaluation of each problem, the corrective surgical steps chosen are illustrated liberally with artful renderings supplemented by clear, step-wise surgical maneuvers. Importantly, surgical outcomes are revealed with follow-up patient images. From the outset, thorough and cogent chapters document the importance and techniques of nasal analysis, functional evaluation, surgical planning, and the utilization of a wide variety of grafts useful in creating nasal support and form. Unlike most texts devoted to revision rhinoplasty, the author discusses his contemporary approaches to a wide variety of nasal injuries, reconstructive techniques following soft tissue loss in various regions of the nose, and management of nasal tissue loss and deformities resulting from systemic diseases.

Nasal function does not suffer from exclusion in this exposition, since preservation or restoration of the normal functions of the nose is emphasized throughout the volume. Newer endoscopic techniques, which aid in functional restoration and surgical dissection, add much to the teaching value of the book.

In summary, all serious rhinoplasty surgeons or students of the art will benefit enormously from adding this sophisticated textbook to their medical library.

M. Eugene Tardy, MD, FACS
Emeritus Professor
University of Illinois Medical Center
Chicago, Illinois, USA

Foreword

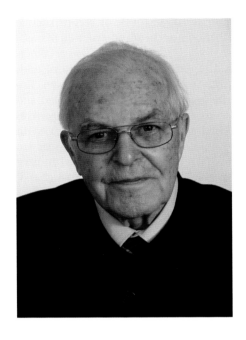

It is an honor for me to have been asked by Professor Behrbohm and his co-authors to introduce their new book on revision rhinoplasty.

The topic of the book is revision rhinoplasties, including all facets of surgery of the nose: aesthetics, functional, and reconstructive surgery of the nose. A special part of this interesting book is reserved at length to discuss secondary corrections of the nose and nasal septum.

The nose is a very difficult part of the face on which to operate because of the anatomy and physiology of the nose and possible allergies influencing the nasal mucosa. Furthermore, the nose contributes a great deal to the harmony of the face. Consequently, its configuration is responsible for psychological disturbances for patients.

In order to perform proper surgical interventions, the surgeon benefits from a three-dimensional view for better judging the components of the face in relation to the nose.

All of these criteria find a synthesis in the different chapters of the book, which are of an excellent quality. In spite of the numerous publications on rhinoplasties since 1900, Professor Behrbohm and his co-authors have published a most interesting compendium of a book dealing with all phases of surgery containing first-quality artist's drawings, beautiful patient photography of the nose during the operation, and excellent written explanations of surgical techniques for or during the surgery.

Considering the importance of the nose in relation to the face, the authors have divided their new book into different sections from reference points in aesthetic facial surgery to pre- and post-operative functional examinations to surgery for nasal defects after trauma and tissue loss.

The book is divided into different chapters, first dealing with aesthetic, functional, and revision surgery and trauma and defect surgery of the nose, and malformations and profile corrections in conjunction with rhinoplasty. A brief discussion and explanation of how to use instruments during the nasal surgery is helpful and unique in the literature. A different chapter of this extraordinary book deals especially with rhinoplasties to require secondary revisions including septal surgery.

As in all the other parts in the book we find here also very well represented figure drawings, photographs, and text to add special knowledge to be able to solve these more complicated cases. The combination of options so well presented is most helpful.

The multitude of hints on how to use different techniques, including grafts, demonstrated in drawings and photographs of different surgical approaches, and different options and combinations of uniquely shown techniques help bring even the worst cases back to normal. The surgeon will find in this book a wide variety of cases seldom presented so extensively.

In my opinion, such a wonderful combination is rarely seen. Due to its perfection, this book will find a special place in the world literature on rhinoplasties and many readers.

Claus Walter, MD, PhD
Emeritus Professor
St. Gallen, Switzerland

Preface

Udo Lindenberg (1946) is a well-known German musician, poet, and painter. After releasing his first LP with English lyrics in 1971, he revolutionized the German language of that time and introduced it into rock music. His talents range from the best German lyrics and most sensitive ballads to the hardest rock 'n' roll. The artist has always been politically outspoken, whether actively working for the fall of the Berlin Wall or launching a "Rock Initiative" against right-wing violence in 2000. I began listening to his music as a young student in the early 1970s, when a schoolmate brought some of Udo's recordings, including the song *Hoch im Norden*, and played them in our shared apartment. Forty years later, it is my wish to have a pictorial metaphor for the title of my book from the artist who had written the soundtrack of my student years. I am grateful to Udo for making my wish come true.

The didactic goal of this book is to confront the reader with various problem situations in patients. Revisions are demonstrated in a range of common and rare presentations in patients who have had previous functional, aesthetic or reconstructive surgery, trauma, tumor resections, or the reconstruction of nasal defects.

Readers are challenged to explore the particulars of each case and consider which solution they would have chosen. The procedure that was actually implemented is then revealed and discussed. The book proceeds systematically from the general to the specific and from the simpler to the more complex, with emphasis on a concise presentation. The applied techniques are presented in easy-to-follow steps. The authors discussed and envisioned the general layout of a "cookbook." The express goal of this book is to steer clear of all schools and current trends. Thus, it covers the gamut of closed, open, and endoscopic approaches and all graft and suture techniques, ranging to complex reconstructions with free tissue transfers. The full armamentarium of rhinoplastic and facial plastic surgical techniques is employed. For the repertoire of the pianist that Udo Lindenberg painted for us, this means "using all the keys." That is precisely our intention.

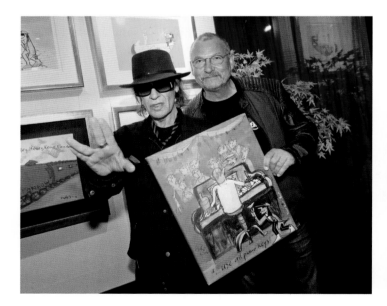 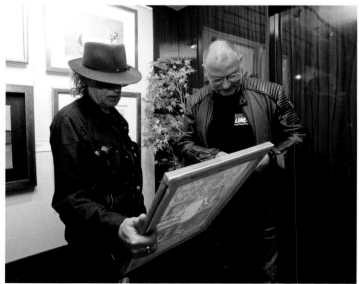

The artist and the author during an exchange of ideas in May 2014.

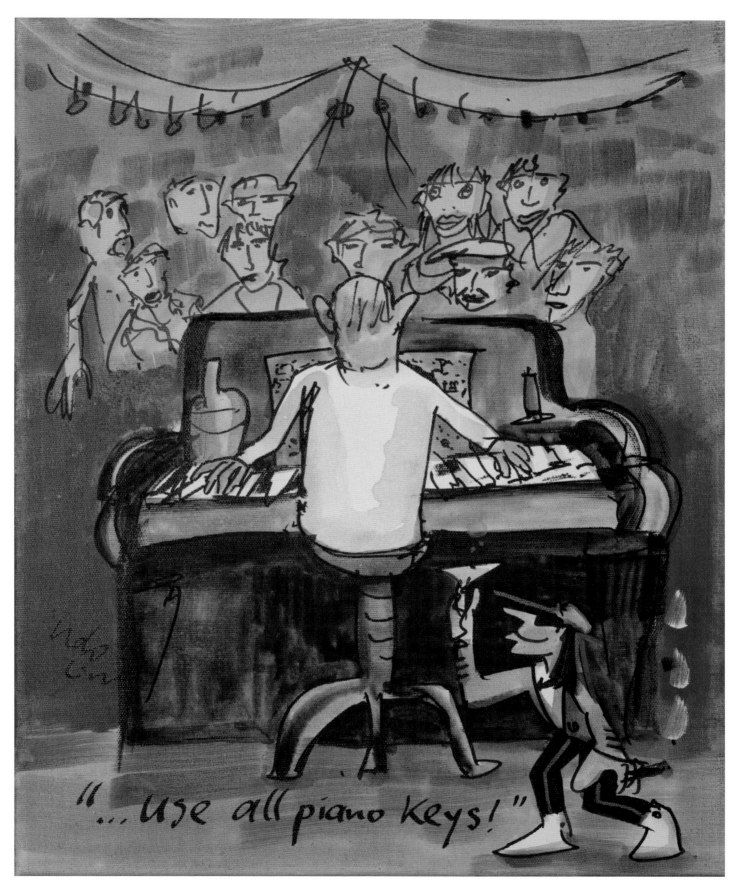

"*. . . use all piano keys!*" by Udo Lindenberg. Original acryrelle on canvas (40 x 50 cm)

Contributors

Hans Behrbohm, MD, PhD
Professor
Department of Otorhinolaryngology
  and Facial Plastic Surgery
Park-Klinik Weissensee
Academic Teaching Hospital of the
  Charité University Hospital
and
Institute of Medical Development and
  Further Education Berlin e.V.
Berlin, Germany

Johanna Brehm, MD, PhD
Department of Otorhinolaryngology
  and Facial Plastic Surgery
Park-Klinik Weissensee
Academic Teaching Hospital of the
  Charité University Hospital
Berlin, Germany

Walter Briedigkeit, MD, PhD†
Emeritus Professor
Department of Pediatric Cardiology
Charité University Hospital
Berlin, Germany

Jacqueline Eichhorn-Sens, MD, PhD
Plastic and Aesthetic Surgeon
Berlin, Germany

Holger Gassner, MD, PhD, FACS
Clinical Professor
Department of Facial Plastic Surgery (ABFPRS)
University Hospital Regensburg
Regensburg, Germany

Wolfgang Gubisch, MD, PhD
Professor and Director
Department of Facial Plastic Surgery
Marienhospital Stuttgart
Stuttgart, Germany

Thomas Hildebrandt, MD, PhD
Limmatklinik AG Zurich
Zurich, Switzerland

Joachim Quetz, MD, PhD
Department of Otorhinolaryngology,
  Head and Neck Surgery
University Clinic Schleswig-Holstein,
  Campus Kiel
Kiel, Germany

Section I

1 Revision Rhinoplasty—An Introduction

> The grand aim of all science is to cover the greatest number of empirical facts by logical deduction from the smallest number of hypotheses or axioms.
>
> —Albert Einstein, *Life magazine*, January 1950

1.1 Revision Rhinoplasty: Why a Separate Topic?

Sooner or later, every surgeon who practices functional and aesthetic nasal surgery must face the issue of revision surgery. Surgeons should be concerned first and foremost with their own revisions. Often they are not dealing with a major disaster but with "minor complaints," which are just as challenging. The more subtle the problem, the greater the importance that the patient attaches to his or her physical appearance. This blurs the distinction between "mild" and "serious" revisions. Every nose is "serious" because rhinoplasty is an all-or-nothing operation. The most important factor in judging its success is the subjective satisfaction of the patient.[1] It is not unusual for the patient and surgeon to disagree in this respect. Everyone wants an optimum result and everyone has an opinion. But what is a realistic expectation when all factors are taken into account? The ability to predict a realistic outcome of revision rhinoplasty and communicate it to the patient beforehand is an important prerequisite for achieving patient satisfaction. Whether and when a surgeon performs a revision or refers it elsewhere will depend on his or her experience and success rates.

Is there really a need for a book on revision rhinoplasty? Do primary rhinoplasties differ from secondary and tertiary operations? We believe the answer is yes! There are psychological, biological, and certainly technical aspects that distinguish revisions from primary operations. Because the expectations of revision candidates were not met in the previous operation, all hopes are centered on the revision procedure and on the surgeon, who must decide whether, when, and by whom the revision should be done based on a precise morphological and psychological evaluation.

1.2 The Myth of Michael Jackson's Nose

The most famous rhinoplasty patient of all time is the "King of Pop," Michael Jackson. He never personally acknowledged having facial and nasal surgery, and we shall not offer analysis or commentary on that point. But the fact remains that his name comes up in almost every consultation visit with a rhinosurgeon; he is "always there." Michael Jackson underwent extreme changes during the course of his life. The dark-skinned youth with an "Afro" became progressively lighter-skinned, his nose more slender. The human being morphed into an art figure. Was it a quest for his personal ideal of beauty? Or did he simply no longer want to look like his father, who often teased the young Michael for having a "wide nose."[2] Perhaps we will never know why this transformation took place. It is certain that Michael Jackson had multiple surgeries and entered a virtual Neverland between all ethnic and aesthetic norms, in the process becoming as unmistakable as his music. **Fig. 1.1a–f** illustrates the phenotypic changes that marked different stages in the life of Michael Jackson.

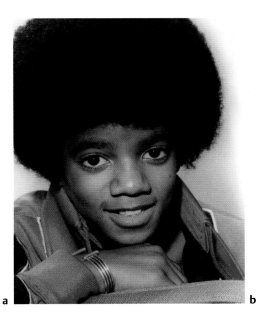
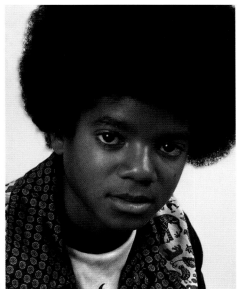
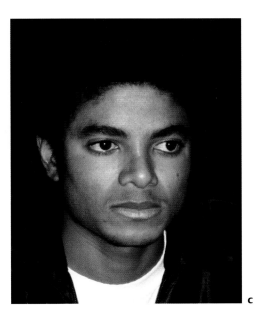

Fig. 1.1 (**a–f**) Portraits of Michael Jackson through the years. (*Continued on next page*)

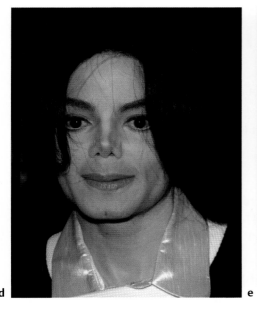 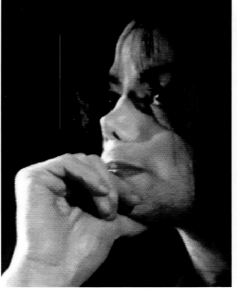 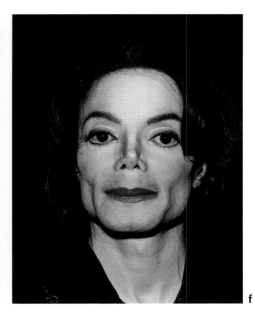

d   e   f

Fig. 1.1 (*Continued*)   (**a–f**) Portraits of Michael Jackson through the years.

1.3 Special Problems of Revision Rhinoplasty

Fundamental differences exist between a primary rhinoplasty and a revision. While the surgeon in a primary septorhinoplasty seeks to locate the "surgical plane" that will afford elegant access with minimal bleeding, this plane is not available in revision surgery because it has been obliterated by scarring (**Fig. 1.2**).

The ideal surgical plane for septal surgery is located between the mucoperichondrium and cartilage of the anterior septum, while the ideal plane for surgery of the nasal dorsum is located below the superficial musculoaponeurotic system (SMAS) of the facial muscles and the perichondrium of the upper lateral cartilage. In revision rhinoplasties these planes are either obliterated or difficult to define. The surgeon is always faced with anatomic changes and a loss of elasticity or stability in cartilage that has been weakened by incisions or excisions. Circulation is usually poorer than in primary rhinoplasties because of scarring, and the soft tissues covering the nose have usually not "forgotten" the trauma of previous surgery.[3] As a result, revision surgery always carries an increased risk for both the patient and surgeon, despite all available options and possibilities.[4] Access requires a sharper dissection technique. Bleeding tends to be heavier and may obscure visibility. The blood flow to scar tissue is relatively poor, areas of soft-tissue elevation may show delayed or asymmetric healing, and repeated undermining of the soft-tissue envelope may lead to cutaneous telangiectasia and trophic changes. As in any rhinoplasty, the surgeon must enter the operation with a well-devised plan of action. But revision surgery also requires a talent for improvisation in cases where, say, anticipated structures are not found or cannot be realigned or trimmed in the usual way. Scars are bradytrophic and hamper the uncomplicated healing of implants. This is why only autologous tissues should be used in revision rhinoplasties. Richard Goode's advice to "replace what is missing with like material" is a sound rule to follow.[5,6] For these and other reasons, revision rhinoplasties belong in the hands of experienced surgeons.[7] **Fig. 1.3** illustrates a hemitransfixion incision for a primary septorhinoplasty. Even this approach can be problematic in revision cases.

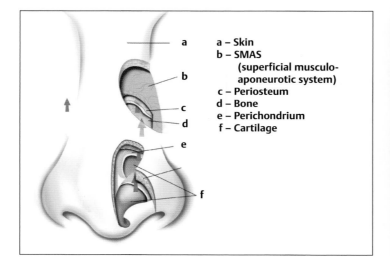

a – Skin
b – SMAS
    (superficial musculo-
    aponeurotic system)
c – Periosteum
d – Bone
e – Perichondrium
f – Cartilage

Fig. 1.2   The ideal surgical plane for rhinoplasty.

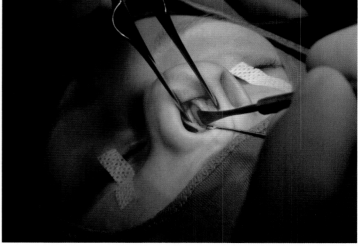

Fig. 1.3   The hemitransfixion incision is the most commonly used rhinosurgical approach. Sharp dissection of the surgical plane between the mucoperichondrium and anterior septal cartilage allows for safe, bloodless surgery.

1.4 What Can We Learn from Revision Surgery?

Of course, a book on revision rhinoplasty is also a book on primary rhinoplasty because it will inevitably raise the question: How can I avoid revision surgery? A second question is: Can I avoid revisions entirely, and if not, to what degree? Are there deformities that are inherently more likely to require later revision? If this happens, is the first operation a failure? Under what circumstances are revisions most likely to be needed? To answer these questions, the surgeon must be fully open to a critical analysis that will show whether a particular revision is traceable to a flawed surgical concept, technical imperfections, a wound healing problem, or an unpredictable deformity.

Regardless of these questions, this book urges every surgeon to make the most of a primary rhinoplasty and accomplish as much as possible in the ideal setting of unaltered tissues. Adamson called rhinoplasty "the thinking man's operation,"[4] and this principle is illustrated in **Fig. 1.4**.

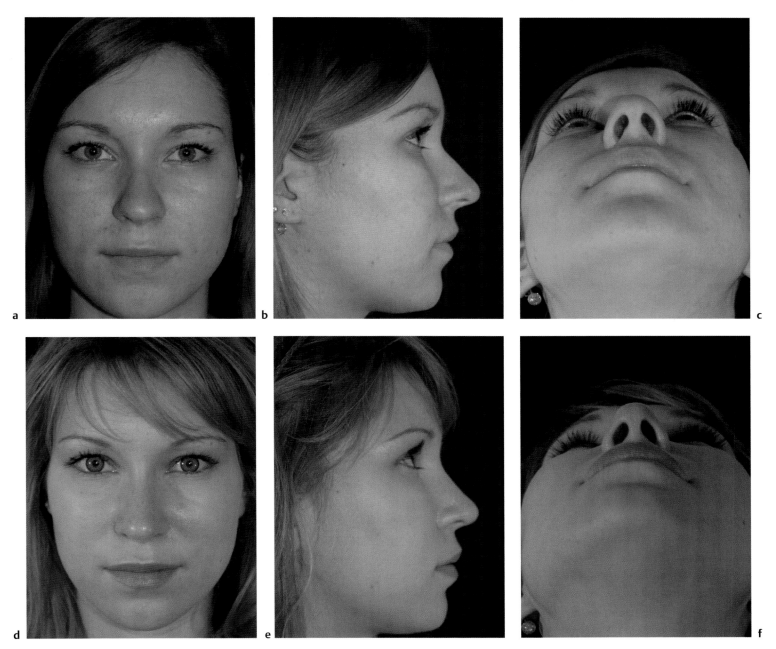

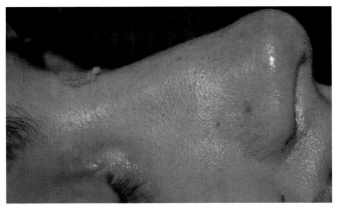

Fig. 1.4 A 21-year-old woman presented with the desire to remove her nasal hump and narrow the nasal tip. "Hump removal" would not have improved the aesthetic outcome, however, and in fact would have worsened it. Analysis of findings: (**a**) Front view shows disproportion between a thin, delicate nasal pyramid and a broad tip. (**b**) Profile view shows a depressed nasal dorsum (nasofrontal angle). (**c**) Basal view shows a boxy tip. Surgical concept: Do not reduce the nasal dorsum! (**g**) Instead, augment the nasofrontal angle with an onlay graft from the nasal septum. Use the delivery approach and a transdomal suture to narrow the tip and decrease the interdomal angle. (**d–f**) Result at 15 months. A targeted, minimally invasive procedure has improved the patient's overall attractiveness and appearance.

1.5 Most Frequent Indications for Revision Surgery

From 5% to 15% of patients who have a primary rhinoplasty will undergo revision surgery, depending on the experience of the first operating surgeon.[4,8] Rates as high as 30% have been reported for complex deformities such as a crooked nose.[9] A special characteristic of nasal surgery is its dual nature: it has both functional and aesthetic goals. Both aspects factor into every nasal operation to some degree. On the one hand, a large percentage of candidates for purely aesthetic rhinoplasties are found, on closer analysis, to have nasal airway problems. On the other hand, primary rhinoplasty is followed by an ~ 10% incidence of surgery-related airway complaints.[10–12] From 60% to 70% of patients who present for a revision rhinoplasty complain of nasal airway obstruction.[13,14] Moreover, the nasal septum is a central structural element that must also be integrated into a purely aesthetic surgical concept.[5,15]

　　Various classifications are used to describe the deformities that may follow a primary rhinoplasty. Usually the nose is divided into an upper, a middle, and a lower third as originally described by Jacques Joseph.[16] Upper-third deformities involve the bony nasal pyramid, middle-third deformities the cartilaginous nose and middle vault, and lower-third deformities the nasal tip, ala, and columella. The upper two thirds are usually considered as a unit due to frequent concomitant deformity of the bony and cartilaginous pyramids. Another classification distinguishes among deformities of the nasal dorsum, nasal tip, nasal base, and caudal septum.

The most common deformities after septorhinoplasties are the following[17]:

- Polly beak deformities involving both the nasal tip and dorsum

- Dorsal nasal deformities: overresection of the nasal dorsum with saddling, dorsal irregularities after hump removal, widening (e.g., open-roof deformity), asymmetries and deviations of the nasal dorsum due to uncorrected lateral disparities or incomplete osteotomies

- Nasal base deformities: underrotation and underprojection of the nasal tip with retraction of the columella, asymmetry or widening of the nasal tip, alar collapse

Although the nose consists of just a few anatomic parts, it displays endless morphological and functional variations (**Fig. 1.5**). Even more important than understanding the anatomy of specific deformities is to have a basic understanding of dynamic changes involving the whole bony and cartilaginous framework of the nose after previous surgery. For example, the nasal tip is not just a composite structure formed by the anatomic components of the cartilaginous and membranous septum and the medial and lateral crura of the alar cartilages. It is an aerodynamic body whose parts are suspended and supported by the soft tissues, the subcutaneous connective tissue, the SMAS, and the skin. Destabilizing the system, by septal surgery, for example, may cause typical complex changes characterized by nasal tip and supratip deformity (**Fig. 1.6**).[15,17] See also Case 1, Chapter 16.

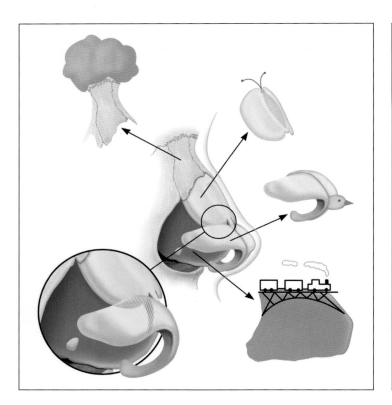

Fig. 1.5　The rhinion marks the site where the flexible cartilaginous nose is attached to the rigid bony nasal pyramid. The septum is the central supporting structure of the nose. The upper lateral cartilages (anatomically, part of the septal cartilage) have the functional mobility of butterfly wings. The lateral crura of the alar cartilages (lower lateral cartilages) determine the property of collapsibility, i.e., resistance to opening of the external nasal valve. Detail: The internal nasal valve represents the narrowest portion of the airway and is the site of greatest elasticity and functional dynamics.

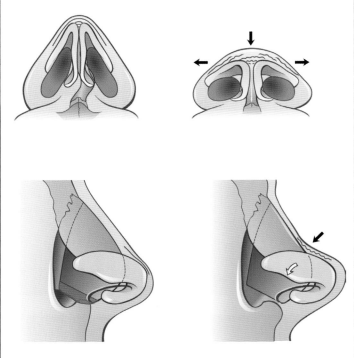

Fig. 1.6　The alar and septal cartilages, superficial musculoaponeurotic system, skin, and subcutaneous and connective tissues combine to give support and shape to the nasal tip. Any settling of the anterior septum or division of the connective-tissue fibers between the domes may cause widening of the nasal tip (after Rettinger, 2007).

References

1. Rettinger G. Risks and complications in rhinoplasty, an update on functional and esthetic surgery of the nose and ear. GMS Curr Top in Otorhinolaryngology Head and Neck Surg 2007;6:73–90

2. Siasios P. Michael Jackson, Der King of Pop in Bildern (1958–2009). Picture Star 2009

3. Adamson PA. The failed rhinoplasty. Curr Ther Otolaryngol Head Neck Surgery 1990;4:137–144

4. Bagal AA, Adamson PA. Revision rhinoplasty. Facial Plast Surg 2002;18(4):233–244

5. Behrbohm H, Tardy ME. Essentials of Septorhinoplasty, Philosophy–Approaches–Techniques. New York, NY: Thieme, 2003

6. Goode RL, Alto P. Surgery of the incompetent nasal valve. Laryngoscope 1985;95(5):546–555

7. Eichhorn-Sens J, Gubisch W. Sekundäre Rhinoplastik. In: Von Heimburg D, Lemperle G, Richter DF. Ästhetische Chirurgie. Heidelberg, Germany: Ecomed; 2010:1–26

8. Kamer FM, McQuown SA. Revision rhinoplasty. Analysis and treatment. Arch Otolaryngol Head Neck Surg 1988;114:257

9. Stal P. Septal deviations and correction of the crooked nose. In: Daniel RK. Rhinoplasty. Boston, MA: Little, Brown and Company; 1993

10. Ballert JA, Park SS. Functional considerations in revision rhinoplasty. Facial Plast Surg 2008;24(3):348–357

11. Beekhuis GJ. Nasal obstruction after rhinoplasty: etiology, and techniques for correction. Laryngoscope 1976;86(4):540–548

12. Courtiss EH, Goldwyn RM. The effects of nasal surgery on airflow. Plast Reconstr Surg 1983;72(1):9–21

13. Bracaglia R, Fortunato R, Gentileschi S. Secondary rhinoplasty. Aesthetic Plast Surg 2005;29(4):230–239

14. Foda HM. Rhinoplasty for the multiply revised nose. Am J Otolaryngol 2005;26(1):28–34

15. Hildebrandt T, Behrbohm H. Functional aesthetic surgery of the nose. The influence of the septum on the aesthetics of the nasal tip. Media Service; 2000

16. Joseph J. Nasenplastik und sonstige Gesichtsplastik nebst einem Anhang über Mammaplastik. Leipzig, Germany: C. Kabitzsch; 1931

17. Rettinger G. Risiken und Komplikationen der Rhinoplastik. Laryngorhinootologie 2007;86(Suppl 1):40–54

2   Basic Rules for Revision Rhinoplasties

After a certain high level of technical skill is achieved, science and art tend to coalesce in aesthetics.

—Albert Einstein, 1923

2.1 Morphologic and Functional Analysis of the Problem

A precise morphologic evaluation is essential. In making this analysis, the surgeon should have access to all previous findings including images before the primary operation, surgery reports, and imaging CDs if available. External inspection, external and internal palpation, and nasal endoscopy will reveal the scope of the problem. Often it is necessary to resect additional tissue from some structures and to augment others. As part of the analysis, then, it should be determined whether there is enough septal cartilage available for grafts or whether conchal or rib cartilage will be needed. Diagnostic maneuvers to assess function are helpful before any type of nasal revision surgery is performed. Standard tests include computed rhinomanometry and a standard olfactory test such as Sniffin' Sticks to determine perception and identification thresholds.

2.2 Functionality and Aesthetics

Every nasal operation has a dual nature. This particularly applies to revision rhinoplasties in cases where functional aspects were poorly assessed and managed initially or the previous surgery itself gave rise to functional problems.[1] The most common problems encountered in rhinoplasty revisions are:

- Stenosis of the external or internal nasal valve
- Inspiratory alar collapse due to overresection of alar cartilage
- Very low lateral osteotomies that constrict the middle vault
- Ballooning effect due to saddling in the supratip area
- Neglected hyperplasia of the inferior turbinate
- Septal deviation

Today it is no longer necessary to sacrifice function to improve nasal aesthetics. Consequently, top priority can be given to the correction of functional problems without compromising aesthetic goals.

2.3 Major Correction or Touch-Up?

Generally speaking, the surgeon always has various options when planning a revision procedure. It is helpful to have the patient rank specific objectionable features in order of their importance. This priority list provides the basis for deciding whether the main problems can be solved by minimally invasive touch-ups through a closed approach or whether an open approach is required. The first option is based on the camouflage principle using selective, circumscribed resections and augmentations, which may be performed through multiple small approaches.[2] The second option is used for the reconstruction of "load-bearing" walls with structural grafts or suture-anchored grafts and implants. Not every patient will require a major revision. The principle of minimally invasive touch-ups targeted at specific flaws can avoid the risks that are associated with large raw surfaces, scars, and vascular disruption.

2.4 Timing of the Surgery

In principle, significant revision surgery should be performed no earlier than 8–12 months after the primary operation. This ensures that a stable result with good scar tissue will be available as a basis for planning the revision. Residual swelling and edema are a contraindication to revision rhinoplasty. Exceptions to this rule would include asymmetries due to faulty or incomplete osteotomies, incomplete profile correction (residual hump), and graft displacement. Revisions in these cases should be scheduled without delay.[2] The surgeon should never take a wait-and-see approach to put off patients. If a definite indication exists for revision surgery, the surgeon must decide on the best timing. Rhinoplasty patients usually have a fairly reasonable expectation of what can and cannot be achieved. Predicting results that do not materialize after swelling has subsided will damage the trusting relationship between the surgeon and patient. The surgeon should always take the initiative in either supporting or discouraging a patient's desire for revision surgery.

References

1. Schultz-Coulon HJ. Rhinoplastik—ein überwiegend ästhetischer oder funktioneller Eingriff. Laryngol Rhinol Otol (Stuttg) 1977;56(3):233–243

2. Tardy ME, Thomas R. Our personal approach and philosophy. In: Becker DG, Park SS, eds. Revision Rhinoplasty. New York, NY: Thieme; 2007:202–222

3 Psychological Evaluation

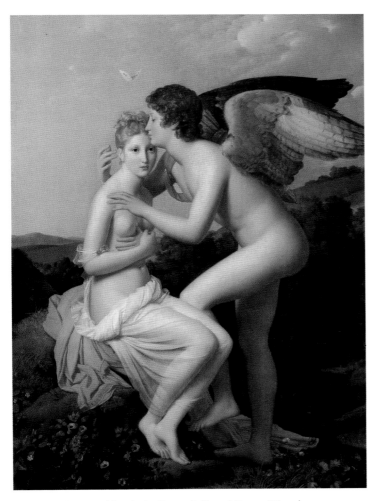

Fig. 3.1 *Amor and Psyche* by François Pascal Simon Gérard.

Patient selection is essential for a successful revision rhinoplasty. The physician will determine whether the patient's desire for surgery is justified and must decide whether a revision will actually solve the patient's problems. More than in any other specialty, the decision to perform or withhold revision surgery in cases with an aesthetic indication will depend on the emotional, conscious, and unconscious motives of the patient (**Fig. 3.1**).[1–3] The task of the physician, then, is to determine the psychosocial context of the desire for surgery independently of the patient's self-will. The mental disorders listed below play an important role.

3.1 Reactive and Adjustment Disorders

Facial deformities that are objectively disfiguring are often associated with reactive mental disorders. They may take the

form of an acute stress reaction or may develop later as a post-traumatic stress disorder. Patients with high vulnerability may develop an adjustment disorder in their attempt to process or overcome disease or disfigurement. Given the severity of the underlying organic problem, plastic reconstructive or cosmetic surgery is appropriate for these patients (see Case 32, Chapter 25) and may lead to a resolution or improvement of psychological symptoms.[4] But if the mental disorder itself is the dominant finding, even a successful operation may cause psychological disturbance in patients who were projecting their emotional distress onto their physical defect and using it as an excuse for that distress.[5]

3.2 Depressive Disorder

Approximately 20% of patients who seek cosmetic surgery have a depressive disorder. The main symptoms are a depressed mood, loss of interest or pleasure in daily activities, apathy, and heightened fatigability.[6] Other symptoms such as body dysmorphic disorder with low self-esteem should be given particular attention in cosmetic surgery because they may create a motive for the operation. The interviewer should ask specifically about suicidal thoughts, which must be excluded. Any evidence in that direction would contraindicate the surgery and prompt an immediate referral for psychotherapy.

3.3 Comorbidity

"Comorbidity" refers to physical symptoms that coexist with a mental disorder. Comorbidities may significantly affect the motivation for and course of aesthetic surgery. Psychological disturbances such as affective disorders (6.3%), anxiety disorders (9%), and somatoform disorders (7.5%) have a high prevalence in the general population. International studies have shown that mental disorders are significantly more prevalent in patients who seek aesthetic surgery.[4,6,7]

3.4 Social Phobias

Anxiety reactions are centered on the fear of being watched and judged by others. Affected individuals tend to avoid social situations, which interferes with relationships, resulting in psychosocial isolation. Primary social phobias in the absence of physical abnormalities are usually associated with a feeling of low self-worth and may cause the patient to seek cosmetic surgery. Eleven percent of patients with social phobia were found to have a body dysmorphic disorder.[8] Cosmetic surgery is not advised in this subset of patients.

3.5 Anxiety Disorders

Increased anxiety scores were found in patients seeking cosmetic surgery.[9] Preoperative symptoms included panic disorders with intense anxiety, palpitations, rapid heart rate and associated autonomic signs, profuse sweating, trembling, shortness of breath, and dizziness.[2]

3.6 Compulsive Disorders

A constant preoccupation with external appearance is characteristic. A distinction is made between compulsive thoughts and compulsive actions. Compulsive thoughts constantly recur, center on the aesthetic aspects of a deformity or operation, and are experienced as intrusive and fraught with anxiety and discomfort. Compulsive actions may be characterized by repetitive rituals, often lasting for hours, or by cosmetic surgery, constant primping, or preoccupation with physical appearance. Surgery is not advised for this subset of patients.

3.7 Somatoform Disorders

These disorders are characterized by recurring physical symptoms combined with a stubborn insistence on medical examinations and treatments despite repeated negative results and physician assurances that the symptoms do not have a physical cause.[9] One particular hypochondriac disorder, body dysmorphic disorder (dysmorphophobia), is important in the setting of cosmetic surgery. Somatoform disorders are a contraindication to rhinoplasty.

3.8 Body Dysmorphic Disorder

The alternate term, "dysmorphophobia," comes from Herodotus' myth about Dysmorphia, the ugliest girl in Sparta.[10] The central feature is an excessive concern about a perceived defect in physical appearance. This defect is either slight or nonexistent and is insufficient to account for the patient's distress. Body dysmorphic disorder (BDD) is one of the leading contraindications to cosmetic surgery and is the most important absolute contraindication.[2,11,12] The stated goal for most candidates is to restore psychological equilibrium, but even a successful operation may not achieve that goal. On the contrary, patients may perceive a successful outcome as a failure because they have attached other expectations to it. The main diagnostic tools are the personal and third-party history and screening instruments such as the Body Dysmorphic Disorder Diagnostic Module with six items or a severity rating scale for BDD. Patients with BDD should be referred to a mental health professional.

3.9 Personality Disorders

Personality disorders are difficult to diagnose. One type is histrionic personality disorder, characterized by excessive emotionality and constant attention seeking. Narcissistic personality disorder is characterized by excessive self-love combined with hypersensitivity to criticism (**Fig. 3.2**). Patients with personality disorders tend to be demanding toward others, lack empathy with others' feelings, and tend to blame others for their failures. Surgery is not advised for this subset of patients.[12,13]

3.10 Surgical Addiction, Munchhausen Syndrome

These individuals have an addiction to medical investigation and treatment that is often focused on cosmetic operations. They seek surgery that is not medically indicated. Patients often have a history of multiple previous operations performed for obscure

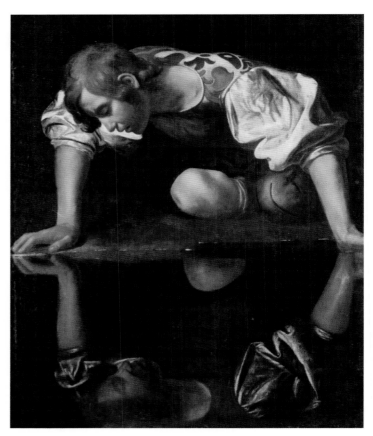

Fig. 3.2   *Narcissus* by Caravaggio.

reasons. The surgeon may become an unwitting instrument in the patient's psychopathological quest to undergo medical procedures. A friendly demeanor will change abruptly to rage if the doctor refuses to operate. These patients are not good candidates for cosmetic surgery.

3.11 Schizophrenia

Schizophrenia is characterized by bizarre delusions and hallucinations, which are often revealed when the patient is questioned about his or her self-perception and motivation to seek surgery. It is an indication for psychiatric treatment. Other features are ego-syntonic, paranoid convictions, and changes in affect and thinking. Cosmetic surgery is contraindicated.[14]

3.12 Psychometric Analysis of Septorhinoplasty Candidates

Effective tools are available for evaluating psychometric parameters in patients who seek functional–aesthetic nasal surgery and for identifying possible psychological contraindications. Of course the most severe potential complication of a rhinoplasty or septorhinoplasty is the death of the patient or surgeon.[12] This would be rooted in a faulty assessment of preoperative psychological status.[5] In one study, validated and standardized questionnaires were used to collect psychometric data such as anxiety, depression, private and public self-consciousness, and general and nose-related life satisfaction in 101 candidates for septorhinoplasty. The patients tended to score higher in the traits of anxiety, public self-consciousness, and dissatisfaction with their nose.[15]

References

1. Adamsen P, Kraus WM. Management of patient dissatisfaction with cosmetic surgery. In: Rhinoplasty 2001, Course Manual. Chicago; 2001:41–46

2. Harth W, Hermes B. Berücksichtigung biosozialer Aspekte vor kosmetischen Operationen. Journal für Ästhet Chir 2011;4:68–73

3. World Health Organization. ICD-10. Internationale statistische Klassifikation der Krankheiten und verwandter Gesundheitsprobleme. Revision 10, Vol. 1. Geneva, Switzerland: WHO; 2001

4. Ishigooka J, Iwao M, Suzuki M, Fukuyama Y, Murasaki M, Miura S. Demographic features of patients seeking cosmetic surgery. Psychiatry Clin Neurosci 1998;52(3):283–287

5. Keck T, Kühnemann S, Ehrat J, Meder G, Dahlbender RW. Patienten mit dem Wunsch nach einer funktionell-ästhetischen Nasenoperation: Psychometrische Parameter. HNO 2012;60(1):55–62

6. Meningaud JP, Benadiba L, Servant JM, Herve C, Bertrand JC, Pelicie Y. Depression, anxiety and quality of life among scheduled cosmetic surgery patients: multicentre prospective study. J Craniomaxillofac Surg 2001; 29(3):177–180

7. Honigman RJ, Phillips KA, Castle DJ. A review of psychosocial outcomes for patients seeking cosmetic surgery. Plast Reconstr Surg 2004;113(4): 1229–1237

8. Hollander E, Aronowitz BR. Comorbid social anxiety and body dysmorphic disorder: managing the complicated patient. J Clin Psychiatry 1999; 60(Suppl 9):27–31

9. Sass H, Wittchen H-U. Zaudig. Diagnostisches und statistisches Manual psychischer Störungen DSM-IV-TR. Berlin, Germany: Hogrefe; 2003

10. Mehler-Wex C, Warnke A. Dysmorphophobie–die Qual mit der eingebildeten Hässlichkeit. MMW Fortschr Med 2006;148(10):37–39

11. Conrado LA, Hounie AG, Diniz JB, et al. Body dysmorphic disorder among dermatologic patients: Prevalence and clinical features. J Am Acad Dermatol 2010;63(2):235–243

12. Rettinger G. Risiken und Komplikationen der Rhinoplastik. Laryngorhinootologie 2007;86:40–54

13. Beck D. Das Koryphäen-Killer-Syndrom. Dtsch Med Wochenschr 1977; 102:303–397

14. Waraich P, Goldner EM, Somers JM, Hsu L. Prevalence and incidence studies of mood disorders: a systematic review of the literature. Can J Psychiatry 2004;49(2):124–138

15. Behrbohm H. Psychometrische Analyse von Septorhinoplastikkandidaten. HNO 2012;60(1):53–54

4 Complications and Risks

The principal risk of a rhinoplasty is the presence of a significant new or residual nasal deformity after the operation (**Fig. 4.1**). This is due to the fact that the definitive result of a rhinoplasty cannot be accurately predicted. When should the definitive result be assessed? At several months, 1 year, or 10 years after the operation?

Healing is a dynamic process that proceeds at different rates in different individuals and may be associated with varying reactions. Moreover, this process involves a variety of tissues such as the skin, subcutaneous tissue, fascia, superficial musculoaponeurotic system (SMAS), nerves, vessels, bone, cartilage, perichondrium, and periosteum. The surgeon should traumatize these tissues as little and as briefly as possible to promote uncomplicated healing. Complications may arise from the individual tissue types or from surgical materials such as sutures, implants, and grafts.[1]

Atraumatic surgery should cause very little swelling. The degree of eyelid hematoma depends on skin and connective-tissue type and on the individual propensity for hematoma formation. Possible early complications include hematoma, local infection, and skin necrosis. Later complications may consist of atrophic skin changes, sensory disturbances, granulomas, or cyst formation.[2,3] Orbital complications may have a traumatic or inflammatory cause. Rhinoplasty may cause injury to the lacrimal ducts or orbital contents.[4] Vascular and intracranial complications are rare but have been described.[5,6] Cerebrospinal fluid rhinorrhea, cerebritis, brain injury, carotid–cavernous fistula, and septic cavernous sinus thrombosis with subdural empyema have all been reported after rhinoplasties.[4,7] Devitalization and discoloration of the anterior teeth may result from osteotomies or surgical manipulations around the nasal floor or piriform aperture.[8] It has also been shown that rhinosurgery may evoke a nasocardiac reflex leading to intraoperative bradycardia or even asystole.[9]

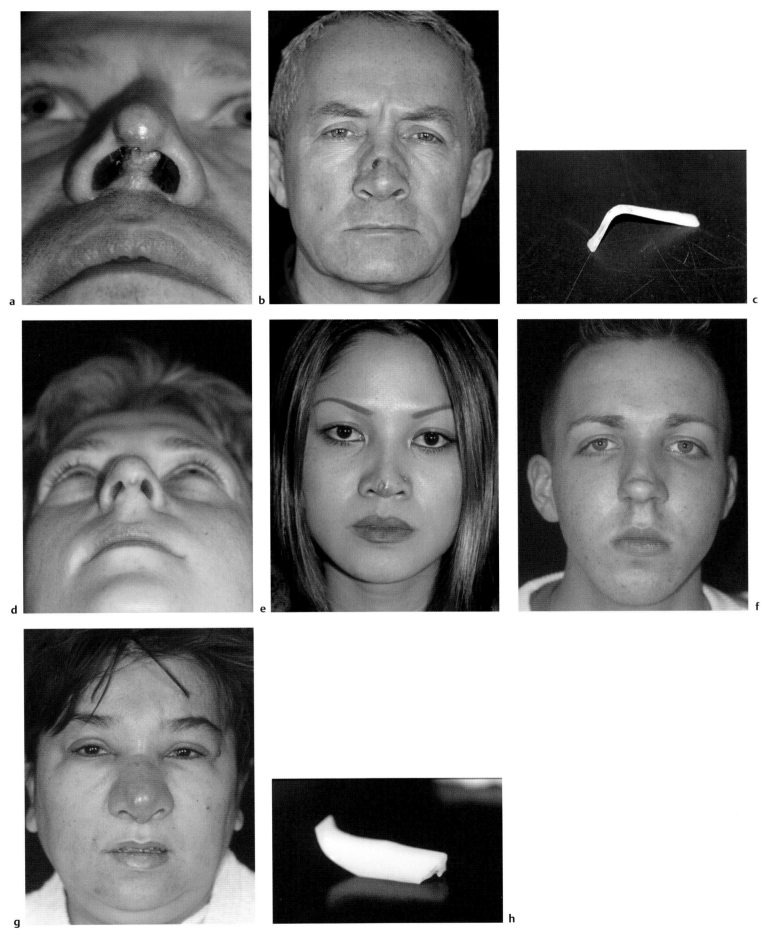

Fig. 4.1 Some typical complications of septorhinoplasty. (**a**) Extrusion of a polyethylene implant 1 year postoperatively. (**b**) Fistula formation over a polyvinyl chloride implant 30 years after implantation. (**c**) The implant in (**b**) after removal. (**d**) Suture fistula 4 months after surgery. (**e**) Extrusion of a silicone implant 3 years after surgery. (**f**) Pressure sore from a nasal cast. (**g**) Infected silicone implant 10 years after insertion. (**h**) The implant after removal.

References

1. Stoll W. Complications following implantation or transplantation in rhinoplasty. Facial Plast Surg 1997;13(1):45–50

2. Kotzur A, Gubisch W. Mucous cyst—a postrhinoplasty complication: outcome and prevention. Plast Reconstr Surg 1997;100(2):520–524

3. Meyer R. Secondary Rhinoplasty. New York, NY: Springer; 1988

4. Rettinger G. Risiken und Komplikationen der Rhinoplastik. Laryngorhinootologie 2007;86:40–54

5. Casaubon JN, Dion MA, Larbrisseau A. Septic cavernous sinus thrombosis after rhinoplasty: case report. Plast Reconstr Surg 1977;59(1):119–123

6. Marshall DR, Slattery PG. Intracranial complications of rhinoplasty. Br J Plast Surg 1983;36(3):342–344

7. Pothula VB, Reddy KT, Nixon TE. Carotico-cavernous fistula following septorhinoplasty. J Laryngol Otol 1999;113(9):844–846

8. Bergmeyer JM. Death of a tooth after rhinoplasty. Plast Reconstr Surg 1994;93(7):1529

9. Russo C, Corbanese U, Della Mora E. Nasocardiac reflex evoking during rhinoseptoplasty. Description of a clinical case [in Italian]. Minerva Anestesiol 1992;58(1-2):63–64

5 Reference Points in Aesthetic Facial Surgery: Part Mathematics, Part Intuition

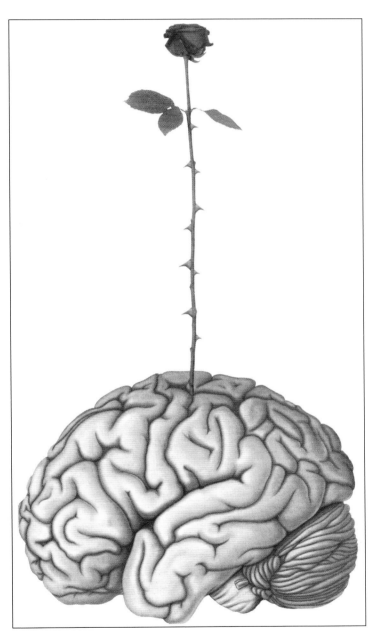

Fig. 5.1 Logo for the "Happiness" exhibit at the German Hygiene Museum, Dresden. (With permission of Stiftung Deutsches Hygiene-Museum, Dresden, Germany.)

5.1 Taking Stock: The Goals of Revision Surgery

The first impression is always an outward one. We perceive the proportions of a face, the skin type, and especially the overall facial appearance and attractiveness. Fine, symmetrical facial features are perceived as more aesthetically appealing than coarse features. But the more time we spend with a person, the more other qualities start to matter: personal charm, voice, and character. These qualities are also important in evaluating candidates for facial revision surgery. Taken as a whole, they may "trump" the external facial features or they may not. A perfect face is not beautiful if it masks an arrogant or narcissistic personality. Inner beauty, then, is ultimately superior to outer beauty while also serving to enhance it.

The question of whether aesthetic surgery can make people happy is disputed. An exhibition titled *Glück welches Glück* ("Happiness What Happiness") opened at the German Hygiene Museum in Dresden in 2008 and dealt with this question (**Fig. 5.1**).[1] It included an exhibit on cosmetic surgery featuring surgical instruments from various periods of history so that visitors could experience the practical side of cosmetic surgery. The instruments designed by Jacques Joseph were of particular interest. Joseph repeatedly cited the great psychological importance of reconstructive and cosmetic surgery in his writings. Going against the mainstream of contemporary professional thought, he was the first to define cosmetic surgery as an aesthetic endeavor.[2]

Everyone has their own definition of happiness. Most candidates for revision rhinoplasty and most of our own patients come to us because they hope to be happier by becoming more attractive. Some are struggling with a sense of being disfigured due to an accident or tumor resection. The hopes of becoming both happier and more attractive are in fact justified, because patients tend to be more self-confident and content following a successful operation. In this sense, a positive result of revision surgery can make people happier.

The present book runs the gamut from major and minor functional–aesthetic corrections to breathtaking reconstructive revision surgery. This is in keeping with the philosophy of Joseph, who wrote:

> The principal motive is not vanity but a sense of being disfigured, or an antipathy toward disfigurement and its psychological effects. The goal of rhinoplasty, then, is to cure mental depression by creating a normally shaped nose. It has an unquestionable social impact and represents a significant branch of surgical psychotherapy.[2]

Figs. 5.2 and **5.3** show two examples of the innovative work of Jacques Joseph illustrating two sides of the same coin: functional–aesthetic surgery and nasal reconstruction.

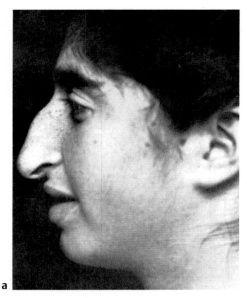

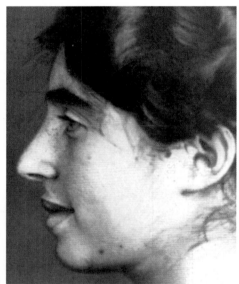

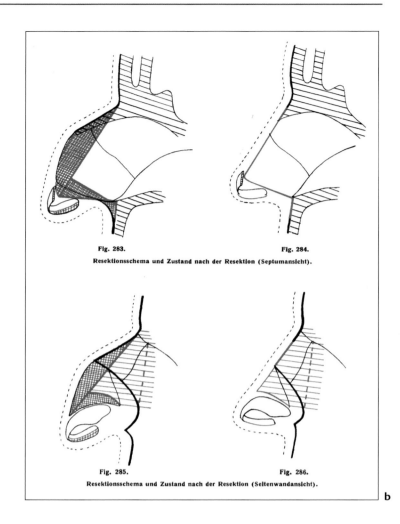

Fig. 283.

Resektionsschema und Zustand nach der Resektion (Septumansicht).

Fig. 284.

Fig. 285.

Fig. 286.

Resektionsschema und Zustand nach der Resektion (Seitenwandansicht).

Fig. 5.2 Case report from Jacques Joseph. (**a**) Patient with a "hanging septum of moderate degree." (**b**) Surgical plan for a reduction rhinoplasty, after Joseph. Resection diagram and status postresection. Above: view of the septum. Below: view of the lateral wall. (**c**) Appearance following bilateral segmental resection (full shortening with hump removal). From J. Joseph, Nasenplastik und sonstige Gesichtsplastik. C. Kabitzsch, Leipzig, 1931.

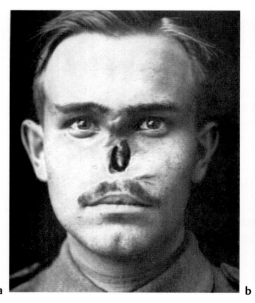

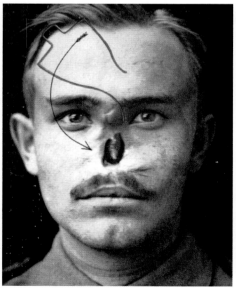

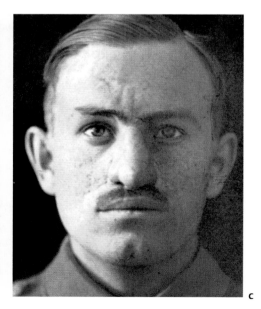

Fig. 5.3 Case report from Jacques Joseph. (**a**) Total nasal defect in a young soldier. (**b**) Forehead incisions for nasal reconstruction (Joseph forehead flap). (**c**) After "surgical modeling and bone implantation." From Joseph J. Nasenplastik und sonstige Gesichtsplastik. Leipzig, Germany: C Kabitzsch; 1931.

5.2 The "Sender" and the "Receiver" in Facial Surgery

While in the planning stage of a revision rhinoplasty, the surgeon should address or readdress the crucial question of in what way and to what extent the revision candidate will actually benefit from another operation.[3] The goal of rhinoplasty is less to create individual "parts" with a pleasing anatomic shape than to contribute to an overall improvement in facial appearance.[4] Simply stated, the nose is the sender and the face is the receiver. Standard formulas, lines, and angles are available for orientation purposes (**Fig. 5.4a**), but the rhinosurgeon must also make intuitive choices based on an appreciation of facial aesthetics (**Fig. 5.4b, c**).

The oldest theorems in geometry presumably originated from Pythagoras (ca. 599 BC), who was quoted as saying "numbers are crucial in nature and in art."[5] The Venetian monk Fra Paciolo di Borgo made a detailed study of proportions and aesthetics during the Renaissance. He published his book in 1509, reporting the discovery of the "golden section." We credit his contemporary, Leonardo da Vinci (1452–1519), with dividing the face into three equal sections by horizontal lines. Albrecht Dürer (1471–1582) was the most important German painter, printmaker, and draftsman of his time. He studied the theory of proportions and what constitutes beauty, which was considered the goal of art.[6] Dürer believed that beauty could be constructed with a "compass and straightedge." The vertical subdivision of the face into five equal portions dates back to Powell and Humphries.[7]

The nose is a central, solitary structure that functions as a bridge joining the upper third of the face to the lower third. It forms the geometric ordinate by which facial symmetry or asymmetry is assessed. Every rhinoplasty will ultimately influence facial anatomy and appearance. Despite its central role, the nose ranks low in the aesthetic hierarchy of facial features. It should showcase the dominant expressiveness of the eyes and brows as well as the lips with their delicately curved Cupid bow, without drawing attention to itself. Nevertheless, the nose should have an individual shape, it should fit the face, and preferably it should contribute to an elegant profile line by harmonizing with the trichion and pogonion. A "standard" type of nose cannot meet these criteria for all individuals.

5.3 Planning by Computer Simulation

In our experience, there are many advantages to simulating one or more possible outcomes of a revision rhinoplasty on a computer. It is an opportunity for the surgeon to spend 30 minutes of concentrated, quality time with the revision rhinoplasty candidate and gather valuable information by addressing the wishes and questions of the candidate. What expectations (realistic or unrealistic) does the patient have? What is his or her main focus? What is the candidate's psychological status, and are there any signs of a mental disorder that would contraindicate surgery? During the simulation process, the surgeon should explain and recommend what will enhance the facial appearance based on existing anatomy. For example, in a patient with a marked "anteface" profile and prominent chin, the nasal dorsum should be lowered

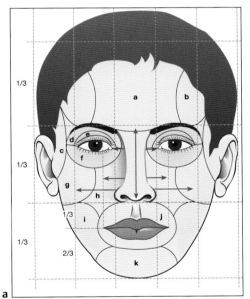
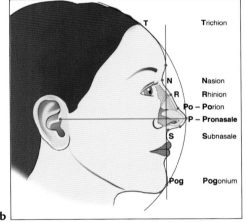
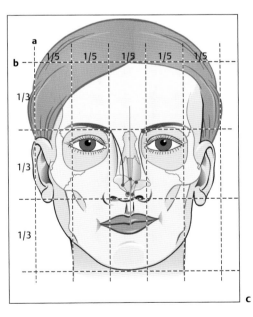

Fig. 5.4 (a) The nose is a central "reference system" for the face: a, frontal region; b, parietal region; c, temporal region; d, eyebrow; e, upper lid; f, lower lid; g, zygoma; h, cheek; i, lower cheek; j, perioral region with upper and lower lip; k, chin. Vertical thirds (Leonardo da Vinci), horizontal fifths (Humphries and Powell), medial vertical line from pupil to oral commissure, medial vertical line from canthus to nasal ala.[11] (b) Geometric points and lines that define the facial profile. T, trichion; N, nasion; R, rhinion; Po, porion; P, pronasale; S, subnasale; Pog, pogonion. (c) Facial disproportions and asymmetries. Left half of face: frequent causes: asymmetrical brow-tip aesthetic line (pseudo-crooked nose); maxillary, midfacial, or mandibular hypoplasia (usually with a crooked mouth); crooked nasal base (cleft lip and palate); asymmetry of individual structural elements; asymmetry of the nasal tip rhomboid (upper and lower lateral cartilages).

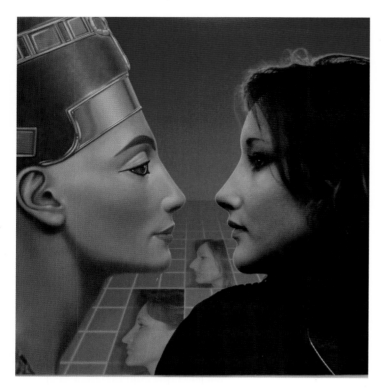

Fig. 5.5 The "virtual nose" aids in the determination of the surgery's objectives and aims at helping the patient to form realistic expectations. The experience of jointly drafting this structure in the discussions with the physician may improve the self-awareness of the patient and prevent preconceived idealistic concepts. The illustration depicts what may go on in the patient's mind prior to surgery: Nefertiti's ideal and attractive features juxtaposed to the patient's "virtual" profile, the result of preoperative counselling. The background depicts pre- and postoperative images of the patient projected onto a two-dimensional matrix, sequences in both time and space.

only slightly because it balances the chin and a concave dorsum would create a Pinocchio effect.[4] Some patients do not know exactly what is bothering them, but they sense a disharmony between the shape of their nose and facial aesthetics: "I would like to have my nose changed. I don't think it fits my face. It is too long, too wide, too narrow, …" In most cases this perception can be visualized, objectified, and resolved in a computer simulation.

The surgeon should demonstrate only what he or she can achieve with surgery and emphasize that simulation is just a tool for preoperative planning, not the standard by which the success of the rhinoplasty will be measured. The simulated pictures should be sketched in the patient's file, not stored as images. A photograph that the patient takes with a smartphone, for example, is allowed. In over 10 years of using this method, we have not had any problems or complaints that the surgical result failed to match the simulation. The goal is to educate the patient about the operation, foster realistic expectations, and illustrate the effect of the nasal surgery on overall facial appearance (**Fig. 5.5**).

5.4 Facial Harmony

The goal of an aesthetic rhinoplasty is to create a nasal shape that will not dominate the face but harmonize with it.[8] At the same time, faces that are dominated by the nose, especially in males, should be changed only after a very detailed analysis, preferably aided by computer animation. The aesthetic indications for rhinoplasty can be grouped into two very broad categories: those that alter facial type and those that preserve it. A type-altering rhinoplasty, such as a reduction procedure that reverses the tip–supratip relationship, may completely alter the physiognomonic appearance of the face. This alteration must be discussed and simulated in advance to avoid problems of identity or identification. Case 32, Chapter 25, shows that an undesired type change or overcorrection may cause the patient to seek another revision aimed at restoring the original nasal shape. This problem is particularly acute when planning the rhinoplasty goal in candidates of different ethnic groups, because the surgery may alter or eliminate the distinctive ethnic characteristics of the nose. Generally speaking, the surgeon should always make an effort to preserve the special and unique qualities of a face or accentuate them with a "tailored correction."

5.5 Basic Questions of Symmetry and Harmony: When Is a Nose "Crooked"?

Many patients will express their concern very succinctly: "My nose is crooked." The surgeon must know how to distinguish a true axial deviation between the reference points of the glabella and philtrum from an asymmetrical contour or brow-tip aesthetic line. Every face consists of two halves that show some degree of physiologic asymmetry. Patients who want to have a "crooked nose" straightened in an asymmetrical face pose a particular challenge. While an axial deviation can be corrected by a septoplasty, with or without release and reattachment of the upper lateral cartilages, by osteotomies, and by shortening the longer side of the nasal pyramid, the correction of asymmetries requires grafting and augmentation.[9–11] The goal in patients with a pseudo-crooked nose is to achieve a "balanced" symmetry, i.e., a result that is not perfectly straight but has the appearance of being so. What Gene Tardy called the "principle of illusion" in rhinoplasty has major practical implications. Straight rarely means "perpendicular," as many noses moved to a true vertical position would look out of place and would accentuate the asymmetry and disharmony of the face. In some cases a slightly crooked nose is better for facial symmetry (**Fig. 5.6**).

5.6 The Classic Hump Removal: A Rare Operation

"I want to have my nose hump (or residual hump) removed." While many patients express this desire, very few surgeons will accommodate it as stated because often it would produce an unsightly Pinocchio effect unless accompanied by tip rotation and/or shortening of the nose. Shortening a too-long infratip triangle will increase the distance from the subnasale to the vermilion border, and this would make a thin, deficient upper lip appear more conspicuous. This will often motivate the patient to seek another change in the adjacent aesthetic unit, such as raising the vermilion border.

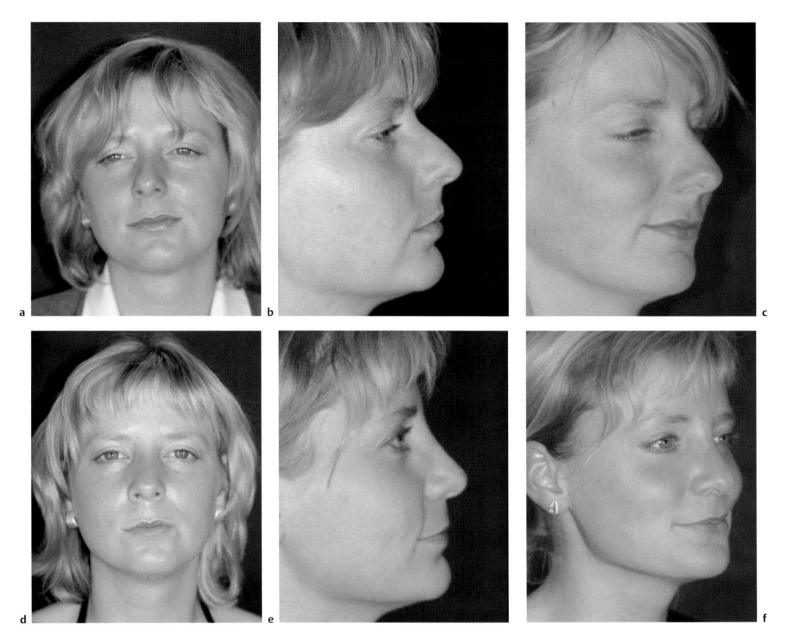

Fig. 5.6 (**a–c**) Preoperative appearance of a patient with a crooked nose in a markedly asymmetrical face with hypoplasia of the left side and a crooked mouth. (**d–f**) Appearance 2 years after a "balanced" rhinoplasty. The nose is not aligned on a true vertical axis, and the nasal base is not straight. Nevertheless, the rhinoplasty has eliminated the impression of a crooked nose and has reduced apparent facial asymmetry.

5.7 Basis for Profile Corrections

The relative positions of the maxilla and mandible, including an analysis of jaw position, occlusal position, and malocclusion (Angle classes), forms the basis for any profile change in septorhinoplasty.[5] This is the only way to distinguish a true abnormality of nasal projection from an apparent abnormality. As a general rule, a primary or revision rhinoplasty—especially one that alters nasal tip projection—should be undertaken only after orthodontic treatment has been completed and the patient has reached skeletal maturity. In a patient with an anteface profile and prominent chin, for example, a reduction of the nasal dorsum would only accentuate the protruding profile. Of course, it should always be determined whether the profile can be improved by rhinoplasty alone or whether a combination of rhinoplasty and mentoplasty would yield better results (**Fig. 5.7**).

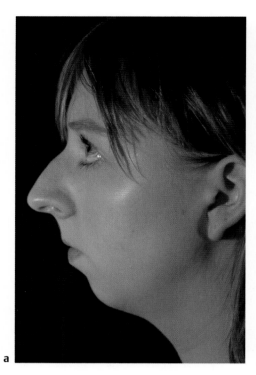
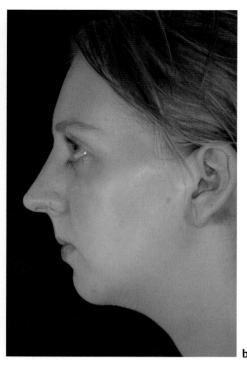

a

b

Fig. 5.7 (**a**) Receding chin with an overprojected nose. (**b**) Appearance 2 years after septorhinoplasty and mentoplasty.

References

1. Glück—welches Glück. Exhibition at the German Hygiene Museum in Dresden and Siemens Arts Program, 2008

2. Joseph J. Nasenplastik und sonstige Gesichtsplastik nebst einem Anhang über Mammaplastik. Leipzig, Germany: C Kabitzsch; 1931

3. Palma P, Khodaei I, Tasman A-J. A guide to the assessment and analysis of the rhinoplasty patient. Facial Plast Surg 2011;27(2):146–159

4. Baud CH. Harmonie der Gesichtszüge. La Chaux-de-Fonds, Switzerland: Clinique de la Tour; 1967

5. Behrbohm H. Septorhinoplastik—klinische Geometrie und virtuelle Op-Planung. HNO-Nach 2001;31:24–29

6. Behrbohm H, Tardy ME. Preoperative Management. In: Behrbohm H, Tardy ME, eds. Essentials of Septorhinoplasty. Philosophy—Approaches—Techniques. New York, NY: Thieme; 2003:90–106

7. Powell H, Humphreys B. Proportions of the Aesthetic Face. Stuttgart, Germany: Thieme; 1984

8. Behrbohm H. Bezugskoordinaten der ästhetischen Gesichtschirurgie—zwischen Mathematik und Intuition. Part 1: Die Nase. Face 2007;4:20–25

9. Mahajan AY, Shafiei M, Marcus BC. Analysis of patient-determined preoperative computer imaging. Arch Facial Plast Surg 2009;11(5):290–295

10. Nouraei SA, Pulido MA, Saleh HA. Impact of rhinoplasty on objective measurement and psychophysical appreciation of facial symmetry. Arch Facial Plast Surg 2009;11(3):198–202

11. Yao F, Lawson W, Westreich RW. Effect of midfacial asymmetry on nasal axis deviation: indications for use of the subalar graft. Arch Facial Plast Surg 2009;11(3):157–164

6 Septorhinoplasty in Different Age Groups

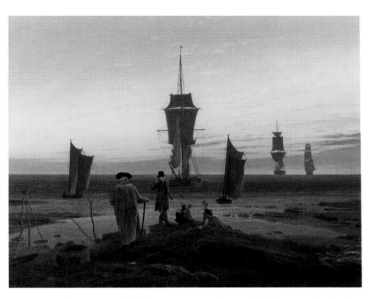

Fig. 6.1 *The Stages of Life* by Caspar David Friedrich (1774–1840). Like all his paintings, this one is neither signed nor dated, and even the title is controversial. Friedrich: "Observe the form exactly, both the smallest and the large, and do not separate the small from the large, but rather the trivial from the important."

Besides the result of the previous operation and the skin and connective-tissue type, the age of the rhinoplasty candidate also has a significant influence on the choice of surgical approach, expected postoperative healing, surgical trauma, and scope of the changes that can reasonably be achieved.[1] The aging process starts at ~ 19–20 years of age with cellular changes and leads to typical changes in the skin (loss of thickness and compliance, atrophy and decreased tone of connective tissues, increased vascular rigidity). As a result, septorhinoplasty in children and adolescents requires a different technique than in adults and the elderly (**Fig. 6.1**). Juveniles also differ from adults in their psychological status, motivations, and expectations from rhinosurgery.

6.1 Septal Surgery in Children

Surgery of the pediatric nose presents special difficulties. The goal of nasal surgery in children is to improve function, but in a way that does not compromise further nasal and midfacial development. The ratio of the bony and cartilaginous components of the nasal skeleton changes in growing children, and it is not until adulthood that a large portion of the nasal septum consists of bone.[2] The cartilaginous nasal septum is currently viewed as the dominant growth center in the developing midface, interacting with the suture-based growth of the bony skeleton. Loss or lesions of the septodorsal cartilage may lead to growth abnormalities of the nose and maxilla.[3] This means that the earlier surgery is performed on the pediatric septum, the greater the

risk of adverse effects on midfacial growth. Injuries to the cranial suture typically lead to saddle nose deformity, while lesions of the inferior suture lead to hypoplasia of the cartilaginous nose with abnormal growth of the premaxilla (Binder syndrome). It is important, therefore, to maintain the integrity of the supportive and growth zones during septoplasty. Particular care should be taken not to separate the cartilaginous septum from the perpendicular plate, as this area is crucial for the support and further growth of the nasal septum and dorsum.[4] Very strict criteria should be applied in selecting children for septal surgery, and this determination should always be made by an experienced surgeon. Submucous septal surgery can be performed for the treatment of severe posttraumatic, congenital, and other deformities in selected children.[5] Great care should be taken, however, to avoid destabilizing any part of the keystone area and to preserve a broad, sturdy cartilage pillar below the cartilaginous nasal dorsum to prevent postoperative saddle deformity. It is seldom justifiable to accept significant nasal airway obstruction before 16–18 years of age.

On the whole, septal deviations are rare in younger children. They most commonly result from growth-related movements of the mosaic components in the medial nasal wall before and during puberty. Deviations in children usually represent deformities involving the anteroinferior portion of the septum. Any corrective surgery should preserve the integrity of the perichondrium and growth zones, e.g., the caudal septum, premaxilla, and the suture with the perpendicular plate and vomer. The surgery should be atraumatic and chondroplastic. Any cartilage pieces that are removed should be straightened and reimplanted at their original site. Septal cartilage will retain its regenerative capacity even after surgical trauma.

Nasal trauma in children can have various effects, typically producing a greenstick fracture of the nasal pyramid. Septal hematomas or abscesses should be excluded or managed appropriately (**Figs. 6.2, 6.3**).

Severe or recurrent trauma may lead to abnormal maxillofacial development as in Binder syndrome, requiring later correction by a reconstructive procedure (**Fig. 6.3**).

6.2 Cosmetic Septorhinoplasty in Adolescents

The nose may be a significant source of distress in teenagers, who may seek rhinoplasty for a large nose, an overprojected nose or tip, a crooked nose, or a saddle nose. With puberty comes a new body awareness, and even minor variants such as a dorsal hump or functional tension nose may prompt a dissatisfaction with personal appearance. As minors, adolescents must be accompanied by parents during their consultation visit. Most are highly motivated to have their nose changed. Most parents are already convinced and either support their child's desire or adopt a neutral attitude. Adolescents are rarely very specific about the desired change, and the surgeon must be able to recognize the problem and state whether the desire for surgery is justified or

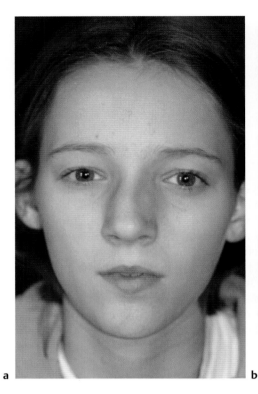
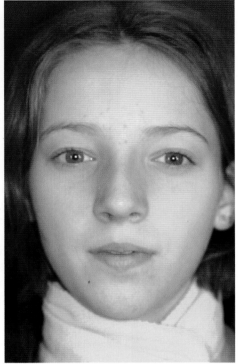
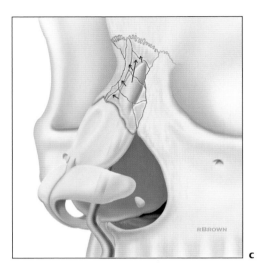

a   b   c

Fig. 6.2 (**a**) Posttraumatic crooked nose in a 13-year-old girl who sustained a nasal fracture. (**b**) Appearance after reduction with the Behrbohm–Kaschke elevator. Greenstick fractures are common in children and are often reducible for up to 10 days after the injury. (**c**) Principle of straightening a nasal fracture with a specially designed elevator.

exaggerated. Most importantly, the surgeon should counsel adolescents and parents in a responsible manner.

6.2.1 Basic Considerations in Septorhinoplasty in Adolescents

Septorhinoplasty should be performed after puberty when the patient is at least 15–16 years of age. Girls should already be having regular menstrual periods, indicating that their skeletal growth is largely complete. Orthodontic treatment with dental braces should be completed as it will significantly affect profile landmarks. The pronasale, subnasale, and soft-tissue pogonion are key reference points in patients with an overprojected nose, for example, in producing a harmonious profile line. Sagittal occlusion defects were graded and classified by Angle in 1907. A convex soft-tissue profile indicates an Angle class II relation, while a concave profile corresponds to Angle class III. The position of the nasal tip is significantly influenced by the position of the jaw and midface. A forward-slanting face, for example, may contribute to nasal overprojection. Very strict criteria should be applied in selecting adolescents for septorhinoplasty because the cartilaginous and bony structures will continue to change with further aging. For example, the skin will become thinner and the nose will narrow. It is essential, then, to take a conservative approach whenever possible and to operate with atraumatic technique. The closed intranasal approach is preferred whenever it

can be applied. Rhinosurgery in children and adolescents should be structure-conserving with an emphasis on cartilage preservation and reorientation.

Orthodontic considerations are important for rhinosurgeons for several reasons:

1. With regard to the timing of a profile-correcting rhinoplasty in adolescents, it should be noted that jaw growth is complete by age 16 years in girls and by age 18 years in boys.
2. Gnathic anomalies lead to typical profile changes:
   - Mandibular prognathism: anterior position of the pogonion
   - Retrognathia: receded position of the pogonion (underbite)
   - Maxillary prognathism: anterior position of the subnasale and upper lip

6.3 Septorhinoplasty in Middle Age

The rhinosurgeon needs to have a particularly large repertoire of surgical techniques and approaches in this age group, as well as an understanding and feel for mechanisms of postoperative wound healing. He should utilize the entire "rhinosurgical keyboard." An incidental advantage of having to acquire this repertoire is the mental exercise available to all rhinosurgeons:

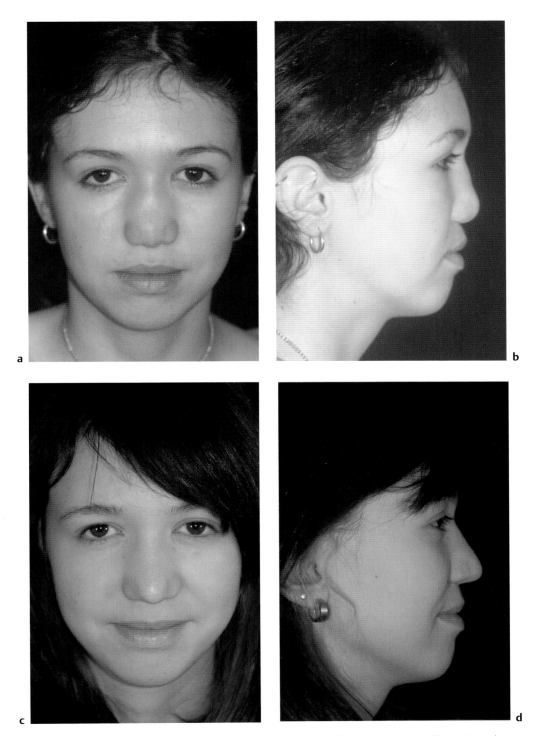

Fig. 6.3 (**a, b**) Young patient with maxillonasal dysplasia (Binder syndrome). The patient has a broad nose with short, thin nasal bones. (**c, d**) Appearance 2 years after augmentation of the maxillary nasal crest and cartilaginous nose with rib cartilage. Low-infracture osteotomies.

they can casually survey the diverse nasal morphologies encountered in restaurants, concert halls, social gatherings, etc., which they are free to analyze and surgically improve in their imagination.

Most septorhinoplasty patients are in their 20s or 30s. Rhinoplasty candidates tend to have a clear motivation, can clearly articulate their goals, and are sensitive in their self-perception. They often place very high expectations on the outcome. The percentage of patients with unrealistic expectations is higher than in other age groups. This is why the preoperative consultation should always include time for recognizing the possible signs of psychological disorders. Typical middle-aged rhinoplasty patients are financially independent, emancipated, and used to living their lives in a proactive way. Some patients seek cosmetic surgery in the wake of a midlife crisis or a change of direction in their private life or professional career.

6.3.1 Biological Age of the Tissues

The biological status of the various tissues should be assessed preoperatively. Discrepancies may have arisen between chronological and biological age due to, for example, lifestyle or nutrition, athletic activity, smoking, or alcohol use. Tissue changes may involve the skin, bone, cartilage, SMAS (superficial musculoaponeurotic system), connective tissues, and blood vessels.

The corium becomes thinner in middle age, and elastic fibers become less abundant. In patients with a thin or intermediate skin type, the nasal tip becomes increasingly narrow while the bony nasal pyramid becomes more prominent. The opposite changes may occur in individuals with a seborrheic skin type. The skin becomes thicker and the pores enlarge as a result of glandular hyperplasia. The cartilage becomes softer and loses some of its stabilizing properties, while portions of the septal cartilage may calcify. The connective tissue attachments between the upper and lower lateral cartilages, for example, become more lax and more yielding to gravity. The nose appears to elongate while the nasal tip becomes ptotic. The bone becomes thinner, more brittle, and demineralized and takes considerably longer to consolidate after an osteotomy. The condition of the blood vessels, along with the coagulation system, becomes an important factor with respect to intraoperative bleeding, postoperative hematoma formation, and the occurrence of wound healing problems.

Analysis of the cutaneous and connective-tissue status of the face should take into account the following criteria:

- Skin type, thickness, texture, and compliance (caution: skin thickness and texture may vary in different areas of the same face)

- Ptosis: e.g., of the eyebrows, eyelids, cheek, or nasal tip

- Skin creases: location, course, depth, cause (mimetic, superficial, gravitational)

- Dermal elastosis: location, degree

- Junction of the chin and neck

Besides expressing a desire for rhinoplasty, patients in this age group also raise questions relating to aesthetic medicine (Botox, filler) and rejuvenation surgery such as blepharoplasty and facial recontouring, usually at specific sites. Simultaneous corrections are therefore not uncommon.

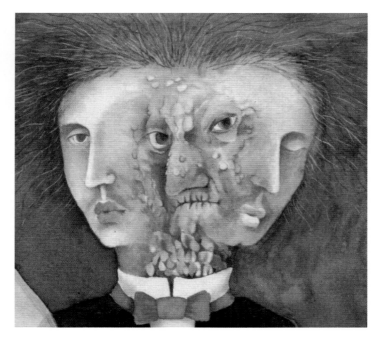

Fig. 6.4   *The Picture of Dorian Gray* (book illustration by K. Müller).

6.4 Septorhinoplasty in Older Patients

As Oscar Wilde noted in *The Picture of Dorian Gray*, "The tragedy of old age is not that one is old, but that one is young." Unlike in the protagonist of his novel, in real life the traces of the biological aging process are manifested overtly in the face (**Fig. 6.4**). But it is precisely the mismatch between a "young mind" and "old face" that motivates older patients to seek cosmetic surgery. Rhinoplasty is an example. Many candidates will have desired this procedure their entire life and, for various reasons, were either unable to act on their desire or did have the surgery, were dissatisfied with the result, and then took years to brave a second attempt.

The tissue changes previously described for middle-aged patients will have advanced markedly with further aging and require a preoperative analysis, thorough counseling, and a cautious approach to surgery. Most older patients undergo subtle, partial rhinoplasties that focus on the correction of specific objectionable features. Small raw surfaces, atraumatic operative technique, and the sparing use of grafts will help prevent wound healing problems. In hump removals, an externally reduced hump can be reused for autologous grafting (**Fig. 6.5**).

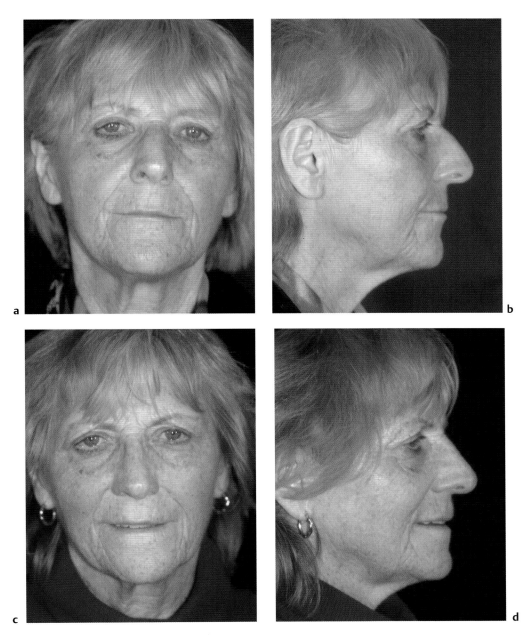

Fig. 6.5   (**a, b**) Preoperative photographs of a woman with thin elastotic skin, a deviated septum, and a bony and cartilaginous nasal hump. (**c, d**) Appearance 3 years after a partial septorhinoplasty using conservative technique, limiting corrections to the primary surgical goal.

References

1. Behrbohm H. Septorhinoplastik in verschiedenen Lebensabschnitten. HNO aktuell 2003;(Pts 1–3):13–17, 59–68, 219–228

2. Pirsig W. Open questions in nasal surgery in children. Rhinology 1986;24(1):37–40

3. Verwoerd CDA, Verwoerd-Verhoef HL. Rhinochirurgie bei Kindern: Entwicklungsphysiologische und chirurgische Aspekte der wachsenden Nase. Laryngorhinootologie 2010;89:46–71

4. Grymer LF, Bosch C. The nasal septum and the development of the midface. A longitudinal study of a pair of monozygotic twins. Rhinology 1997;35(1):6–10

5. AMWF online. Leitlinie Funktionsstörungen der inneren und äußeren Nase bei funktionellen und ästhetischen Beeinträchtigungen. Nr. 017/070. 2010. www.awmf.org/leitlinien/detail/ll/017-070.html

6. Behrbohm H, Tardy ME. Essentials of Septorhinoplasty. Philosophy—Approaches—Techniques. New York, NY: Thieme; 2003

7 Identity and Aesthetics: Ethnic Aspects of Rhinoplasty

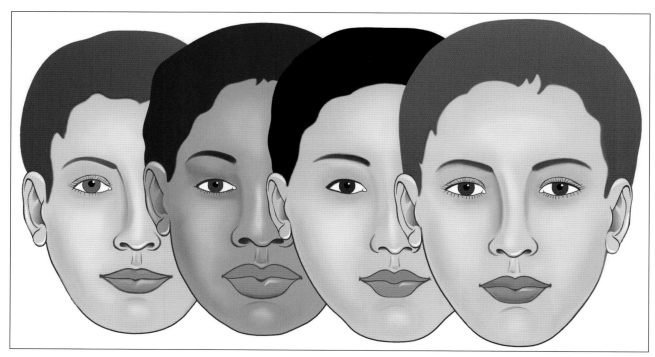

Fig. 7.1 If the faces of European, African, and Asian women are blended into a composite face on a computer, the result is a face (illustrated on the right) with no distinguishing features.

7.1 The Mainstream and the Individual

Where different cultures, religions, and ethnic groups converge in the metropolitan regions of the world, new questions are arising with regard to facial plastic surgery (**Fig. 7.1**).

The problem of altering the size and shape of the nose becomes particularly acute in planning rhinoplasties for patients of different ethnic origins because the surgery may either eliminate or preserve key ethnic features.[1] An Asian nose may be changed to a European type, with considerable impact on the face, or its Asian character may be preserved despite the rhinoplasty. Aside from any desire to alter ethnic features, there is no such thing as an "ideal nose." Yet there are aesthetic features that transcend all ethnic and cultural boundaries, such as a straight nasal dorsum or a harmonious brow-tip aesthetic line.[2]

The rhinosurgeon should have an appreciation for the distinctive features of ethnic nasal variants and for the motivations and desires of the candidates who seek rhinoplasty. Intensive counseling is essential, preferably with visualization aids that will show patients the often-underestimated effect of the rhinoplasty on facial appearance. The risk of a postoperative identity crisis because a technically successful outcome nevertheless proves unacceptable must be avoided. It always stems from a lack of preoperative communication.

Patients who are dissatisfied with their profile, for example, after a primary rhinoplasty pose a special challenge. It is our ex-perience that some of these patients will want to refine the appearance of their nose while preserving their ethnic traits, while others will seek improvement without regard for those traits. As an example, we were once consulted by a set of twins. The brother wanted to keep his distinctive ethnic features while the sister did not. **Fig. 7.2** shows a patient who wanted her profile changed by rhinoplasty but also wanted to preserve her convex nasal dorsum as a desired ethnic trait.

7.2 Nose Types

7.2.1 European Nose

The European or leptorrhine (long, thin) nose is typical of people of European origin. One feature is the relationship of the nasal tip and supratip point. With a well-defined tip, a line drawn along the dorsum to the supratip point will rise to the tip-defining point, make a double break at the lobule–columella junction, then continue on to the subnasale and vermilion border.[3]

7.2.2 Middle Eastern Nose

The Middle Eastern nose has a high, narrow, usually convex dorsum. The supratip point is located above the tip-defining points. The nasolabial angle is smaller than in the European nose (**Figs. 7.3, 7.4**).[4]

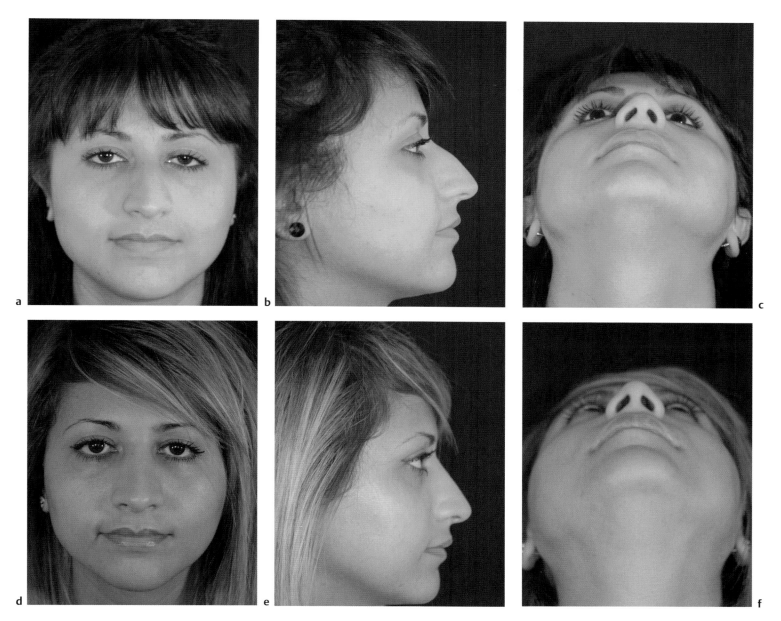

Fig. 7.2   (**a–c**) A 23-year-old woman sought to have her nasal hump removed while retaining a convex nasal profile. She did not want a "European" profile. (**d–f**) The patient 2 years after rhinoplasty, with her ethnic characteristics preserved.

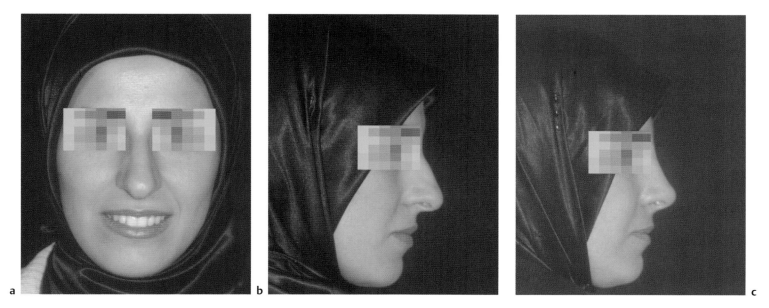

Fig. 7.3   (**a, b**) Frontal and profile views of a young Turkish woman who wanted her nose changed to a more European shape. (**c**) Appearance 1 year after rhinoplasty documents reduction of the nasal dorsum, cephalic tip rotation, and an altered tip–supratip relationship (supratip break).

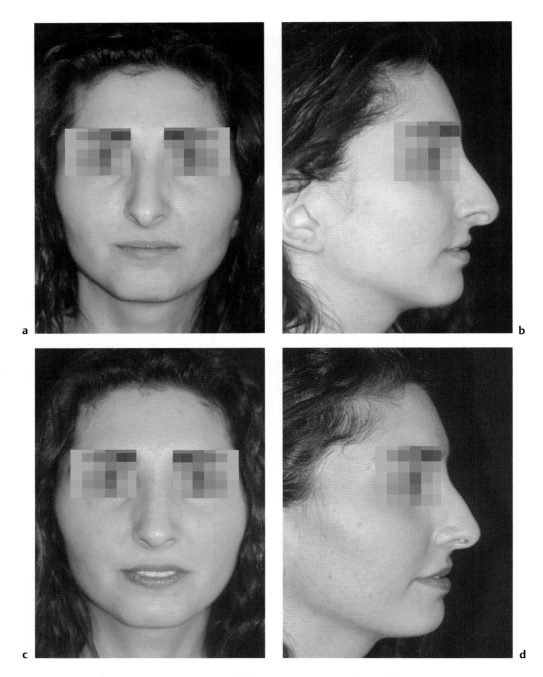

Fig. 7.4 (**a, b**) Young woman with a Middle Eastern–type nose desired shortening of the infratip triangle and hanging columella. The patient expressly desired to maintain the characteristic slight convexity of her profile line. (**c, d**) Appearance 1 year after rhinoplasty documents shortening of the infratip triangle and correction of the columella–lobule–upper lip complex.

7.2.3 African Nose

The platyrrhine nose (broad and flat) is usually found on people of African descent. It is typically distinguished by a deep nasal root, a short concave dorsum, broad separation of the canthi, a bulbous and underprojected nasal tip, flared alae with round nostrils, and thick skin. The nasofrontal angle is often in the range of 130–140°. Ethnic mixing has also given rise to subgroups of the platyrrhine nose. Unlike the African-type nose, the Afro–European nose typically has a longer and more prominent dorsum, an occasional hump, moderately flared alae, and a fine nasal tip.

7.2.4 Hispanic Nose

The terms "Hispanic nose" or "Latino nose" are often used in reference to people of Spanish, Portuguese, and South and Central American descent, as well as those from Caribbean countries such as Cuba, Puerto Rico, or Costa Rica. Daniel classified the Hispanic nose into four major subtypes: Castilian, Mexican American, Mestizo, and Creole.[5] A Mestizo nose, for example, is thicker and more sebaceous and has a smaller osseocartilaginous vault, a weak caudal septum, and a wide alar base with rounded nostrils, a short medial crus, and a short columella (**Fig. 7.5**).[5,6]

7.2.5 Asian Nose

The mesorrhine nose (intermediate, Asian) displays features of both the European and the African nose. The skin is moderately thick and the nasal dorsum is deep and broad. The nasal tip is underprojected. The columella appears short and the nostrils have a round or oblong shape (**Fig. 7.6**).

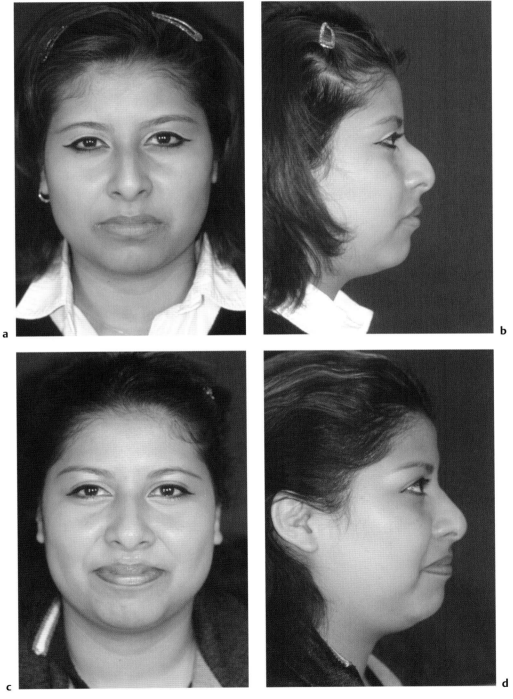

a

b

c

d

Fig. 7.5 (**a, b**) Latin American woman with a pronounced nasal hump. She wanted to have the predominantly bony hump removed while preserving her ethnic character. (**c, d**) Frontal and profile views 7 years after rhinoplasty.

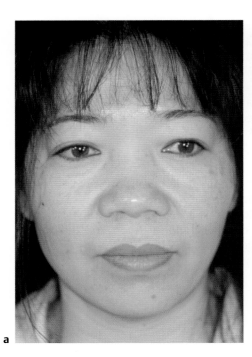 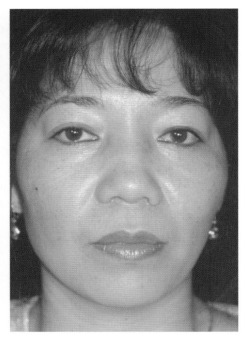

a   b

Fig. 7.6 (**a**) Young woman with an Asian-type nose desired to have the dorsum raised. (**b**) The same patient 5 years after elevation of the nasal dorsum with a static columellar strut and an autologous onlay rib graft.

References

1. Behrbohm H. Ethnische Gesichtspunkte bei der Rhinoplastik— zwischen Identität und Ästhetik. HNO Nach 2006;1:28–30

2. Meneghini F. Clinical Facial Analysis. Elements, Principles, Techniques. New York, NY: Springer; 2005

3. Papel ID, Capone RB. Facial proportions and esthetic ideals. In: Behrbohm H, Tardy ME, eds. Essentials of Septorhinoplasty. Principles— Approaches—Techniques. New York, NY: Thieme; 2003:66–87

4. McCurdy JA Jr, Lam SM. Cosmetic Surgery of the Asian Face. New York, NY: Thieme; 2005

5. Daniel RK. Hispanic rhinoplasty in United States, with emphasis on the Mexican American nose. Plastic Reconstr Surg 2003;112:244–256

6. Hiquera S, Hatef DA, Stal S. Rhinoplasty in Hispanic patient. Semin Plast Surg 2009;23(3):207–214

8 The Nose As an Aerodynamic Body

8.1 The Physics of the Nose and the Patient's Subjective Complaints

The nose shares several aerodynamic properties in common with a turbine or jet engine. A comparison will aid in understanding the nose as an aerodynamic body and how its function can be improved by surgery (**Fig. 8.1**).

In a jet engine, a gas or fluid stream is drawn into the front intake, is compressed, and then slowed in a diffusor before being accelerated and redirected. Air flowing through the nose is directed and modified in a similar way.

In the nasal vestibule, the constricted lumen accelerates and laminates the inspired air on its way to the internal orifice. The concave internal orifice acts like a concave lens in optics: the air stream is dispersed and directed into the expanding anterior nasal cavity, which is analogous to a diffuser.[1] Next it enters the functional cavity of the nose with the nasal turbinates. Aerodynamically, this cavity functions as a partitioned space that can perform its tasks of warming, filtering, and humidification (also olfaction) only when all portions of the cavity are reached by a slowed, turbulent stream of air. On entering the posterior nasal cavity, the now-conditioned air is accelerated and becomes less turbulent.[2] It then reaches the convex-shaped choana, which further converges the flow so that it can be delivered to the lower airways with the least possible resistance.

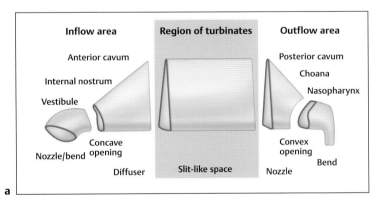

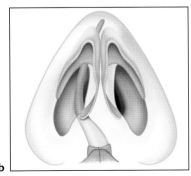

Fig. 8.1 (**a**) The nasal "jet" (explanation in text). (**b**) The nose as an aerodynamic body during inspiration.

Aside from functional diagnostic tests, it is important in everyday practice to have an algorithm that can "interrogate" specific functional and morphologic structures and can actually select patients who require surgical modification of one or more functional problem zones.[3] In a study on the long-term results of septoplasties, Mlynski found that nasal breathing was improved in only 68% of the patients operated.[4] One approach to solving this problem may lie in a more complex consideration of the nose as an aerodynamic body.

8.2 Evaluating Dynamic Functional Elements

The dynamic functional elements discussed below play a role in the pathogenesis of impaired nasal breathing and should be evaluated before every operation.[4,5]

8.2.1 Nasal Septum

All septal deviations are not the same. Small curves and pronounced ridges or spurs may have no functional significance. Sites of narrowing in the nasal airway have highly variable functional (aerodynamic) implications. From a functional standpoint, a centered septum is more important than a straight septum.[4] The height of the septum is also of functional importance (**Fig. 8.2**).

8.2.2 Nasolabial Angle

The curvature of the nasal vestibule is a critical factor for optimum nasal airflow. It must be between 90° and 100°. A simple test is to rotate the nasal tip upward to see whether this maneuver improves nasal breathing. The correction of tip ptosis during septoplasty of the aging nose is appropriate for functional reasons if the nasolabial angle is less than 90°. Angles greater than 100° lead to decreased airflow through the upper functional space and impaired function.

8.2.3 Inferior Turbinates

The nasal turbinates form the air passages and functional space of the nasal cavity and provide the necessary morphology for normal airflow. Along with the septal cavernous tissue, they increase flow resistance and turbulence to promote greater contact between the air and mucosa. Overresection of the inferior turbinates, for example, cause flow to follow the path of least resistance and pass through the nose much too rapidly without adequate mucosal contact. The other portions of the nose are no longer ventilated, and important components of nasal respiratory function are lost. Consequently, any resection of the inferior turbinates should be done very sparingly. Overresections are irreparable. The goal of functional nasal surgery is not to maximize the cross-sectional area of the nasal airway, but to promote an optimum flow distribution (**Fig. 8.3**).

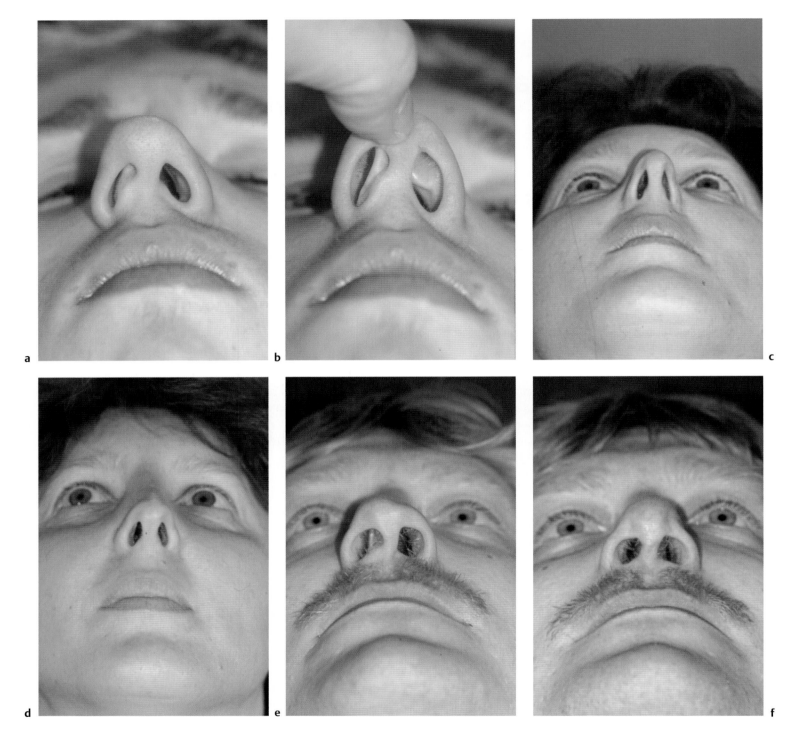

Fig. 8.2 Diagnostic evaluation of the nasal vestibule. (**a**) Subluxation of the septum. (**b**) Degree of deformity is assessed by upward rotation of the nasal tip. (**c**) Functional tension nose with typical tense, narrow nostrils and stenosis of the internal and external nasal valves. (**d**) Tension has been relieved by shortening the anterior septum. (**e**) Dislocation of the anterior septum. (**f**) After submucous septoplasty.

8.2.4 Nasal Valves

In the past, there have been inconsistencies in the nomenclature used for the nasal valves. The nasal valve area is subdivided into the external nasal valve and internal nasal valve. The *internal* nasal valve described by Mink,[6] called also the "internal nasal orifice," is located between the caudal end of the upper lateral cartilage and the medial border of the septum.[7] The *external* nasal valve is formed by the inferior rim of the lateral alar cartilage, the connective tissue of the nasal ala, and medially by the medial crus of the alar cartilage and the membranous and cartilaginous septum.[8] From the standpoint of physiologic airflow resistance, the valves function as the *flow-limiting segment* because they form the narrowest part of the nasal airway. An endoscope can detect stenosis in a functional tension nose, for example, as well as ballooning of the nasal valve due to saddle nose deformity. The normal internal nasal valve has an aperture angle of 15°. The Cottle maneuver can detect functional stenosis. In the Bachmann test, the uppermost part of the internal nasal valve is expanded and rounded with a small cotton ball. If the patient reports subjective improvement of nasal breathing with this maneuver, the test is positive for an internal nasal valve problem. Numerous surgical techniques have been described for expanding and stabilizing the nasal valve (**Fig. 8.4**).[9–11]

It is important to preserve the caudal border of the upper lateral cartilage whenever possible and ensure a concave shape of the internal orifice to maintain good valvular function.[10,12,13] Even when a valid indication exists for enlarging the nasal valve, it should still remain narrow enough to act as a flow limiter.

8.2.5 Inspiratory Collapse

Functional endoscopy of the nasal vestibule with a rigid endoscope can detect alar collapse during inspiration. This phenomenon may have various causes. "Collapsibility" refers to the force that the alar cartilage can exert against the suction produced by inspiration to keep the vestibule open. Inspiratory alar collapse is a common problem that may result from a functional tension nose (**Fig. 8.5**), excessive cephalic trimming of the alar cartilage, weakened cartilage, or anterior septal deviation or subluxation.[14]

8.2.6 Middle Vault

The nasal roof may be too narrow to permit adequate ventilation of the upper nasal cavity. By analogy with a sharp-pointed Gothic arch, it may be appropriate to widen and stabilize the middle vault of the nose. This can be accomplished with spreader grafts, for example, which expand the space from the rhinion to the nasal valve and neutralize axial deviations.[10,12,15,16] In spreader flaps, the dorsal border of the upper lateral cartilage is turned over medially and fixed with a mattress suture.[17]

8.2.7 Posttraumatic Changes

Posttraumatic functional disturbances may result from cartilaginous or bony fractures of the nasal septum, organized hematomas, or displaced fragments from the bony pyramid. Infractured

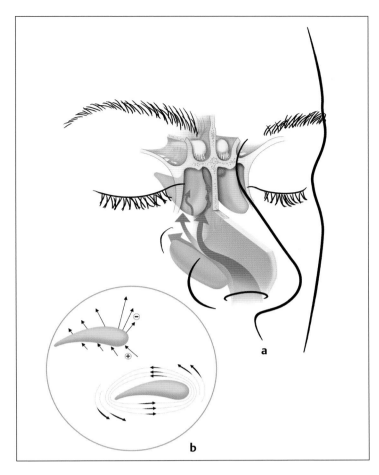

Fig. 8.3 Function of the inferior turbinate. The inferior turbinate is the "thermostat" of the nose. Its mucosa warms the inspired air and directs a portion of it toward the middle turbinate and olfactory groove.

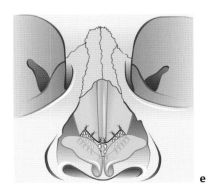

Fig. 8.4 Some surgical measures to enlarge or stabilize the internal nasal valve. (**a**) Flaring sutures. (**b**) Alar batten grafts of autologous cartilage, used to treat stenosis of the internal (*circled a, circled b*) and external nasal valve (*circled c*). (**c**) Butterfly grafts keep the nasal valve patent. They are placed on the dorsal border of the septum and pushed beneath the dorsal alar cartilage. (**d**) Horizontal mattress bending sutures. (**e**) The Wengen titanium Breathe Implant.

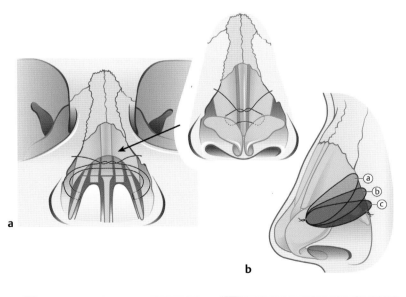

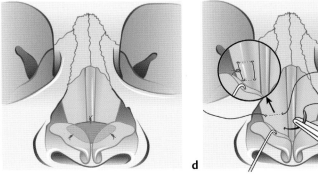

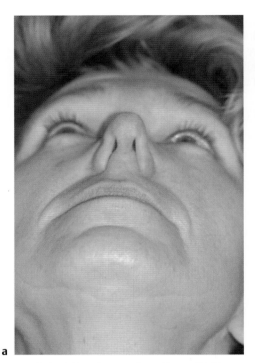
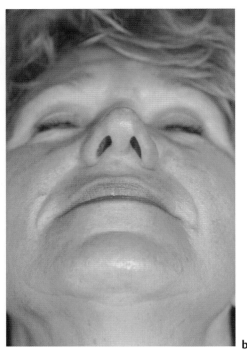

a   b

Fig. 8.5   (**a**) Inspiratory alar collapse. (**b**) The external nasal valve is stabilized with alar rim grafts.[18,19]

nasal bones, especially when relatively long, may cause airway obstruction in the keystone area, middle vault, or nasal valve area and should be osteotomized and reduced. Postoperative saddle nose can often lead to various problems with functional relevance such as dilatation of the internal nasal valve (ballooning), separation of the bony nose from the cartilaginous nose, displaced or sequestered bone fragments, lateralization of the upper lateral cartilage, a hanging columella, or cephalic rotation of the nasal tip. Most of these cases require a complex reconstruction based on a detailed analysis.

8.2.8 Hidden Columella

The anterior septum may be absent as a result of previous surgery, infection, or trauma. The diagnosis is quickly made by internal palpation of the nose. The examiner should also determine whether nasal projection (tip recoil phenomenon) is impaired and whether nasal tip position has been changed. Septal or conchal cartilage is particularly well suited for reconstructing the anterior septal cartilage.

References

1. Mlynski G. Physiology and pathology of nasal breathing. In: Behrbohm H, Tardy ME, eds. Essentials of Septorhinoplasty. Stuttgart, Germany: Thieme; 2003:76–87
2. Behrbohm H. Funktionell-ästhetische Chirurgie der Nase, Reparatur an einem Strömungskörper. Face 2012;(1):12–15 http://www.oemus.com/de/publikationen/archiv.php?p=sim/fa/2012/fa0112
3. Ballert JA, Park SS. Functional considerations in revision rhinoplasty. Facial Plast Surg 2008;24(3):348–357
4. Mlynski G. Gestörte Funktion der oberen Atemwege. Wiederherstellende Verfahren bei gestörter Funktion der oberen Atemwege. Nasale Atmung. Laryngorhinootologie 2005;84:101–124
5. Forkel P. Untersuchungen an Nasenmodellen zum Einfluss rhinochirurgischer Massnahmen auf die Atemströmung [inaugural dissertation]. Greifswald, Germany: Ernst-Moritz-Arndt-Universität; 2009
6. Mink PJ. Physiologie der oberen Luftwege. Leipzig, Germany: Vogel; 1920
7. Mink PJ. Le nez comme voie respiratoire. Presse Otolaryngol (Belg) 1903;21:481–496
8. Bloching MB. Disorders of the nasal valve area. GMS Curr Top Otorhinolaryngol Head Neck Surg 2007;6:Doc07 http://www.egms.de/static/en/journals/cto/2008-6/cto000041.shtml
9. Apaydin F. Nasal valve surgery. Facial Plast Surg 2011;(2):179–189
10. Apaydin F. Nasal valve surgery. Facial Plast Surg 2011;27(2):179–191
11. Rhee JS, Kimbell JS. The nasal valve dilemma: the narrow straw vs the weak wall. Arch Facial Plast Surg 2012;14(1):9–10
12. Gassner HG, Friedman O, Sherris DA, Kern EB. An alternative method of middle vault reconstruction. Arch Facial Plast Surg 2006;8(6):432–435
13. Toriumi DM, Josen J, Weinberger M, Tardy ME Jr. Use of alar batten grafts for correction of nasal valve collapse. Arch Otolaryngol Head Neck Surg 1997;123(8):802–808
14. Bull TR, Mackay IS. Alar collapse. Facial Plast Surg 1986;3(4):267–276
15. Sheen JH. Spreader graft: a method of reconstructing the roof of the middle nasal vault following rhinoplasty. Plast Reconstr Surg 1984;73(2):230–239
16. Sykes JM, Tapias V, Kim JE. Management of the nasal dorsum. Facial Plast Surg 2011;27(2):192–202
17. Oneal RM, Berkowitz RL. Upper lateral cartilage spreader flaps in rhinoplasty. Aesthet Surg J 1998;18(5):370–371
18. Boahene KD, Hilger PA. Alar rim grafting in rhinoplasty: indications, technique, and outcomes. Arch Facial Plast Surg 2009;11(5):285–289
19. Sufyan A, Ziebarth M, Crousore N, Berguson T, Kokoska MS. Nasal batten grafts: are patients satisfied? Arch Facial Plast Surg 2012;14(1):14–19
20. Pedroza F, Anjos GC, Patrocinio LG, Barreto JM, Cortes J, Quessep SH. Seagull wing graft: a technique for the replacement of lower lateral cartilages. Arch Facial Plast Surg 2006;8(6):396–403

9 Evaluation and Analysis

9.1 Visual Inspection

Visual inspection of the patient is done to evaluate the face and external nose. Questions of overall assessment are paramount: Are there gnathic abnormalities? Is there significant facial asymmetry or facial scoliosis? Is the nose over- or underprojected? In making these determinations, the surgeon relies not just on classic facial geometry formulas but also on his or her aesthetic sense (**Fig. 9.1**).[1]

Does the nose look too long, too short, too broad, or too narrow? Does it distract from the attractiveness of the eyes? In previously operated cases, does the current nose fit the patient's face or personality? Once these determinations have been made, attention is directed toward local findings in the external nose. We have had good experience with photographing rhinoplasty candidates on their initial visit, then using modern graphic software to jointly analyze the photo on the computer screen and simulate possible changes (**Fig. 9.2**). This process generates

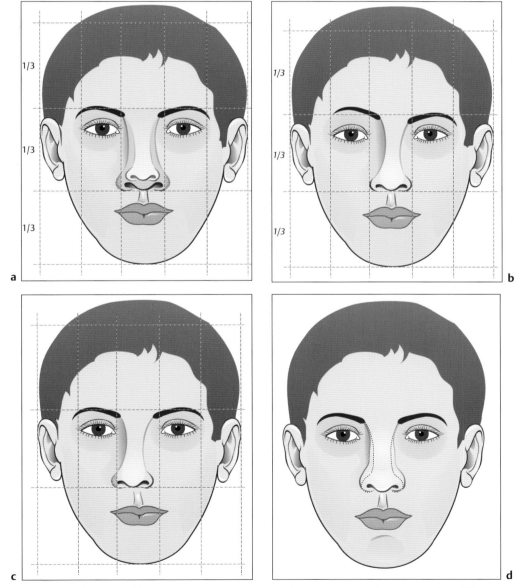

Fig. 9.1 (**a**) Measured by reference lines, a nose may be too short, too long, or too broad for the face. (**b**) Straight nose with asymmetric brow-tip aesthetic lines creates the impression of a crooked nose. (**c**) Bony crooked nose with distortion of the philtrum and true axial deviation to the right. (**d**) The nose appears too wide in a narrow face. This is only an impression and is not measurable.

sketches, diagrams, and interview notes that document both the findings and the consultation and will ultimately direct surgical planning.

9.2 Palpation

Visual inspection is followed by palpation. But before touching the nose, the surgeon should tell the patient that only palpation can supply essential information on the tension and elasticity of the various structural components of the nose.[2,3] Some problems are easier to palpate than to see (**Fig. 9.3**). There are five areas in which palpable findings are particularly important:

1. The nasal dorsum. The junction of the bony and cartilaginous nasal dorsum is palpated to detect any roughness, irregularities, appositional bone growth after previous surgery, or an open roof.

2. Protection. Finger pressure is applied to the nasal tip and anterior septal angle to assess tip and supratip recoil, which will indicate the quality of protection in both areas. The height and tension of the anterior septal cartilage can be assessed over the anterior septal angle.

3. Length of the nasal bones. The relationship of the bony and cartilaginous portions of the nasal pyramid will influence surgical planning. Short nasal bones, or a short nasal pyramid, are a frequent indication for the use of spreader grafts.

4. The nasal vestibule. The shape and tension of the anterior septum and the size of the nasal spine and premaxilla can be assessed by palpation.

5. The alar cartilages. The shape, size, and elasticity of the alar cartilages can be assessed by bimanual palpation.

9.3 Nasal Endoscopy

Nasal endoscopy is useful for detecting any intranasal pathology.[4,5] A logical, consistent routine should be followed to ensure complete and systematic coverage (**Fig. 9.4**). With endoscopy, the examiner can explore the internal anatomy of the nose and evaluate the lateral nasal wall, the "sluice" leading to the paranasal sinuses, and the general appearance of the nasal mucosa.[6] The mucosa is scrutinized for mucous or pus tracks, edema, and polyps. The function of the internal and external nasal valves during inspiration and expiration can also be assessed endoscopically (**Fig. 9.4**).

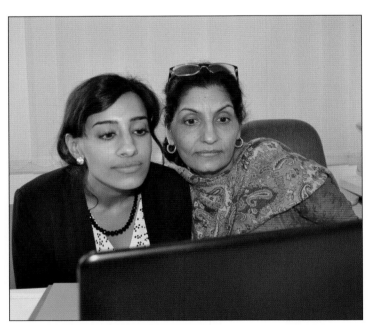

Fig. 9.2 The potential results of a revision rhinoplasty are simulated by computer animation during a consultation visit.

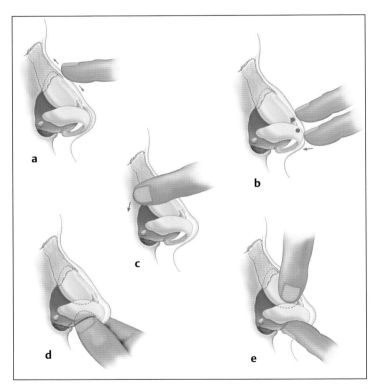

Fig. 9.3 Palpation of the nose. (**a**) Bimanual palpation of the bony and cartilaginous nasal dorsum to assess elasticity, skin thickness and texture, irregularities, bony boundaries and to detect a possible open roof. (**b**) The tip recoil maneuver is a useful indicator of tip support (*arrow*). The anterior septal angle is palpated to assess the size and tension of the anterior septum. (**c**) Exploring the length and strength of the bony nasal pyramid. The relationship of the bony and cartilaginous portions is particularly important. (**d**) Palpation of the caudal septum, vestibules, and nasal spine. The surgeon gains information on the tension, width, and strength of the anterior septum; the size and shape of the nasal spine; and the tension of the medial crura, the membranous septum, and the footplates. (**e**) Bidigital evaluation of the shape, size, and elasticity of the upper and lower cartilages, especially the cephalic and caudal edges.

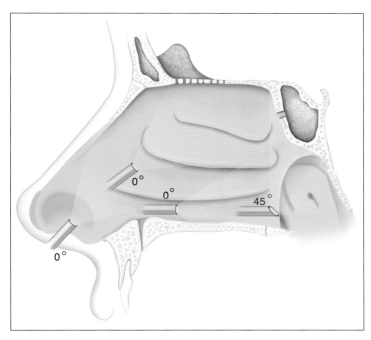

Fig. 9.4 Algorithm for systematic endoscopic exploration of the nose.

Algorithm for nasal endoscopy (**Fig. 9.5**):

1. Start with a 0° scope 3 or 4 mm in diameter. Advance the endoscope over the nasal floor to the choana. The inferior turbinate, caudal nasal septum, choana, and pharyngeal tubal orifice can be visualized in the same sagittal plane as the posterior extension of the inferior turbinate (**Fig. 9.5**).

2. Retract the endoscope to inspect the nasal vestibule and valve area during normal and forced inspiration and expiration. The middle meatus is visualized.

3. Switch to a 30° or 45° scope with a 3- or 4-mm diameter. Advance the endoscope with the field of view directed upward, passing beneath the middle meatus. Inspect the sphenoethmoid recess and the sphenoid sinus ostium. Look into the olfactory rim. Angle laterally after passing the choana. Tell the patient to swallow, and evaluate the opening mechanism of the eustachian tube.

4. Withdraw the endoscope and evaluate the inferior meatus with the orifice of the nasolacrimal duct several millimeters behind the head of the inferior turbinate.

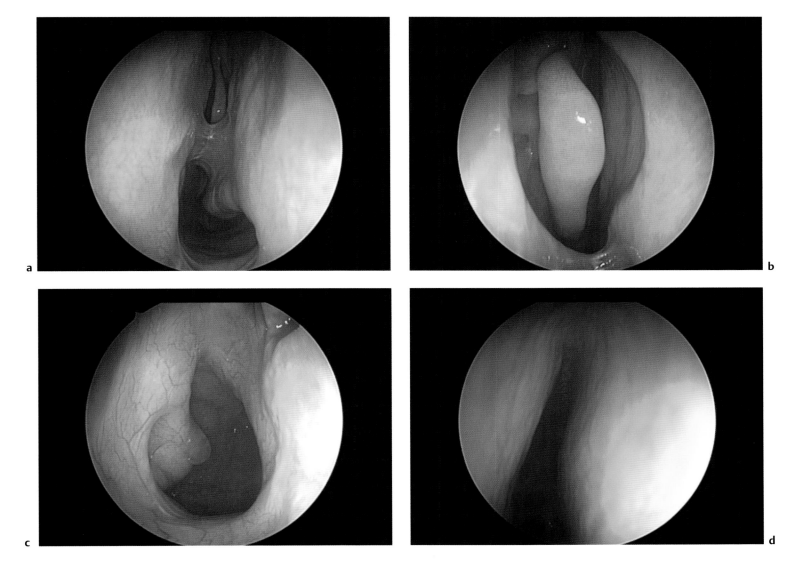

Fig. 9.5 Typical key areas in nasal endoscopy: (**a**) View from the vestibule into the nasal cavity. The examiner assesses the inferior and middle turbinates, the position of the septum, the nasal valve, and mucosal color and congestion. (**b**) View into the middle meatus, the "bellwether" of the paranasal sinuses. Possible findings include mucous and pus tracks, edema, polyps, or tumors. (**c**) View into the choana with the pharyngeal tubal orifice. The opening mechanism of the tube is observed during swallowing. (**d**) The nasal valve area is evaluated at rest and during forced inspiration.

9.4 Function Testing

9.4.1 Computed Rhinomanometry

Computer-assisted rhinomanometry can provide objective evidence for the subjective feeling of obstructed nasal breathing. The principle involves the synchronous recording of the pressure differential (DΔ) between the nasal vestibule and choana (measured in pascal, Pa) and the airflow (V) measured in cubic centimeters per second (**Fig. 9.6**).[7–10] An improved technique called four-phase rhinomanometry determines not only intranasal pressure and flow at 150 Pa but also the log peak resistance (log VR) and log effective resistance (log R_{eff}) for the quantitative analysis of nasal obstruction.[11] In practice, active anterior rhinomanometry with a decongestion test (using decongestant nose drops) is most commonly used in selecting patients for nasal surgery. The test aids in differentiating stenosis with an anatomical cause from dynamic stenosis (mucosal disease, hyperreactivity) and pseudostenosis (e.g., in rhinitis sicca) (**Fig. 9.6**).

9.4.2 Acoustic Rhinometry

Acoustic rhinometry determines cross-sectional areas in the nasal cavity by analyzing the reflections from an acoustic signal introduced into the nose.[12] By generating a graph of nasal cross-sectional areas at different distances from the nostril, acoustic rhinometry can accurately map the internal geometry of the nasal cavity. This test is not as widely used in practice as computed rhinomanometry, however.

9.4.3 Olfactometry

Subjective and objective tests are available for the assessment of olfactory performance. Sniffin' Sticks is a standard test that is widely used in dysosmia patients. The cap is removed from the pen-like dispensing device, and the pen is held under the patient's nose for 3 second Several types of odorants are used:

- Pure odorants: cinnamon, lavender, vanilla, peppermint oil, turpentine

- Odorants with a trigeminal component: ammonia, acetic acid

- Odorants with a gustatory component: pyridine, chloroform

An olfactory test consists of three parts:

1. Screening identification test. The patient is presented with different suprathreshold odorants and must choose one odorant from among four possible answers.

2. More detailed threshold and discrimination test. In the threshold test, the patient is presented with 16 odor triplets. Each triplet consists of two odorless pens and one pen with *n*-butanol in 16 different concentrations (*n*-butanol has a characteristic pungent smell). The object is to determine the threshold of odor detection, i.e., the concentration at which the patient can smell something.

3. Discrimination test. The patient is presented with 16 different sets of suprathreshold odor triplets, two identical and one different. The patient must identify the one that is different.

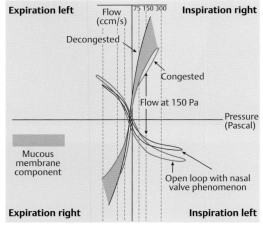

	Log10R (VR, REFF)	Flow (ccm/s) ln 150 Pa	Obstruction, resistance
1	<= 0.75	> 500	very low
2	0.75 – 1.00	300 – 500	low
3	1.00 – 1.25	180 – 300	moderate
4	1.00 – 1.50	60 – 180	high
5	> 1.50	< 60	very high

b

a

Fig. 9.6 Four-phase rhinomanometry, illustrated in a patient with septal deviation. Right side: high flow at low pressure. Left side: limited. Open loops indicate a movable nasal vestibule ("nasal valve phenomenon"). The distance between the plots for the first and second measurements (green area) represents the contribution of the mucosa to total airway resistance. (**b**) Level of nasal obstruction.

9.5 Assessment of Nasal Breathing—Problems and Modern Solutions

T. Hildebrandt, S. Zachow, S. Bessler, L. Goubergrits

The pressure drop in the nose during respiration is determined mainly by the geometry of the nasal airway. This geometry results from the anatomy of the bone and cartilage framework and from the variable morphology of the tissues lining the nose. Changes in the functional and reactive state of the nasal mucosa and turbinates lead to relatively large physiologic variance in the nasal airway.

Even a very experienced rhinosurgeon often finds it difficult to interpret preoperative findings and to predict with adequate precision how changes in the internal and/or external nose will affect airflow.

Frequently, discrepancies between the doctor's and the patient's assessment of nasal breathing have to be noted, and unsatisfactory results of functional nasal surgery are quite common.[13] One reason for this may be that our understanding of nasal breathing is still fragmented. The current scientific focus on the inhaled air and nasal patency possibly does not give sufficient credit to the complexity of the physiologic processes that occur in conjunction with nasal breathing. The question arises whether nasal airflow during respiration can and should be viewed as being part of endonasal self-regulatory mechanisms.[14,15]

Today, about the only tool available for the objective analysis of impaired nasal breathing is determination of total nasal airway resistance. However, technological developments suggest that methods of numerical flow simulation (computational fluid dynamics, CFD) could one day become important in the evaluation of transnasal airflow. Used in industry for years, CFD methods make it possible to calculate or map flow parameters with a high degree of spatial and temporal resolution. This offers a high analytical potential that could be of major importance in the progress of nasal surgery.

9.5.1 Principles of Physiologically Based Nasal Surgery

Every septorhinoplasty causes a certain degree of structural change in the bony and cartilage framework of the nose. Even seemingly minor alterations in tissue structures carry a risk of compromising nasal breathing, possibly also resulting in flow-related morphologic changes in the mucosa and disturbances in the internal milieu of the nasal cavity. An extreme example of the latter is empty nose syndrome.

Physiologic or near-physiologic airflow conditions are essential for a functionally competent nasal organ and not least for a comfortable subjective perception of breathing. Respiratory resistance is only one aspect of this issue.[14,16]

An important anatomical prerequisite for a functioning nose is approximate symmetry of the nasal cavities combined with a variable, slitlike airway (**Fig. 9.7**).[14,15,17,18] The ability of the nasal turbinates, especially the inferior turbinate, to alternately congest and decongest plays a major role in this regard and is the basis for the nasal cycle. Therefore, a routine turbinotomy, which is often common practice with intention of easy reduction of nasal resistance, cannot be justified. Careful analysis will usually reveal alternative surgical interventions that can adequately decrease nasal resistance while preserving the original configuration of the nasal airway.

The greatest pressure drop in the nose (up to 80% according to Wexler) occurs in the isthmus nasi (**Figs. 9.8, 9.9**).[19,20] Any additional narrowing in that area will have a particularly marked effect on nasal resistance. This area is also crucial for producing an optimum airflow pattern in the nasal cavity.[14,16,17,19] Hence it merits close attention during evaluation and surgery of the nasal framework. It is not uncommon to find septal deviations in the isthmus nasi that are barely detectable rhinoscopically but are the actual cause of an initially unexplained impairment of nasal breathing. Not only for this reason, palpation of the septum or the nasal framework is necessary.

Essential components of the nasal cavity's wall are elastic structural elements that interact with the airflow, resulting in

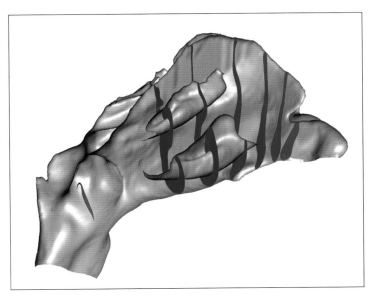

Fig. 9.7 Reconstructed 3D geometry of the nasal cavity derived from CAT scan: visualization of the right nasal airway with the turbinates decongested by medication. View through the transparent nasal wall. Image kindly provided by Dr. Leonid Goubergrits. Software: Amira.

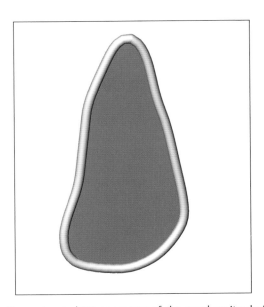

Fig. 9.8 Reconstructed 3D geometry of the nasal cavity derived from CAT scan: cross section of the isthmus nasi on the right side. The average size is according to Huizing 50–70 mm2.22 Image kindly provided by Dr. Leonid Goubergrits. Software: ZIBamira.

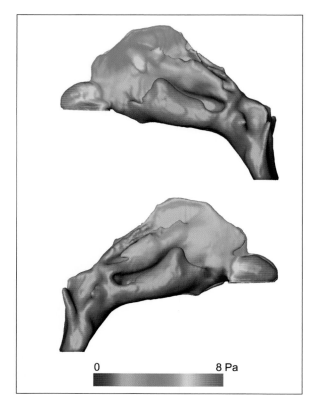

Fig. 9.9 Computational Fluid Dynamics: visualization of the pressure drop in the nasal cavities during the inspiratory phase (average flow in the respiratory cycle). View of the lateral nasal wall. Image kindly provided by Dr. Leonid Goubergrits. Software: Amira Fluent.

morphological fluctuations with retroaction on the airstream. This behavior is called fluid–structure interaction, which is characteristically represented by the nasal valve function. The purpose of the valve mechanism is not yet clarified; it may serve to protect the olfactory region during forced inspiration. According to Bridger and Proctor, the nasal valve is comparable with a Starling resistor.[21]

Normally, the elastic components of the nasal wall are all individually matched to one another in their rigidity. This balance must be considered in the use of grafts and in resections, especially of the alar cartilages, so that it will not be seriously tipped in one direction or the other. Postoperative scarring is also a significant factor in this regard.

The surgeon should be aware that the nose is the main contributor to airway resistance in the upper respiratory tract. Huizing and De Groot state that nasal airway resistance accounts for 50–60% of the total.[22] Like other authors, they believe that this relatively high nasal resistance is essential for the nasopulmonary and nasocardiac reflexes. Swift (quoted by Drettmer) has emphasized its importance in the maintenance of lung capacity.[23] Accordingly, radical surgical strategies for minimizing airway resistance may adversely affect not only the internal milieu of the nasal cavity, but also systemic body functions.

9.5.2 The Dilemma of Conventional Resistance Tests

The implementation and further development of physiologically optimum nasal surgery requires an accurate and detailed knowledge of the flow field or flow parameters within the nasal cavity. But currently available clinical methods for the assessment of nasal breathing can at best determine only the integral airway resistance or airflow capacity of the nose.

According to a study by Bermüller and colleagues, even this value cannot be reliably determined in relation to complaints and findings. Approximately 25% of patients with subjective nasal airway obstruction and related anatomical findings had no detectable abnormalities either by rhinomanometry or by the determination of peak nasal inspiratory flow.[24]

Nasal valve dysfunction can be detected based on the typical shape of the flow-versus-pressure curve. Some false positives could occur, however, due to the unilateral measurement and associated increase in nasal valve responsiveness.[14] Conversely, the mask pressure causes some lateralization of the buccal soft tissues that may mask a possible nasal valve collapse.

We know from experience that rhinomanometry is best at detecting obstructions that are already apparent clinically.

The German Society of Otorhinolaryngology has stated that rhinomanometry is only "occasionally useful" as a preoperative investigation.[13] On the other hand, comparative rhinomanometry with provocative testing is definitely rewarding in the evaluation of allergy patients.

Generally speaking, even the most accurate resistance measurement is of only limited value. Low-resistance respiration is not always synonymous with a well-functioning nose. Moreover, the normal values that have been established for flow physiology cannot be uniquely correlated with a particular anatomic configuration of the nasal cavity. This means that, in theory, there are a range of different nasal geometries that allow for normal volume flow. This may explain the certain arbitrariness that exists in the current practice of functional rhinosurgery.

At present, the criterion of integral pressure drop is the only objective measure available in the diagnosis and treatment of nasal airway disorders. This criterion can provide only a limited, qualitative assessment of nasal breathing, however.

9.5.3 Added Benefit of Numerical Flow Simulation

Methods of numerical flow simulation have made it possible to investigate the dynamics of arbitrary parameters in nasal airflow. Of course this includes nasal airway resistance and the associated pressure drop, which are traditionally determined by rhinomanometry (**Fig. 9.9**).

First, CT data are used to reconstruct the three-dimensional geometry of the nasal airway. Next the flow space is discretized with finite elements (e.g., tetrahedrons). This creates a computational grid that, when combined with physical and mathematical modeling, provides the basis for the computation. The solution process will finally yield the desired flow parameters for every linking node of finite elements and for every point in time during the respiratory period. The correct interpretation of those data is very challenging and also depends on the type of visualization that is used (**Fig. 9.10**).

In the case of complex nasal airflow, it has always proven very difficult to distinguish between characteristic features and random phenomena. Thus, special theoretical approaches and concrete working hypotheses are needed to perform goal-directed analyses.

An example is the recently developed concept of rhinorespiratory homeostasis. This proposal of a universal, trans-species model of nasal respiration implies that wall shear stress is a primary consideration, especially from the standpoint of comparative animal physiology.[14,15]

Wall shear stress is a kind of meta-parameter that represents the degree of functionally relevant interaction between the nasal mucosa and flowing air. Accordingly, the distribution patterns of this quantity in the nasal cavity may carry important rhinologic information.

Wall shear stress or related value patterns differ markedly between the inspiratory and expiratory phases, even when nasal valve effects are disregarded. This is relatively independent of the flow and therefore similar to the characteristic of a Tesla valve device which, based only on its geometry, facilitates different flow paths for each direction.[14,16,25,29] The background of this phenomenon is unclear. Possibly there are resulting effects on endonasal heat and water balance. For certain mammals nasal breathing even plays an essential role in regulating body or brain temperature.[30,31]

Figure 9.11 displays the different inspiratory and expiratory wall shear stress patterns in a left nasal cavity. While the peak wall shear stresses during inspiration are concentrated in a band along the middle meatus starting from the isthmus nasi, the wall shear stress pattern during expiration shows a more homogenous distribution at lower levels. The pictured partial exclusion of the inferior turbinate during inspiration is not in accordance with its commonly attributed role for warming and moistening the inhaled air. However, several authors have also reported about this specific feature.[14,16,26-28] Therefore, it should be discussed and clarified as far as possible.

Numerical simulation provides a noninvasive means of generating flow data within the narrow confines of the geometrically complex nasal cavity. Realistic results require an accurate geometric reconstruction, an adequate computational grid, coherent boundary conditions, and sound physical and mathematical modeling. Currently, it is still very difficult to include the elastic properties of portions of the nasal cavity wall in the computational model. Nevertheless, the good agreement of calculated and measured flow-pressure values in one and the same test subject still supports the basic validity of these nasal airflow calculations even when fluid–structure interaction is not taken into account.[14,32]

Numerical flow simulation permits a differentiated analysis of nasal breathing. This process still involves huge technological hurdles, which can be overcome only through interdisciplinary collaboration with engineers. But the experience of various groups of authors[18,26,32-39] proves that numerical simulation is a very promising approach to improving the diagnosis and management of nasal airway disorders. One advantage over experimental flow studies is its potential application to individual patients.

A particular benefit of numerical simulation is its ability to provide spatial and temporal quantification of flow effects along the nasal wall or mucosa by means of wall shear stress analysis (**Fig. 9.11**). This application in itself may well create a new impetus for scientific research on the physiology of nasal breathing.[14]

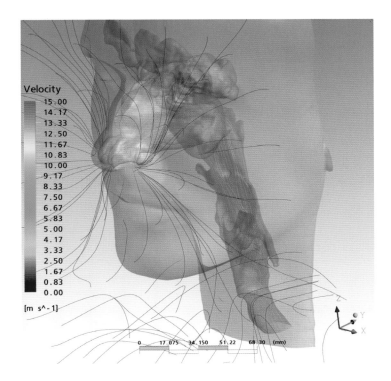

Fig. 9.10 Computational Fluid Dynamics: flow lines in the nose and pharynx with color-encoded velocity during inspiration. Image kindly provided by Dr. Stefan Zachow and Dr. Alexander Steinmann. Software: CFX.

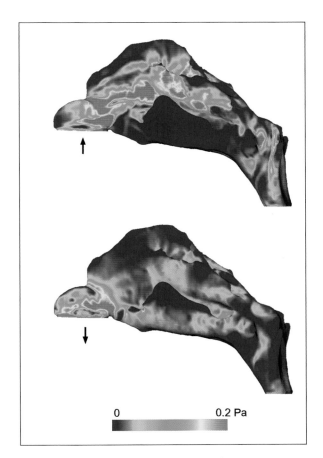

Fig. 9.11 Computational Fluid Dynamics: wall shear stress pattern in the left nasal cavity during the inspiratory and expiratory phases (peak flow in the respiratory cycle). View of the lateral nasal wall. Image kindly provided by Dr. Leonid Goubergrits. Software: Amira Fluent.

References

1. Behrbohm H, Kaschke O, Nawka T. Erfassen und Bewerten von visuellen Organbefunden on der Otorhinolaryngologie. Tuttlingen, Germany: Endopress; 2005

2. Constantian MB. The two essential elements for planning tip surgery in primary and secondary rhinoplasty: observations based on review of 100 consecutive patients. Plast Reconstr Surg 2004;114(6):1571–1581, discussion 1582–1585

3. Tardy ME. Rhinoplasty, The Art and the Science, Vol. I and Vol. II. Philadelphia, PA: Saunders; 1997:69–81

4. Messerklinger W. Endoscopy of the nose [in German]. Monatsschr Ohrenheilkd Laryngorhinol 1970;104(10):451–456

5. Messerklinger W. Die Rolle der lateralen Nasenwand in der Pathogenese, Diagnose und Therapie der rezidivierenden und chronischen Rhinosinusitis. Laryngol Rhinol Otol (Stuttg) 1987;66(6):293–299

6. Behrbohm H, Tardy ME. Essentials of Septorhinoplasty. Philosophy—Approaches—Techniques. New York, NY: Thieme; 2003

7. Bachmann W. Differential diagnosis in patients with nasal obstruction: rhinomanometric indications for surgery. Facial Plast Surg 1990;7:274

8. Behrbohm H, Kaschke O, Nawka T. Endoskopische Diagnostik und Therapie in der HNO. Jena, Germany: Gustav Fischer; 1997

9. Behrbohm H, Kaschke O, Nawka T. Kurzlehrbuch HNO. 2nd ed. Stuttgart, Germany: Thieme; 2012

10. Pallanch JF. Objective measures of nasal function. In: Kennedy DW, Hwang PH. Rhinology. Diseases of the Nose, Sinuses and Skull Base. New York, NY: Thieme; 2012

11. Vogt K, Jalowayski AA. Four-phase rhinomanometry, basics and practice. Rhinology 2010; Suppl. 21

12. Cakmak O, Tarhan E, Coskun M, Cankurtaran M, Celik H. Acoustic rhinometry: accuracy and ability to detect changes in passage area at different locations in the nasal cavity. Ann Otol Rhinol Laryngol 2005;114(12): 949–957

13. Mlynski G, Beule A. Diagnostik der respiratorischen Funktion der Nase. HNO 2008;56(1):81–99

14. Hildebrandt T. Das Konzept der Rhinorespiratorischen Homöostase—ein neuer theoretischer Ansatz für die Diskussion physiologischer und physikalischer Zusammenhänge bei der Nasenatmung [dissertation]. Freiburg, Germany: Albert-Ludwig-Universität; 2011

15. Hildebrandt T, Heppt WJ, Kertzscher U, Goubergrits L. The concept of rhinorespiratory homeostasis—a new approach to nasal breathing. Facial Plast Surg 2013;29(2):85–92

16. Hildebrandt T, Goubergrits L, Heppt WJ, Bessler S, Zachow S. Evaluation of the intranasal flow field through computational fluid dynamics. Facial Plast Surg 2013;29(2):93–98

17. Mlynski G. Physiologie und Pathophysiologie der Nase: In: Behrbohm H, Tardy ME, eds. Funktionell-ästhetische Chirurgie der Nase: Septorhinoplastik. 1st ed. Stuttgart, Germany: Thieme; 2004:73–84

18. Tan J, Han D, Wang J, et al. Numerical simulation of normal nasal cavity airflow in Chinese adult: a computational flow dynamics model. Eur Arch Otorhinolaryngol 2012;269(3):881–889

19. Fischer R. Die Physik der Atemströmung in der Nase [dissertation]. West Berlin, West Germany: Freie Universität; 1969

20. Wexler DB, Davidson TM. The nasal valve: a review of the anatomy, imaging, and physiology. Am J Rhinol 2004;18(3):143–150

21. Bridger GP, Proctor DF. Maximum nasal inspiratory flow and nasal resistance. Ann Otol Rhinol Laryngol 1970;79(3):481–488

22. Huizing EH, De Groot JAM. Functional Reconstructive Nasal Surgery. 1st ed. Stuttgart, Germany: Thieme; 2003

23. Drettner B. Physiologie und Pathphysiologie der Nase. In: Naumann HH, Helms J, Herberhold C, Kastenbauer E, eds. Oto-Rhino-Laryngologie in Klinik und Praxis. Vol 2: Nase, Nasennebenhöhlen, Gesicht, Mundhöhle und Pharynx, Kopfspeicheldrüsen. 1st ed. Stuttgart, Germany: Thieme; 1992:40–48

24. Bermüller C, Kirsche H, Rettinger G, Riechelmann H. Diagnostic accuracy of peak nasal inspiratory flow and rhinomanometry in functional rhinosurgery. Laryngoscope 2008;118(4):605–610

25. Bailie N, Hanna B, Watterson J, Gallagher G. A model of airflow in the nasal cavities: Implications for nasal air conditioning and epistaxis. Am J Rhinol Allergy 2009;23(3):244–249

26. Hahn I, Scherer PW, Mozell MM. Velocity profiles measured for airflow through a large-scale model of the human nasal cavity. J Appl Physiol (1985) 1993;75(5):2273–2287

27. Proctor DF. The upper airway. In: Proctor DF, Anderson IB, eds. The Nose, Upper Airway Physiology and the Atmospheric Environment. New York, NY: Elsevier Urban & Fischer; 1982:23–43

28. Wen J, Inthavong K, Tian ZF, Tu JY, Xue CL, Li CG. Airñow patterns in both sides of a realistic human nasal cavity for laminar and turbulent conditions. 16th Australasian Fluid Mechanics Conference, Gold Coast, Australia, 2007

29. Tesla N, inventor. US patent 1,329,559. February 3, 1920

30. Schmidt-Nielsen K, Bretz WL, Taylor CR. Panting in dogs: unidirectional air flow over evaporative surfaces. Science 1970;169(3950):1102–1104

31. Schmidt-Nielsen K. Physiologie der Tiere. 1st ed. Heidelberg, Germany: Spektrum; 1999

32. Zachow S, Muigg P, Hildebrandt T, Doleisch H, Hege H-C. Visual exploration of nasal airflow. IEEE Trans Vis Comput Graph 2009;15(6):1407–1414

33. Doorly DJ, Taylor DJ, Gambaruto AM, Schroter RC, Tolley N. Nasal architecture: form and flow. Philos Trans A Math Phys Eng Sci 2008;366(1879): 3225–3246

34. Doorly DJ, Taylor DJ, Schroter RC. Mechanics of airflow in the human nasal airways. Respir Physiol Neurobiol 2008;163(1-3):100–110

35. Elad D, Naftali S, Rosenfeld M, Wolf M. Physical stresses at the air-wall interface of the human nasal cavity during breathing. J Appl Physiol (1985) 2006;100(3):1003–1010

36. Hildebrandt T, Zachow S, Steinmann A, Heppt W. Innovation in der funktionell-ästhetischen Nasenchirurgie: Rhino-CFD. Face Int Mag of Orofacial Esthetics 2007;2:20–23

37. Keck T, Lindemann J. Strömungssimulation und Klimatisierung in der Nase. Laryngorhinootologie 2010;89:1–14

38. Zachow S, Steinmann A, Hildebrandt T, Weber R, Heppt W. CFD simulations of nasal airflow: Towards treatment planning for functional rhinosurgery. Int J CARS 2006;1(1):165–167

39. Zachow S, Steinmann A, Hildebrandt T, Heppt W. Understanding nasal airflow via CFD simulation and visualization. Proc Computer Aided Surgery 2007;173–176

10 Tissue Replacement in the Nose

Three main types of graft material are used in revision rhinoplasties: autologous grafts, allografts, and alloplastic implants.[1] Autologous grafts are always preferred.[2] They can be used in various ways as structural and contouring grafts in nasal revision surgery.[3]

10.1 Autologous Grafts

10.1.1 Septal Cartilage (First Choice)

Cartilage from the nasal septum has good stability and elasticity. The Rubin cartilage morselizer can be used to squeeze cartilage with careful, controlled pressure to alter its bending properties without damaging the cartilage tissue. The cartilage remains pressure-stable and changes its bending properties without fraying when worked by gentle pressure (**Fig. 10.1**). Generally speaking, the properties of the cartilage should be altered as little

as possible. The cartilage can be harvested through a hemitransfixion incision or a posterior endoscopic endonasal approach.

10.1.2 Alar Cartilage

Pieces of alar cartilage, usually from the upper lateral crura, can be used for augmentation of the nasal dorsum or tip. Because of their thinness, they are excellent grafts for superficial contouring.

10.1.3 Conchal Cartilage (Second Choice)

As Tardy observed, "the external ear exists as a marvelous storehouse of skeletal spare parts for the nose."[2] Conchal cartilage is dimensionally stable, resilient, and provides good mechanical support for applications in the nose. It can be harvested quickly and easily (**Fig. 10.2**).

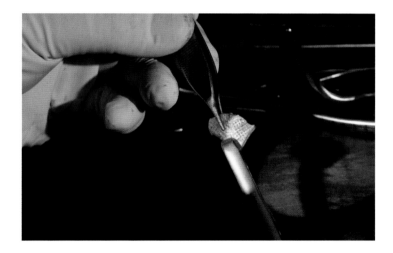

Fig. 10.1 Gentle compression of septal cartilage.

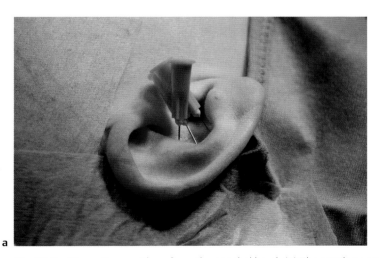

a

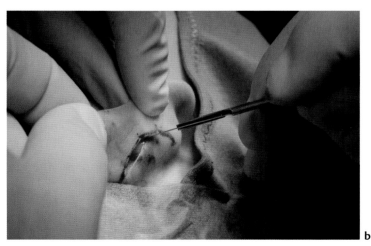

b

Fig. 10.2 Harvesting cartilage from the conchal bowl. (**a**) The cartilage resection line is marked below the postauricular sulcus. (**b**) The skin is incised along the marked line.

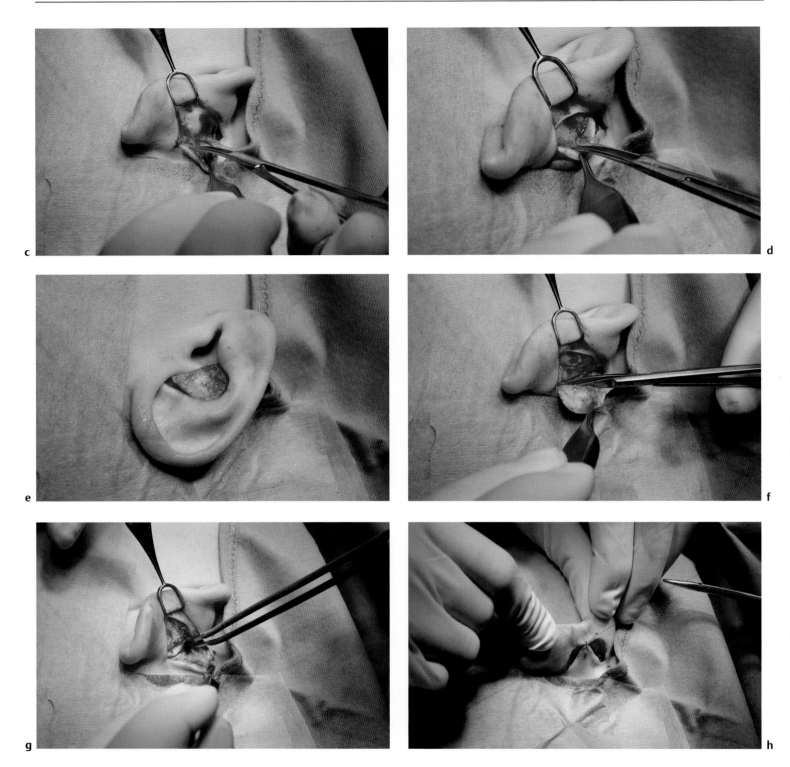

Fig. 10.2   Harvesting cartilage from the conchal bowl. (**c, d**) Cartilage dissection on the (**c**) posterior and (**d**) anterior side of the auricle. (**e**) A relatively large cartilage implant can be obtained. (**f**) The cartilage is de-tached. (**g**) Meticulous hemostasis is necessary to prevent postoperative hematoma formation. (**h**) Wound closure.

One advantage of conchal cartilage is its varieties of convexities and concavities, which can be matched as needed to specific recipient sites in the nose.[4] Conchal cartilage can be used for the replacement of septal cartilage, upper lateral cartilage, and alar cartilage. It can be used in the form of a shield graft, tip graft, alar button graft, or columellar strut (**Fig. 10.3**). It is often recom-mended that connective tissue be left on the cartilage when the graft is harvested, as that will be helpful for reconstructing larger defects in the nasal dorsum. Conchal cartilage is easy to carve with a scalpel. It is extremely difficult to compress, however, as the slightest pressure will cause it to fray. The implanted graft should heal without difficulty and is highly resistant to resorption.

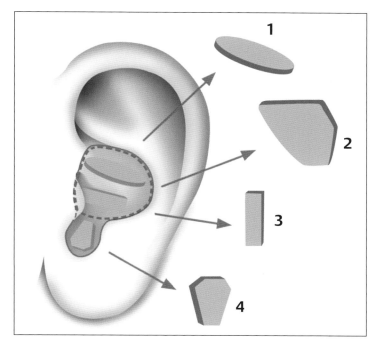

Fig. 10.3 The auricle is a rich source of cartilage implants for nasal surgery. The cartilage is available in a variety of thicknesses and curvatures: 1, onlay graft; 2, septal graft; 3, columellar strut; 4, shield or tip graft.

10.1.4 Tragal Cartilage

Tragal cartilage is harvested through an incision made with a No. 15 blade just behind the anterior border and directed toward the ear canal. It can be harvested along with two small perichondrial flaps, which can be dissected quickly and easily. The cartilage is thin but very strong. The perichondrium undergoes less postoperative swelling than fascia.

10.1.5 Costal Cartilage

Costal cartilage is used in cases that require a stable reconstruction due to extensive loss of structural support. It is harvested from the sixth or seventh rib through a 4- to 5-mm skin incision, which in women is placed in the inframammary crease (**Fig. 10.4**). The perichondrium is incised, and the costal cartilage is harvested within a perichondrial sleeve. Rib cartilage should be "balanced," meaning that only the central portions of the cartilage should be used for grafting. One disadvantage of costal cartilage is its unnatural consistency in the nasal dorsum, for example. It makes the nose stiff, and even a perfectly healed graft may create a foreign-body sensation.

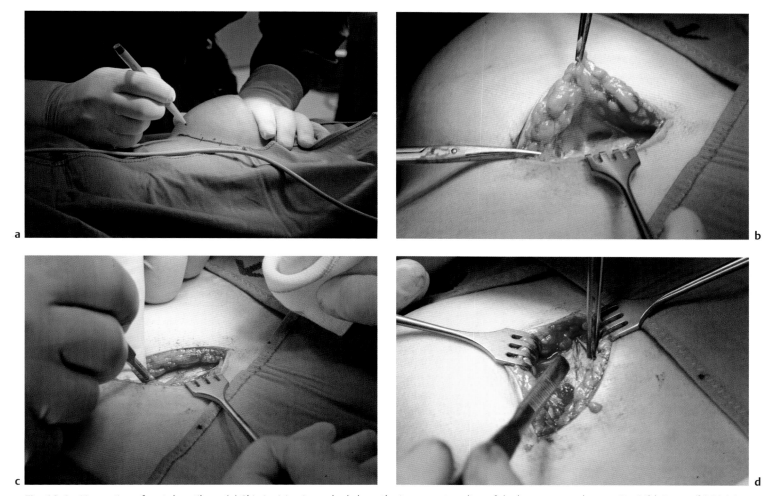

Fig. 10.4 Harvesting of costal cartilage. (**a**) Skin incision is marked along the inner contour line of the breast to produce an "invisible" scar. (**b**) Division of the skin and subcutaneous tissue. (**c**) Incision of the perichondrium. (**d**) Reflection of the perichondrium.

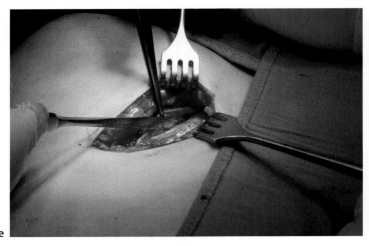

e

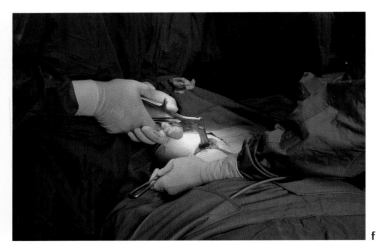

f

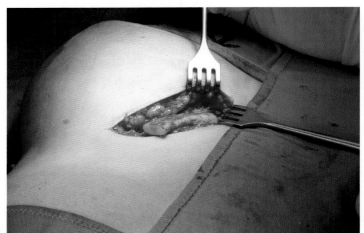

g

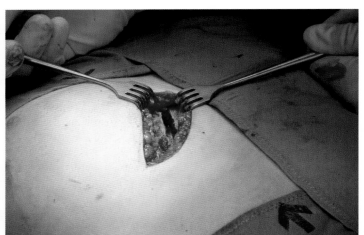

h

Fig. 10.4   Harvesting of costal cartilage. (**e**) Dissection of the rib carti-lage in a perichondrial pocket. (**f**) Division of the rib. (**g**) Removal of the rib. (**h, i**) Closure of the perichondrium and wound.

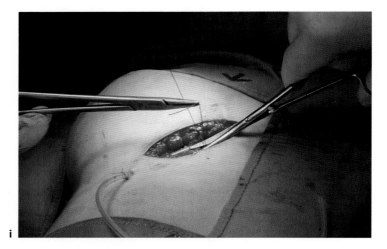

i

10.1.6 Fascia

Sufficient amounts of autologous temporal fascia or fascia lata can be quickly harvested through an incision made in the hair-bearing scalp or lateral thigh. Fascia lata is the strongest fascia in the body. It consists of an ~ 5-cm-wide strip extend-ing between the greater trochanter and the lateral epicondyle of the femur (**Fig. 10.5**). The course of the fascia lata should be considered in the harvesting of graft material. After the fascia is removed, the defect should always be closed to prevent her-niation of muscle tissue.

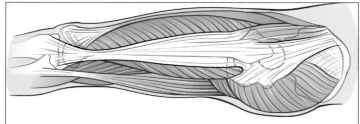

Fig. 10.5   Fascia lata is the strongest fascia in the body. It runs from the outer lip of the iliac crest to the lateral femoral condyle and to the patellar retinaculum on the lateral side of the thigh.

10.1.7 Bone

For decades, bone was the most commonly used tissue for the correction of saddle nose deformity. The harvesting of iliac bone is a painful procedure. Bone grafting to the nose requires a stable, well-vascularized recipient bed or else the graft will be resorbed. In our view, bone grafting is no longer necessary in rhinoplasty owing to the availability of other materials.

10.2 Alloplastic Materials

The development of new synthetic materials for tissue replacement in the human body has made progress in recent years. One problem remains, however: an "ideal" prosthetic material does not exist, especially in the previously operated nose.[5] Whenever possible, it is best to avoid the use of alloplastic materials in revisions and use autologous tissue instead. Since autologous material is almost always available in sufficient quantities at one or more sites, we see very little reason to use alloplastic implants. Nevertheless, here is an update on available options:

Gold and silver were the first implant materials (1828), followed later by paraffin, ivory, cork, marble, and acrylic.[1] Until a few years ago, rhinoplasty patients who had been treated by Jacques Joseph came to us because an ivory implant was causing problems after years of trouble-free service. Joseph procured the ivory from the Bechstein piano factory in Berlin, where it was used for making piano keys (a musical nasal implant, one might say).

Alloplastic implants must meet very rigorous requirements.[3] They must be chemically and thermally stable, autoclavable, and dimensionally stable. Other requirements are a minimal foreign-body reaction and the absence of cytotoxic, antigenic, and carcinogenic properties.

10.2.1 Cements

Cement materials (biocement, ionomeric cement, e.g., aluminum oxide ceramic, hydroxyapatite cement) cannot be used in the flexible nose because of their brittleness. They have proven useful, however, for bone replacement in areas such as the forehead and glabella (**Fig. 10.6**).

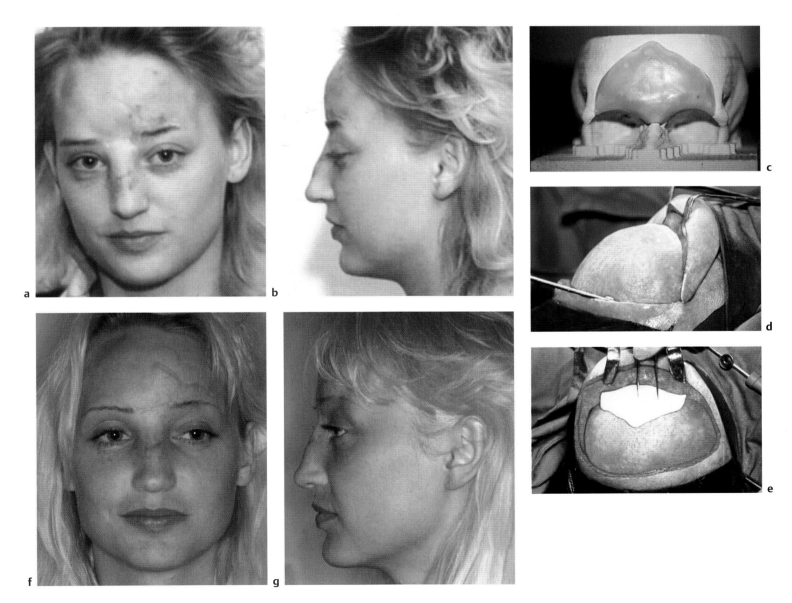

Fig. 10.6 (**a, b**) Young patient with a posttraumatic wide nose and absence of the outer table of the frontal sinus on both sides. (**c–e**) Frontal contour is reconstructed with a bioceramic implant fabricated by com-puter-aided design and manufacturing technology and inserted through a bicoronal incision. (**f, g**) The patient 10 years after reconstruction of frontal contour and septorhinoplasty to close the posttraumatic open roof.

10.2.2 Silicone

Silicone is sometimes used for augmentation of the nasal dorsum, particularly in Asia. There is a substantial risk of early or late extrusion. A fibrous tissue layer forms around the silicone implant, which does not establish a strong attachment to surrounding tissue. Microtrauma, especially in the cartilaginous nose, may lead to microhemorrhages, edema, and inflammatory reactions around the implant, with an associated risk of infection and extrusion. Silicone is unsuitable for use in the cartilaginous nose.

10.2.3 PTFE (Teflon), ePTFE (Gore-Tex), and Porous Polyethylene (Porex)

Some materials such as polytetrafluoroethylene (PTFE) (Teflon, Proplast), expanded polytetrafluoroethylene (ePTFE) (Gore-Tex), and porous polyethylene (Porex) are receptive to permeation by fibrous tissue ingrowth when used in the form of thin-walled implants. This tissue ingrowth depends on the porosity of the plastic. Large pore sizes in the range of 100–150 μm are favorable.

PTFE has proven unsatisfactory for reconstructive nasal surgery due to problems of stability and tissue compatibility. The FDA revoked its approval of Proplast implants in 1990. The material is easy to shape.

Gore-Tex (ePTFE) is used mainly for volume replacement and is less suitable for providing structural support. It has good biocompatibility, although a 10.6% incidence of infection with fistulation and extrusion has been reported.[6-8]

Porous polyethylene (Porex) is a porous plastic used to replace cartilage that provides mechanical support. When heated, it can be shaped, cut, and perforated. Its tissue compatibility is good. The material is receptive to tissue ingrowth and is becoming increasing popular in rhinosurgery.[9,10]

10.2.4 Turkish Delight and DCF Transplants

"Turkish delight" is diced cartilage mixed with blood and antibiotic and wrapped in methylcellulose (Surgicel). The graft remains moldable, even days or weeks after the operation. The Surgicel wrap is resorbed in ~ 2 weeks. Fascia can be used as an alternative to Surgicel. A diced cartilage in fascia transplant (DCF transplant) is recommend for the repair of large defects of the nasal dorsum.[11]

10.3 Allografts

10.3.1 Fascia and Dura

Fascia lata and dura mater are used in the form of lyophilized or dehydrated banked material. The tissue is rehydrated before implantation. It is broken down by resorption and replaced by connective tissue. This transformation depends on the size of the graft and the properties of the recipient bed (scarring, mechanical stresses, blood supply).

10.3.2 Cartilage

Cartilage tissue from the septum, concha, or rib can be preserved by various methods (e.g., with thiomersal [Merthiolate], Cialit, alcohol, freeze-drying, dehydration, gamma irradiation). Its bio-logical properties are comparable to those of autologous cartilage. Cartilage preserved with thiomersal behaves like devitalized tissue. It is partially resorbed at its edges and is also replaced and ensheathed by connective tissue.[12-14]

10.3.3 AlloDerm

AlloDerm is banked human skin from which the epidermis and cellular components have been removed. The remaining protein matrix is freeze-dried.[15,16] The material can be used to augment the nasal dorsum or for camouflage.

10.3.4 Fibrin Glue

The principle of the physiologic two-component fibrin glue is based on the final stage of blood coagulation. Fibrinogen is polymerized by thrombin to produce fibrin. The latter is cross-linked by factor XIII to form a stable fibrin clot. The glue contains a small amount of aprotinin to protect the fibrin clot from premature breakdown in vivo. Fibrin glue is excellent for attaching onlay grafts and for the "sealing" of raw surfaces and access incisions.

References

1. Behrbohm H. Autologous grafts & allografts. In Behrbohm H, Tardy ME. Essentials of Septorhinoplasty. Approaches—Techniques—Philosophy. New York, NY: Thieme; 2003:214–217

2. Tardy ME. Rhinoplasty, the Art and the Science. Vol II, Cartilage Autograft Reconstruction of the Nose. Philadelphia, PA: Saunders; 1997:649–723

3. Gassner HG. Structural grafts and suture techniques in functional and aesthetic rhinoplasty. GMS Curr Top Otorhinolaryngol Head Neck Surg 2010;9

4. Jovanovic S, Berghaus A. Autogenous auricular concha cartilage transplant in corrective rhinoplasty. Practical hints and critical remarks. Rhinology 1991;29(4):273–279

5. Neumann A, Kevenhoester K. Biomaterials for craniofacial reconstruction, technology for quality of life. Implants and biomaterials in otorhinolaryngology. GMS Curr Top Otorhinolaryngol Head Neck Surg 2009;8:Doc07

6. Berghaus A. Implants for reconstructive surgery of the nose and ear [in German]. Laryngorhinootologie 2007;86(Suppl 1):S67–767

7. Berghaus A. An update on functional and aesthetic surgery of the nose and ear. GMS Curr Top Otorhinolaryngol Head Neck Surg 2007;6:Doc07

8. Berghaus A. Implants for reconstructive surgery of the nose and ear. GMS Curr Top Otorhinolaryngol Head Neck Surg 2007;6:Doc06

9. Berghaus A, Stelter K. Alloplastic materials in rhinoplasty. Curr Opin Otolaryngol Head Neck Surg 2006;14(4):270–277

10. Romo T III, Sclafani AP, Sabini P. Use of porous high-density polyethylene in revision rhinoplasty and in the platyrrhine nose. Aesthetic Plast Surg 1998;22(3):211–221

11. Daniel RK, Calvert JW. Diced cartilage grafts in rhinoplasty surgery. Plast Reconstr Surg 2004;113(7):2156–2171

12. Gammert C, Masing H. Long term experience of using preserved cartilage in reconstructive surgery of the nose [in German]. Laryng Rhinol Otol (Stuttg) 1977;56:650–656

13. Hellmich S. Fehler und Gefahren bei der freien Knorpeltransplantation im Gesichtsbereich. HNO 1982;30:140–144

14. Strauch B, Wallach SG. Reconstruction with irradiated homograft costal cartilage. Plast Reconstr Surg 2003;111(7):2405–2411, discussion 2412–2413

15. Sclafani AP, Romo T III, Jacono AA, McCormick SA, Cocker R, Parker A. Evaluation of acellular dermal graft (AlloDerm) sheet for soft tissue augmentation: a 1-year follow-up of clinical observations and histological findings. Arch Facial Plast Surg 2001;3(2):101–103

16. Winter, M. Verwendung von Alloderm in der Rhinoplastik. HNO Aktuell 2004;12:383–388

11 Principles of Nasal Implantology

The successful transplantation of autologous or allogeneic cartilage tissue is influenced by the following factors[1,2]:

- The type of cartilage tissue
- Its preservation and storage
- Surface area and volume of the graft
- Methods used to harvest and prepare the graft
- Biological characteristic of the recipient bed
- Location of the recipient bed (rigid or flexible part of the nose, deep or superficial)
- Condition of the operative field, connective tissue type
- Surgical technique and postoperative mechanical stresses acting on the graft

The principal dangers of cartilage grafting in the nose are graft resorption, deformation due to cartilage warping, infection, and extrusion. The graft material of first choice in revision rhinoplasties is always viable autologous tissue. If it is not available, allograft tissue should be used.

11.1 Harvesting Graft Material

Atraumatic tissue harvesting is essential for successful grafting. Septal cartilage should be dissected in the subperichondrial plane, conchal cartilage in the supraperichondrial plane. The tissue should not be injured or crushed when harvested.

Perichondrium does not protect the graft from resorption and should therefore be dissected off the cartilage.[3] For grafting in children, however, the perichondrium should remain on the graft so that it can provide a chondroplastic function. Meticulous, definitive hemostasis is important after graft harvest to prevent hematoma formation in the septum or ear. Not infrequently, this complication may become the main problem during postoperative care. The conchal cavity should be packed with ointment-impregnated cottonwool after graft harvest to promote adhesion of the skin layers. The harvested material is prepared for use on a small carving bench with a millimeter scale (**Fig. 11.1**).

After the size of the recipient defect has been measured with a plastic surgical caliper (Karl Storz, Tuttlingen, Germany), the size and shape of the graft are precisely marked with a color marker[4] while the graft is held with a blunt Adson forceps. Either that instrument or a Rubin cartilage squeezer can be used to work on the cartilage. Tension can be removed from the graft by cross-hatching or incising its concave side to prevent graft deformation at the recipient site.

11.2 Recipient Bed

The quality of the recipient bed is crucial for the fate of the graft and the long-term success of the rhinoplasty. In principle, the recipient bed should be just large enough to accommodate the graft, as this will help prevent subsequent displacement. A tight or even slightly undersized recipient bed is helpful for maintaining graft tension to stabilize sites such as the nasal valve or alar rim. Deep implants in the nasal dorsum perform a supporting function while also providing tissue replacement for cartilage or bone defects (**Fig. 11.2**).

These grafts should be placed between the perichondrium and the vascularized SMAS layer (superficial musculoaponeurotic system), from which they will derive their blood supply. Injuries to the superficial masculoaponeurotic system (SMAS)

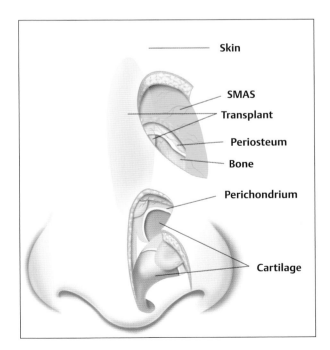

Fig. 11.2 Deep and superficial nasal grafts and their topographic relationship to the various structures and planes of the nose. SMAS, superficial musculoaponeurotic system.

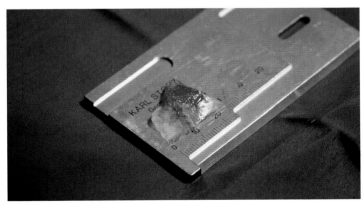

Fig. 11.1 Fabrication of a cartilage graft on a cutting bench.

layer lead to bleeding. Hematomas carry a risk of graft infection and may also cause heavy scarring that will jeopardize graft healing. Superficial grafts are used for contouring the external nose, and this application requires a direct subcutaneous graft placement. The decision whether to attach grafts with sutures or fibrin glue is made on a case-by-case basis. We mainly use absorbable suture material—usually polydioxanone (PDS) and occasionally polypropylene (Prolene). In revision rhinoplasties, care should be taken to dissect the tissues in such a way that little or no scar traction will act upon the graft.[2]

References

1. Adams JS. Grafts and implants in nasal and chin augmentation. A rational approach to material selection. Otolaryngol Clin North Am 1987; 20(4):913–930

2. Behrbohm H, Tardy ME. Essentials of Septorhinplasty. Approaches—Techniques—Philosophy. New York, NY: Thieme; 2003

3. Tardy ME. Rhinoplasty, the Art and the Science. Vol. II. Philadelphia, PA: Saunders; 1997

4. Behrbohm H. Caliper for plastic surgery, Endoworld 2004; ORL 58–2-E/12

12 Lateral Osteotomies

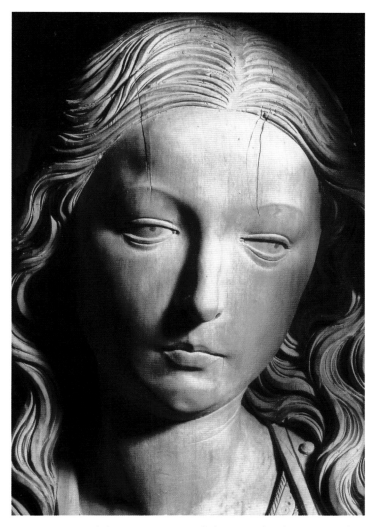

Fig. 12.1 Detail from *Assumption of the Virgin* by the German late Gothic master Tilman Riemenschneider. There are parallels between the sculptor's chisel and the surgeon's osteotome. There is no going back: each step creates an irreversible change.

In 1898, Jacques Joseph described his technique for performing a lateral osteotomy with a saw. Later, in the 1920s, chisels and osteotomes became the instruments of choice for lateral osteotomies. The trend in later decades was toward a low-to-high osteotomy. Webster[1] and Farrior[2] described the high-low-high osteotomy as a technique for preventing functional stenosis of the nasal airway. The introduction of micro-osteotomes by Tardy[3] contributed greatly to minimizing tissue trauma by helping to preserve the periosteum and intranasal mucosa in lateral osteotomies. Nowadays, powered instruments are available.

The selective division and repositioning of the bony nasal pyramid is an essential step in rhinoplasty. Every bone cut should be carefully planned and executed, because a technically flawed osteotomy is extremely difficult to correct. Thus, the selection of osteotomes and optimum technical proficiency will greatly influence the success of a rhinoplasty.

It is often said that an aesthetic rhinoplasty should never improve appearance at the cost of function. Osteotomies do affect nasal breathing, however, and may significantly alter the width of the nasal valve region.

Guyuron[4] was able to show that lateral osteotomies almost always cause narrowing of the nasal airway. The length of the nasal bones, the degree of medialization of the osteotomized fragments, the position of the inferior turbinate, and the type of osteotomy are key factors that determine the functional result. In this regard, low-to-low osteotomies tend to have a better functional outcome than low-to-high osteotomies.

The principal risks of lateral osteotomies are postoperative asymmetry, instability of the fragments, nasal valve stenosis, and inward displacement of the lateral nasal wall.[5] This should motivate the surgeon to preserve as much periosteum as possible to give support to the mobilized fragments. Whether this is achieved better with continuous endonasal micro-osteotomies[3] or percutaneous perforating osteotomies[6] is open to discussion and depends on the above requirements and the technical proficiency of the surgeon.

12.1 Technically Flawed Osteotomies

The following examples show typical problems after osteotomies (**Fig. 12.2**, **Fig. 12.3**, **Fig. 12.4**) and one clinical case (**Fig. 12.5**).

12.2 Revision Osteotomies

12.2.1 Case Report

Young lady two years after septorhinoplasty. We see a removal of higher cartilages from the nasal pyramid on the right side after an incomplete lateral osteotomy, steep position of both osteotomized fragments, open roof (**Fig. 12.6a–e**).

12.2.2 Surgical Procedure

Osteotomies and rhinoplasties in general require an individualized approach. It is important to consider the length of the nasal bones, the thickness of the bone, the age of the patient, and the expected brittleness of the bone. With these factors in mind, the surgeon can select the osteotome that is most suitable for a particular osteotomy.[7]

In principle, bone can be divided with chisels or osteotomes. Chisels are beveled on one side only and tend to deviate toward the beveled side. Osteotomes have two beveled surfaces. If the bevels are equal on both sides, the osteotome will tend to cut in a straight line.

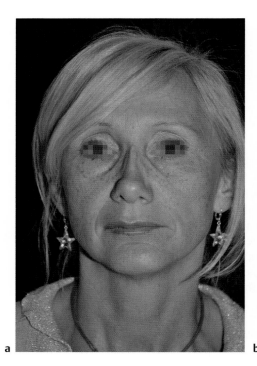
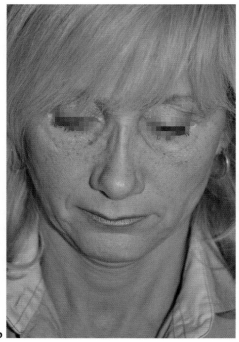
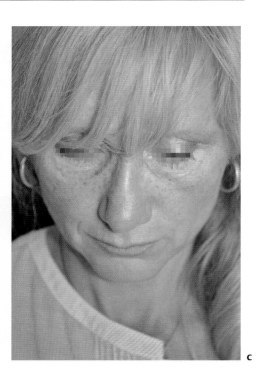

a b c

Fig. 12.2 (**a**) Patient 10 years after rhinoplasty with almost complete loss of the bony nasal pyramid in frontal view. (**b**) Nasal dorsum of the same patient viewed from above. (**c**) Appearance one year after reconstruction of the nasal pyramid with conchal cartilage and connective tissue.

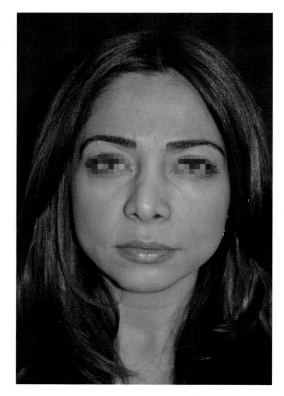

Fig. 12.3 Young woman several years after rhinoplasty. The groove at the level of the nasal pyramid on the right side is caused by a lateralized fragment that was incompletely osteotomized. The open-roof deformity is on a continuum with an inverted V.

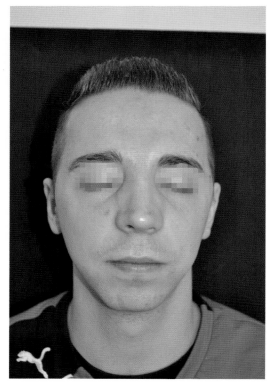

Fig. 12.4 This young man underwent a rhinoplasty in which the osteotomy lines were placed too high. A low-to-low osteotomy in this case could improve the transition.

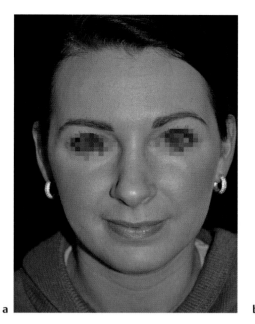
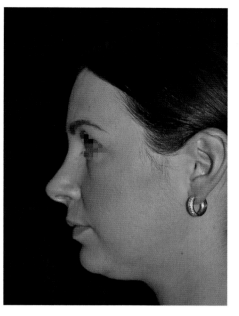
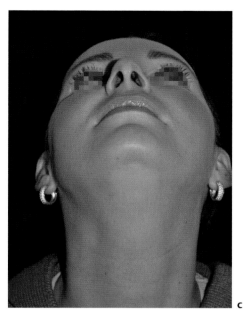

a   b   c

Fig. 12.5 (**a–c**) Young woman 2 years after aesthetic rhinoplasty. The right nasal pyramid is still swollen after the osteotomy. The problem is that persistent periosteal reactions are often associated with new tissue formation and do not completely resolve. The surgeon has limited options: external taping, injecting small amounts of triamcinolone 10%, or revision osteotomy.

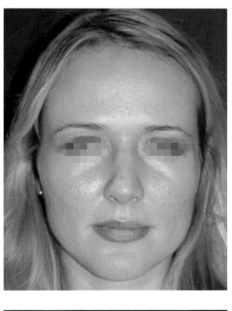
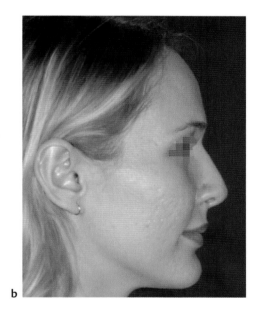
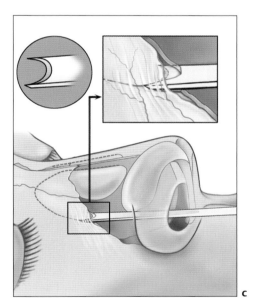

a   b   c

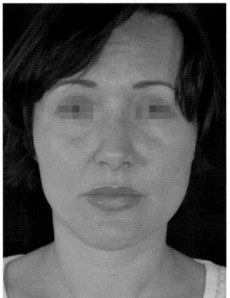
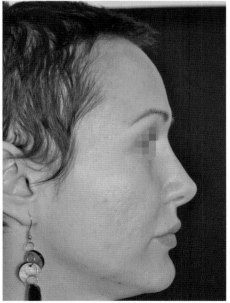

d   e

Fig. 12.6 (**a**) Frontal view. (**b**) Profile view. (**c**) Principle of the mini-osteotome. The bone cut is made within the periosteal layers. The double concave tip, for example, is suitable for thin and hard bone because it give the osteotome a secure grip on the bone edge and permits an accurate cut. (**d**) Frontal view. (**e**) Profile.

The bevel angles should ensure that the osteotome produces an optimum cutting action in the bone without grabbing and without splintering the bone.

Equal bevels allow the osteotome to glide straight ahead. By varying or fine-tuning the lengths of both cutting edges, a variable "curved track" can be designed into the osteotome blade.[8]

We have adopted this concept from speed skating. The speed-skate blade is not straight but has a certain radius of curvature. Speed-skate blades have a different curvature than figure skates, for example. We have adopted and modified this concept in creating the directional bevel osteotome (**Fig. 12.7** and **Fig. 12.8**).[9]

Our task group in Berlin has been working with Karl Storz Endoscopes for many years to develop improved and innovative osteotome designs. The search for the ideal osteotome is a fascinating challenge (**Fig. 12.9a, b**).

Smooth, atraumatic bone cuts are the most important prerequisite for an ideal result. Most "salvage operations" after rhinoplasties and most indications for revision rhinoplasty are based on irregularities, asymmetries, and deformities of the nasal skeleton or nasal dorsum.[9]

Incompletely mobilized fragments should never be "pried out" because this would tear the periosteum, leading to protracted swelling and ecchymosis over the nasal pyramid. The stronger the periosteal and soft-tissue reactions, the greater the tendency for scarring, persistent induration, or callus formation. The designated fragment should therefore be circumscribed and mobilized as accurately as possible.[10]

The cutting action of an osteotome depends critically on the composition and hardness of its steel. The steel should be hard but not brittle so that it can glide "elastically" through the bone—a difficult concept to picture. Brittle steel tends to become chipped or pitted along its cutting edge. The hardness of steel depends on its alloy composition and can be measured on the Rockwell scale. The alloying process and specific production steps are the "stuff that dreams are made of" and, like the formula for Coca-Cola, are secret.

12.2 Types of Osteotomy

12.2.1 Low-to-Low Osteotomy

This osteotomy starts with a vertical, percutaneous transverse osteotomy with a 2-mm osteotome using postage-stamp technique, initiating the cut from the medial canthus. The next, caudal cut runs straight from the nasal process of the piriform aperture to the level of the medial canthus (**Fig. 12.10**).

12.2.2 Low-to-High Osteotomy

This osteotomy starts at the maxillary nasal process of the piriform aperture and runs tangentially from there to the nasofrontal suture, cutting partially through the nasal bones. It leaves a bony bridge that is then infractured by thumb pressure like a greenstick fracture.

12.2.3 High-Low-High Osteotomy

The osteotomy line curves upward from the piriform aperture. This is done to reduce the functional sequelae of medializing the inferior turbinate, the inferolateral fragment, and the soft tissues.

12.2.4 Continuous versus Postage-Stamp

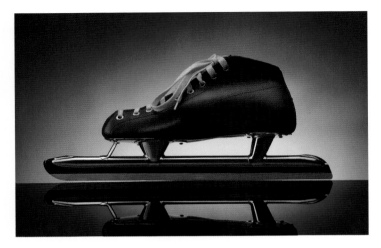

Fig. 12.7   Blade of a speed skate. The radius of curvature is ground into the blade.

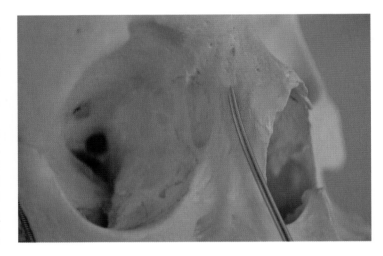

Fig. 12.8   Principle of the directional bevel osteotome, with two different bevels and a curved shaft.

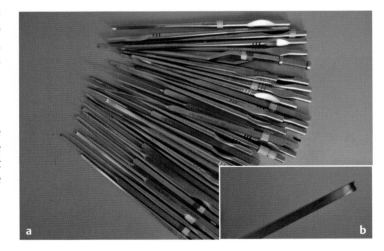

Fig. 12.9   (a) Osteotomy "jackstraws." Many different osteotomes are produced with ever-changing details of shape, bevel, hardness, and steel alloy composition until an optimum is found. (b) Curved cutting edge after testing on a model (inset).

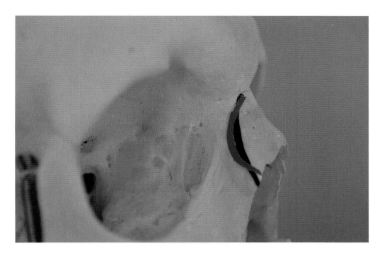

Fig. 12.10 Black, high-to-low osteotomy. Red, high-low-high osteotomy. Yellow, low-to-low osteotomy.

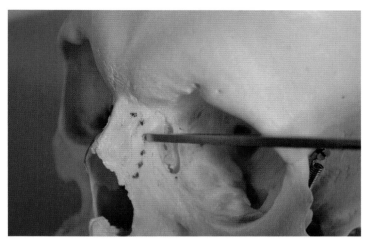

Fig. 12.11 Postage-stamp osteotomy on the left side. The surgeon had to hold the osteotome in very flat position. Percutaneously, a continuous osteotomy is also possible.

Osteotomy

Today, transnasal osteotomies are performed with continuous straight or curved osteotomy lines. The instruments of choice are micro-osteotomes 3–4 mm wide. The problem is that the micro-osteotome should describe an ideal line between the internal and external periosteal layers without injuring both layers. The osteotome is not palpable during the osteotomy. The surgeon must develop a kind of "seventh sense" for the osteotomy, as he can neither see nor palpate the cutting edge (**Fig. 12.11**).

12.2.5 Ship's Bow Osteotomes

To compensate for the problem of an uncontrolled osteotome position while avoiding injuries to the periosteal layers, we added a prominence over the cutting edge, which enables the surgeon to locate the cutting edge by palpation. The prominence is shaped like a "bulbous bow" of a ship, which forces water to flow up over the bulb, optimizing the flow along the hull. A similar effect occurs between the bone and periosteum, as the bulb lifts the periosteum and protects it from injury. The bulbous bow glides beneath the intact periosteum (**Fig. 12.12a, b**).

12.2.6 Double-Click Technique

This is a technique for performing a transnasal osteotomy. It requires practiced teamwork between the surgeon and an assistant. The first click is a test strike in which the assistant taps the head of the osteotome to test the resistance and hardness of the bone. The second click is an action strike that is applied with measured force to drive the osteotome into the bone. The

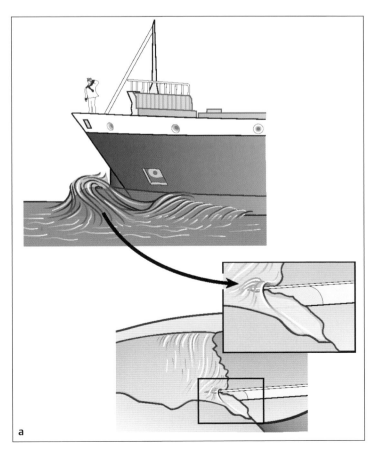

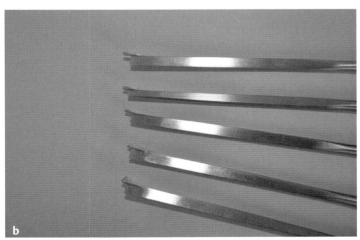

Fig. 12.12 (**a**) Principle of the ship's bow osteotome with a "bulbous bow." (**b**) Various bulbous-bow osteotomes.

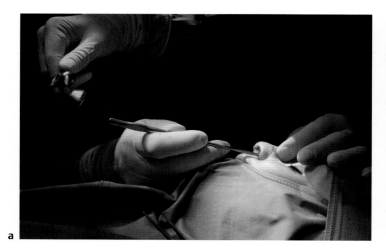
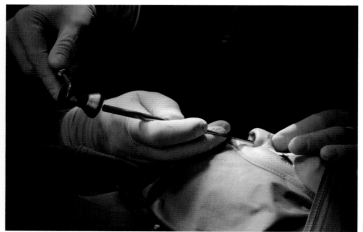

a

b

Fig. 12.13 (**a, b**) The double-click osteotomy technique. The first tap tests to see how much force is needed to drive the osteotome through the bone. The second tap is then delivered with "measured" force to make the definitive cut.

surgeon defines the direction of the osteotome while protecting the eye with his finger or thumb (**Fig. 12.13a, b**).

12.2.7 Percutaneous Osteotomy by the Postage-Stamp Technique

Percutaneous osteotomies are most commonly done in an outside-in direction. The osteotome should be held as close to the facial plane as possible, in an almost horizontal position. After the tip perforates the skin, it is delicately maneuvered to push aside small blood vessels. As a rule, three or four osteotomies can be performed through two perforations on each side. The goal is the complete mobilization of the circumscribed fragment. Immediately cooling the site with ice water will significantly reduce swelling and ecchymosis.

Byrne et al[5] described the inside-out technique of lateral osteotomy involving an outfracture with medialization of the fragments. The osteotomy is performed through intranasal transmucous perforations using the postage-stamp technique. The external periosteum can be largely preserved (**Fig. 12.14**).

12.3 E = mc²

Mass influences the momentum that can be transmitted to the cutting edge of an osteotome. For this reason, Karl Storz also offers mallets of assorted weights, with or without a shock absorber. We have tested a variety of mallet and osteotome weights and volumes over the years and plan to offer "optimal sizes" for practical use in the near future (**Fig. 12.15a, b**).

12.4 Grip and Handling

A mini-osteotome is very prone to slipping when used on thin, hard bone. With the double concave-tip osteotome, the tip design gives the osteotome a very firm grip on a hard bony edge. This allows for a secure cut without slipping (**Fig. 12.16**),

The simplified diagrams in **Fig. 12.17** show the basic variants of the lateral osteotomy. A proven technique is a paramedian

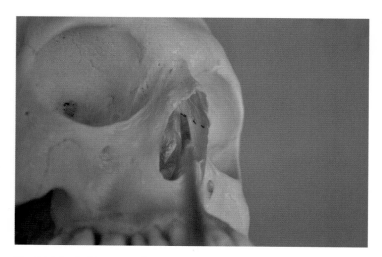

Fig. 12.14 Inside-out and postage-stamp osteotomy.

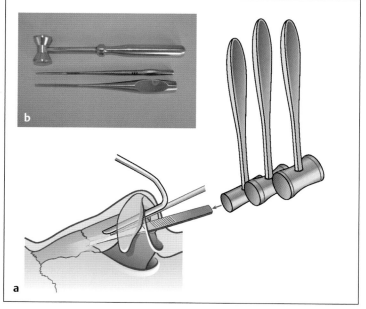

b

a

Fig. 12.15 (**a**) Osteotomy mallets of different weights, with and without shock absorbers. (**b**) Osteotomes of different weights and volumes.

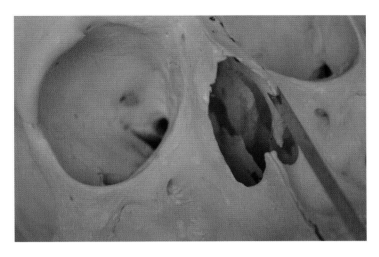

Fig. 12.16 Double concave-tip osteotomes provides a secure grip on thin, hard bone.

oblique osteotomy with the cut directed ~ 30 degrees laterally combined with a laterally curved osteotomy. Both osteotomy cuts intersect at almost a single point. Leaving an ~ 1-mm residual bony bridge is helpful for fixing the fragment at one point.

12.5 Innovations and Essentials

Sharp osteotomes are an essential requirement for precision cutting. Every operating table should have a small Arkansas stone for sharpening and deburring the osteotome. The cutting edge is placed flat against the stone to preserve the bevel angle and is sharpened with backward strokes under moderate pressure. The goal is to smooth away the burs that form during every cut (**Fig. 12.17a, b** and **Fig. 12.18**).

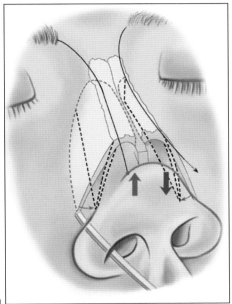

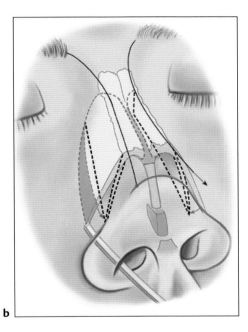

Fig. 12.17 (a) Paramedian oblique osteotomy plus a laterally curved osteotomy. In the outfracture technique, the mobilized fragments are lateralized. The bone cut in this case is made with a directional bevel osteotome with an asymmetrical bevel that cuts in a medially upward curve. In the infracture technique, the mobilized fragments are medialized. The infracture and outfracture techniques can be combined. Green arrow, push-up osteotomy; blue arrow, let-down osteotomy. (b) The more precise the osteotomy cut, the better the results of multiple osteotomies or wedge excisions, which can be used to correct an asymmetrical nasal pyramid in a patient with a bony or bony-and-cartilaginous crooked nose deformity.

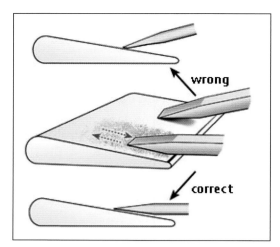

Fig. 12.18   Manual sharpening of an osteotome.

References

1. Webster RC, Davidson TM, Smith RC. Curved lateral osteotomy for airway protection in rhinoplasty. Arch Otolaryngol 1977;103(8):454–458

2. Farrior RT. The osteotomy in rhinoplasty. Laryngoscope 1978; 88(9 Pt 1):1449–1459

3. Tardy ME, Denney JC. Micro-osteotomies in rhinoplasty. Facial Plast Surg 1984;3:137–145

4. Guyuron B. Nasal osteotomy and airway changes. Plast Reconstr Surg 1998;102(3):856–860, discussion 861–863

5. Byrne PJ, Walsh WE, Hilger PA, Orten TS. The use of "inside-out" lateral osteotomies to improve outcome in rhinoplasty. Arch Facial Plast Surg 2003;5(3):251–255

6. Murakami CS, Larrabee WF. Comparison of osteotomy techniques in the treatment of nasal fractures. Facial Plast Surg 1992;8(4):209–219

7. Behrbohm H. Essentials of Septorhinoplasty, Philosophy—Approaches—Techniques. Stuttgart, Germany: Thieme; 2003

8. Behrbohm H. Aesthetic and Reconstructive Facial Plastic Surgery Selected Aspects and Novel Instruments. Tuttlingen, Germany: Endo-press; 2005

9. Behrbohm H. Ästhetische-funktionelle Rhinoplastik: Laterale Osteotomie—ein Update, Face, inderdisziplinäres Magazin für Ästhetik 2014;3/2004, 9:26–30

10. Diamond HP. Rhinoplasty technique. Surg Clin North Am 1971; 51(2):317–331

Further Reading

Joseph J. Nasenplastik und sonstige Gesichtsplastik nebst einem Anhang über Mammaplastik und weitere Operationen auf dem Gebiet der äusseren Körperplastik. Leipzig, Germany: Kabitzsch; 1931

13 Sutures and Structural Grafts in Secondary Nasal Tip Surgery

Jacqueline Eichhorn-Sens and Wolfgang Gubisch

Aesthetic correction of the nasal tip is the most demanding aspect of a rhinoplasty. A vast and diverse range of techniques and methods have been described in the literature. Moreover, the names given to techniques and grafts are not uniform. This already suggests that in most cases a uniform technique is not certain to succeed. On the contrary, experienced rhinosurgeons should always have a wide variety of techniques at their disposal so that the optimum therapeutic approach can be determined based on a detailed analysis of individual anatomy. Besides a comprehensive aesthetic analysis, it is also essential to consider the functional tasks of the anatomical structures of the nasal tip.

If tip-support mechanisms have been weakened by previous surgery, this may combine with postoperative scarring to cause conspicuous and undesirable iatrogenic deformities of the nasal tip in addition to functional problems.

13.1 Analysis

The first prerequisite for a successful operation is an analysis of the problem:

- Symmetry of the dorsal aesthetic lines
- Projection and protection of the nose
- Nasolabial angle and nasofrontal angle
- Width of the nasal tip
- Shape and texture of the lower lateral cartilage. Thin, soft lower lateral cartilages cannot tolerate major structural sacrifice. They lose their stability very easily. In this case, stable long-term results can be achieved only by using additional grafts, struts, and appropriate suture techniques.
- Length of the nose in relation to facial proportions
- Relationship of chin and forehead projection to nasal tip projection in the lateral view
- Facial asymmetry (should be considered in planning the nasal axis)
- Length and width of the columella
- Assessment of the depressor septi muscle
- Quality and thickness of the skin
- The septum. Unrecognized deviation or kinking of the septum will affect the aesthetic outcome of the nasal tip and may lead to functional problems. Note also the length of the nasal septum, which may affect tip rotation and the configuration of the columella.
- Size and position of the anterior nasal spine
- Assessment of the nasal base, including the shape of the nostrils

- Any external and internal nasal valve dysfunction, which must be detected before surgery[1]

13.2 Approach

Especially in secondary rhinoplasties, the open approach is preferred for tip corrections because it gives excellent visualization of the cartilaginous framework of the nose. Often this is necessary for an accurate assessment of cartilage status after previous surgery.

With asymmetries of the nasal tip, especially after a previous closed rhinoplasty, we often find that the cartilages were not worked in the same way on both sides (iatrogenic asymmetry). In some cases we also see an overreduction or complete resection of the caudal cartilage. Secondarily, there are congenital malformations of the caudal cartilage, especially at the medial and intermediate crus, which were not recognized during the previous operation and therefore were not corrected (residual asymmetries).

Previously placed grafts can also be clearly visualized through an external approach. An inverted-V incision is recommended for the open approach. When placed in the narrowest part of the columella, this incision leaves a very inconspicuous scar. However, especially in secondary rhinoplasties, the preexisting scar may not be in an optimum position. In most cases we use the old scar to avoid compromising the blood supply to the columella by incisions at different levels. We also have the opportunity to perform a scar revision at that time (**Fig. 13.1**).

Extensive scarring of the nasal tip is very common after prior surgery, so the dissection must be done in a way that does not injure the skin or delicate cartilage structures. Another drawback of scarring is that it often increases diffuse bleeding during the dissection.

13.3 Intra-, Inter-, and Transdomal Sutures

Intradomal and dome-defining sutures can narrow the single dome precisely (**Fig. 13.2**). Interdomal sutures approximate the domes at the desired distance (**Fig. 13.3**). Sometimes a preexisting underprojection of the nasal tip might not have been adequately corrected during the previous surgery. To reinforce the projection, the domes can be redefined and sutured together by transdomal suturing. Transdomal sutures can simultaneously narrow the domes and move them closer together (**Fig. 13.4**). Thereby overcorrection should be avoided. Otherwise this limits the function because of reducing the angle between columella and nostrils. Even properly placed sutures often cause some degree of pinching in very soft lateral cartilages. In these cases the lateral alar cartilage can be reinforced with thin cartilage grafts such as batten grafts, underbatten grafts, or lateral crural strut grafts.[2]

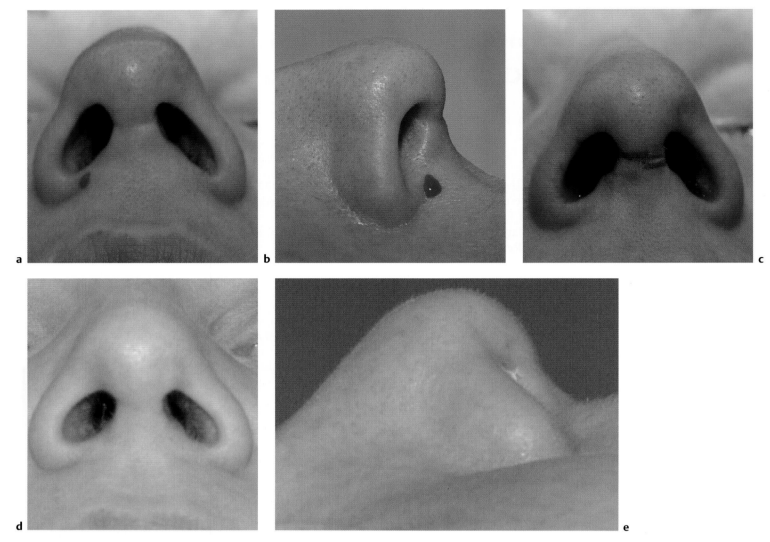

Fig. 13.1 (a) Preexisting scar does not have an optimum horizontal orientation. (b) The resulting scar contracture is most obvious in the lateral view. (c) Stair-step incision removes the old scar tissue and allows for scar correction over time. (d, e) Inconspicuous scar 9 months after secondary rhinoplasty and revision of the old contracture.

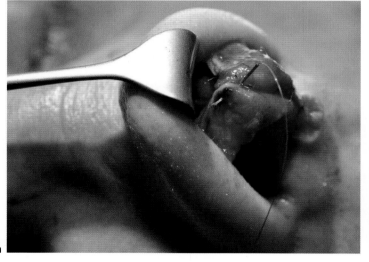
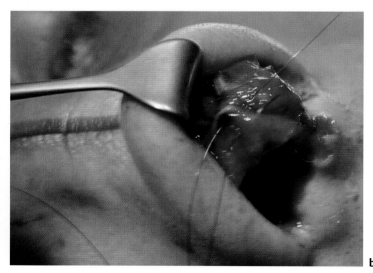

Fig. 13.2 How (a, b) intradomal sutures are applied.

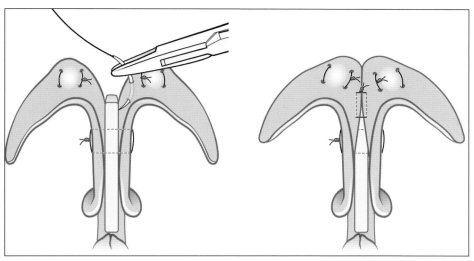

Fig. 13.3 The interdomal suture is a vertical suture placed between the domes of the middle crura to set the desired interdomal distance.

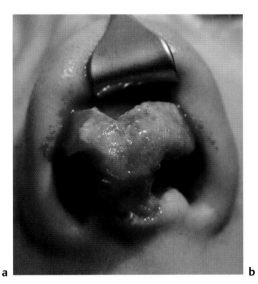
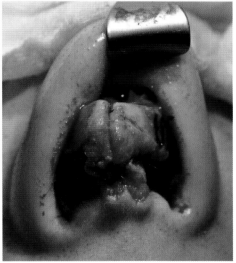
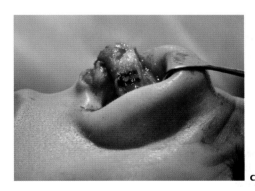

a   b   c

Fig. 13.4 (**a**) The distance between the domes after previous surgery was still very wide. Also, the cephalic portions of the lower lateral cartilages had not been resected equally. (**b**) After trimming of the lower lateral cartilages, intra- and transdomal sutures were placed to move the

domes closer together and refine the nasal tip shape. (**c**) Because the tip still deviates to the right due to excessive length of the left lateral crus, a lateral sliding technique is performed on the left side to restore symmetry.

13.4 Domal Equalization Suture

The domal equalization suture is placed through the cephalic domal segments and moves them closer together (**Fig. 13.5**). The suture ensures tip symmetry and lowers the cephalic portion of the rim below the tip-defining points.[3]

13.5 Spanning Suture

Lateral convexity or "flaring" of the alar cartilages can be effectively corrected with a spanning suture placed through the lateral crura (**Fig. 13.6**), using 5–0 material.

13.6 Tip Suspension Suture

Ptosis of the reconstructed nasal tip is prevented by passing a thread beneath a tip suspension suture fixed through the dorsal septal border (**Fig. 13.6**). This technique will prevent drooping of the tip. Nasal tip rotation and position are optimized and secured with a tip suspension suture. A modification is the suspension suture with an anterior sling for shortening the nose.[4] With the

aid of a cannula, the suture ends are brought anteriorly to the medial crura and tied together (**Fig. 13.7**).

13.7 Horizontal Mattress Suture Technique (Gruber)

Nonabsorbable mattress sutures placed in the lateral crus can balance both concave and convex bulbous deformities, depending on the direction of suture placement.[5] The vestibular skin on the undersurface of the cartilage is carefully undermined in the area of the deformity. Bulbous alar cartilages are corrected by placing the first stitch perpendicular to the length of the alar cartilage, then placing a second stitch perpendicular to the first and 6–8 mm from it. The knot is tied posterior to the lateral crus. A concavity is corrected with basically the same mattress suture placed on the undersurface of the lateral crus. In a modification described by Gruber, which also allows corrections of concave deformities, the cartilage is held in the desired shape with a forceps and the knot is tied posterior to the lateral crus, applying a carefully controlled amount of tension (**Fig. 13.8**).[1]

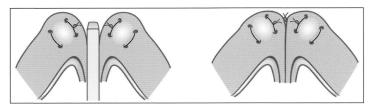

Fig. 13.5 Domal equalization suture approximates the cephalic edges of the two convex domal segments to establish tip symmetry.

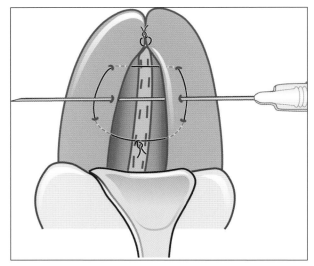

Fig. 13.6 Flaring of the alar cartilages is controlled with a spanning suture that is reinforced with a tip suspension suture through the dorsal septal border. These sutures are made using 5–0 nonabsorbable material.

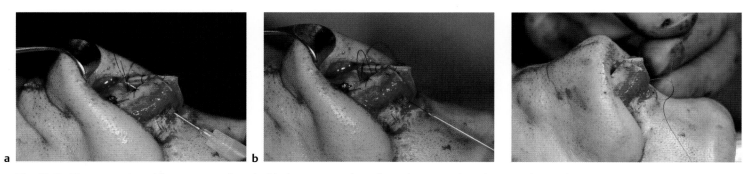

Fig. 13.7 Tip suspension with an anterior sling. (**a, b**) The suture ends are brought anteriorly with a cannula. (**c**) The ends are tied to shorten the nose.

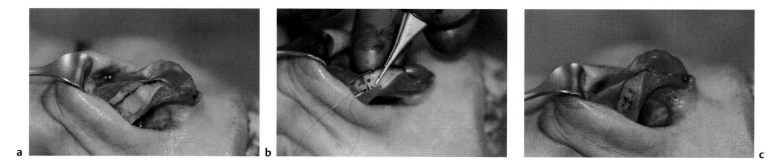

Fig. 13.8 (**a**) Concave deformity at the lateral crus. (**b, c**) The vestibular skin is carefully elevated from the undersurface of the cartilage, and the concave deformity is corrected with a modified horizontal mattress suture technique while the cartilage is held in the desired shape and tension with a forceps.

13.8 Lateral Crural Reversal Technique, Upside-Down Technique

Concavity of the lower lateral cartilages not only may be aesthetically objectionable but may also cause functional problems by pushing the convex undersurface into the vestibule. The deformed portion of the lower lateral cartilage is removed and turned 180° after separation of the vestibular skin from the cartilage. It is then sutured back into place (**Fig. 13.9**). Aiach recommended leaving a thin cartilage strip at the edge of the crus so that the lateral crus could be fixed more easily and securely after the reversal maneuver.[1]

13.9 Lateral Crural Overlay Technique

This technique also corrects concave deformities of the lower lateral cartilages. The cephalic edges of the lateral crura are separated from the vestibular skin (**Fig. 13.10a**) and are incised but not excised (**Fig. 13.10b**). The cephalic edges are then folded over the remaining portion of the lateral crura (**Fig. 13.10c**) and secured at the edges with fine sutures. The formerly concave cartilage is now convex and functionally stable.

13.10 Lateral Crural Underlay Technique

This technique provides another option for correcting concave deformity of the lateral crus. First the underlying vestibular skin is elevated from the cartilage. Then the cephalic portion is incised but left attached to the inferior perichondrium and passed beneath the remaining lateral crus. Fine sutures fix the position (**Fig. 13.11**). A modification is turn-in folding, in which the underlying vestibular skin remains and the cephalic edges of the lateral crura are simply incised and folded downward and reinforced with a spanning suture. Because of the caudal folding, however, the patient may complain of an unusual palpable finding within the nose, especially when the cartilage is of adequate width and thickness.[1]

13.11 Cephalic Trim

A sparing cephalic resection of the lower lateral cartilages will narrow the supratip area while also producing some cephalic tip rotation. The resection should not be parallel to the cartilage edge over the entire length of the cartilage, and the lateral third should be left wider than the medial third (**Fig. 13.12**). The cartilage should be left at least a minimum of 4–5 mm wide to preserve the neces-

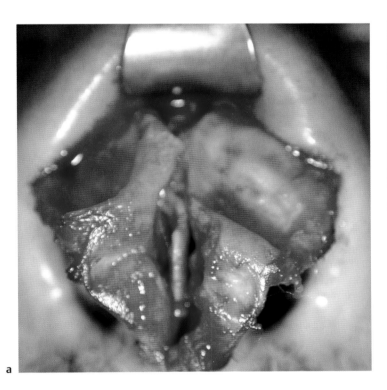

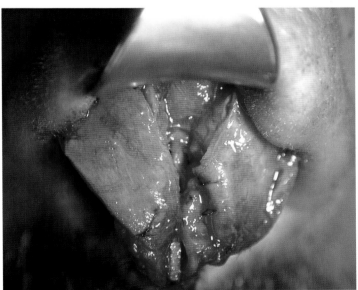

Fig. 13.9 (**a**) There is a concave deformity at the lateral crus. (**b**) The vestibular skin is separated from the cartilages, and the deformed concave portions of the lower lateral cartilage are removed and turned 180 degrees.

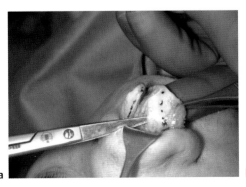
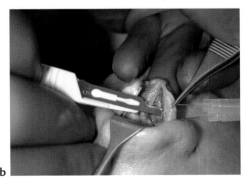
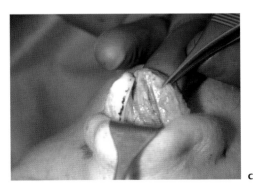

Fig. 13.10 (**a**) The cephalic portion of the lateral crus is separated from the underlying vestibular skin. (**b**) The cephalic edge of the lateral crus is incised only on the underside of the cartilage. (**c**) The cephalic portion overrides the remaining lateral crus and will be fixed in that position with fine nonabsorbable sutures.

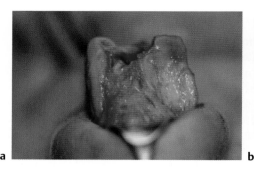
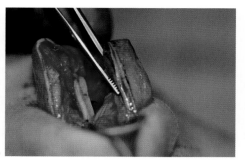
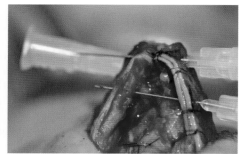

Fig. 13.11 (a) The right lateral cartilage shows a concave deformity. (b) After the underlying vestibular skin is separated from the cartilage, the cephalic portion is marked and incised. Still based on the inferior perichondrium, it is passed beneath the remaining lateral crus. (c) Fine nonabsorbable sutures fix the position.

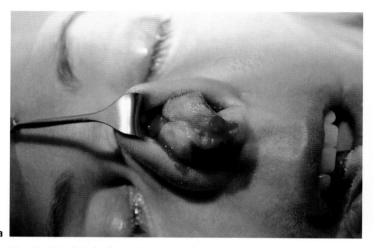
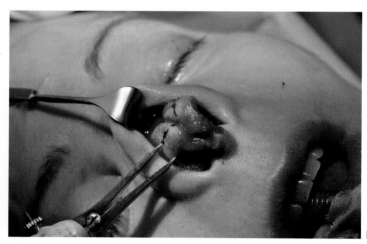

Fig. 13.12 (a) The lower lateral cartilages and supratip area are very broad. (b) The cephalic margin of the lower lateral cartilage is sparingly resected to narrow the supratip area.

sary functional stability of the caudal cartilage framework. Trimming too much cartilage from the lateral third may lead to pinching and collapse of the lower lateral cartilage with subsequent nasal airway constriction. This may even become accentuated over time.

The nose can be precisely analyzed and corrected through an open approach. An asymmetrical cephalic trim of the lower lateral cartilages can be corrected if necessary by resecting additional cartilage from a too-wide lateral crus or by reconstructing an overresected cartilage with batten grafts.

13.12 Dome Division Technique

The dome division technique is most suitable in thick-skinned patients.[6–9] The concept of dome division was first described by Goldmann[10,11] as a universal tip correction technique. Dome division affects both the projection and configuration of the nasal tip. Originally the technique involved incising not just the cartilages but also the vestibular skin at the dome, but today this is obsolete.

Although Goldmann illustrated his technique as a vertical cartilage-splitting incision at the angle of the lobular dome, the term "vertical dome division" was not used at that time and did not appear in the literature until the 1980s.[9,12]

The dome is divided by a vertical incision and reapproximate the cartilage edges with sutures, thereby increasing the tip projection (**Fig. 13.13**). Resecting a vertical cartilage strip causes deprojection. The exact amount of tip deprojection and derotation cannot be accurately predicted, however. Consequently, we recommend this technique only in very thick seborrheic skin and only if increased projection is desired. Dome division in thin-skinned patients may produce a sharp, narrowed tip with potential collapse of the alar sidewalls.[1]

13.13 Sliding Techniques

Familiarity with the "tripod" concept is crucial to fully understanding the principles of nasal tip correction. Anderson introduced this concept of tip surgery in the 1960s.[13] The anterior leg of the tripod is formed by the conjoined medial crura and columella, and the posterior legs are formed by the lateral crura. Changing one or more legs of the tripod will alter the position of the nasal tip. Shortening the anterior leg will decrease tip projection and rotation, while shortening the posterior legs

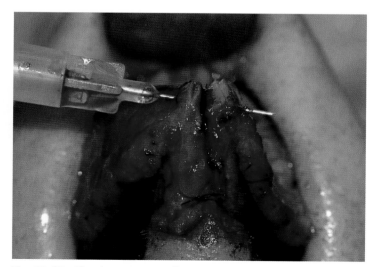

Fig. 13.13 The dome is vertically incised, and the cartilage edges are temporarily apposed with a needle. Then the edges are sutured together, increasing the tip projection.

will increase or support cephalic rotation and decrease projection. According to the tripod theory, shortening the medial crura causes loss of tip projection and slight caudal rotation. Shortening the lower lateral cartilages causes deprojection and cephalic rotation.

13.13.1 Lateral Sliding

An initial mark is placed on the dome, and a second mark is drawn 10 mm from the first (**Fig. 13.14a**). A third mark is placed at a distance that depends on the degree of sliding that is required. After the vestibular skin is dissected from the lateral crus, an incision is made at the second mark and the cartilage is brought down to the third mark. The overlapped edges of the crus are fixed provisionally with small needles and definitively with 6–0 nonabsorbable nylon sutures (**Fig. 13.14b**). A columellar strut can be added to support the anterior leg of the tripod. The effects of lateral sliding include cephalic rotation and deprojection of the nasal tip. Cephalic rotation can be prevented by turning the axis of the slide rather than keeping the edges parallel. The resulting cartilage excess should be trimmed (**Fig. 13.14c**).

The tip must be reconfigured due to the widening of the domes that occurs with lateral sliding. A good way to narrow the domes is by transdomal suturing. A spanning suture will control flaring of the lower lateral cartilages.[14]

13.13.2 Medial Sliding

The dome is premarked, and a second mark 5–6 mm from the first defines the site where the cartilage will be cut. A third mark is drawn at a distance that depends on the amount of sliding required (**Fig. 13.15a**). The rest of the procedure is similar to the lateral sliding technique (**Fig. 13.15b**). Medial sliding results in deprojection and caudal rotation of the tip. Minor malformations at the junction of the medial and intermediate crura can be simultaneously corrected.[14] The caudal rotation effect can be avoided by changing the axis of the dome complex cranially, so that the cartilages are not placed parallel to each other. The excess cartilage at the caudal border of the transposed cartilage should be resected.

After the cartilaginous framework has been reduced, it may be necessary to adapt the skin envelope by excising excess skin at the columella incision.[1]

The sliding techniques can provide accurate deprojection of the nasal tip with long-lasting stable results. Lateral sliding can shorten the length of the lateral crura, while a medial sliding technique can shorten the medial crura. A combination of both techniques is also possible. The sliding techniques do not involve cartilage removal. After division of the lateral or medial crus, the cartilage edges are overlapped and fixed with a nonabsorbable 6–0 suture, increasing the stability of the alar cartilage framework.

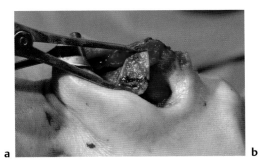
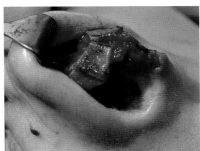
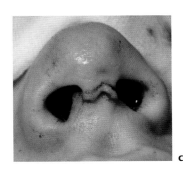

Fig. 13.14 (**a**) The dome is marked after cephalic trimming of the lower lateral cartilage, and a second mark is drawn 10 mm from the first. The position of the third mark depends on the desired amount of sliding. (**b**) After dissection of the vestibular skin from the lateral crus, an incision is made at the second mark and the cartilage is brought down to the third mark. The result is stabilized with nonabsorbable sutures. (**c**) A skin envelope remains after reduction of the cartilage framework. The redundant excess skin is marked for excision.

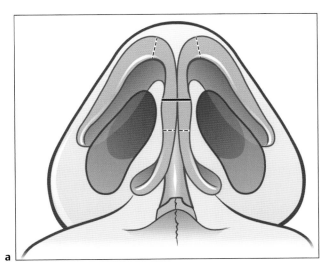
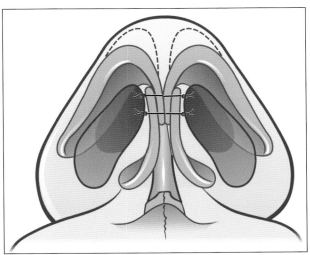

Fig. 13.15 (**a**) The dome is already marked (*pecked lines*), and a second mark 5–6 mm from the first defines the site where the cartilage will be cut (*solid line*). A third mark (*pecked line*) is drawn at a distance that depends on the amount of sliding required. (**b**) After the vestibular skin is dissected from the medial crus, an incision is made at the second mark and the cartilage is brought down to the third mark. The desired position is fixed temporarily with small needles and definitively with 6–0 nylon sutures.

Unequal dome heights can be adjusted by a unilateral sliding maneuver (see **Fig. 13.4**).[1] If there is a concave deformity of the lateral crus in addition to overprojection, both can be corrected simultaneously with this technique alone by overlapping and stabilizing the cartilages.

13.14 Lateral Crural Steal

Various lateral crural steal techniques can be used when the original dome is too low, creating the appearance of an under-projected tip. Lateral crural steal can improve tip projection and rotation while preserving the continuity of the cartilaginous structures (**Fig. 13.16**). It can also improve the contour of a flattened nasal base and change the nostrils from a more horizontal shape to a more natural-looking vertical orientation.[15,16] The vestibular skin is carefully separated from the undersurface of the alar cartilages in the dome area, and the lateral crura are sutured together cephalad to the former dome position. The newly defined domes are then stabilized with an inter- or transdomal suture. The previous undermining of the vestibular skin helps to prevent permanent retraction. This technique also shortens the lower lateral cartilages, causing cephalic rotation of the nasal tip. To prevent this cephalic rotation, Kridel et al recommend separating the entire lateral crus from the piriform aperture and the vestibular skin.[17] The lateral crus is then advanced anteriorly, resulting in increased projection. A columellar strut is recommended in these cases to reinforce the tip support mechanisms. This technique is less advantageous in patients with thin nasal skin because the transposed cartilage edges may be visible through the skin.[17]

13.15 Tongue-in-Groove Technique

With a septum of sufficient length, the anterior border of the septum can be positioned between the medial crura and both structures fixed to each other with fine sutures. This tongue-in-groove technique reliably prevents postoperative loss of tip projection. It not only is effective for controlling nasal length and tip projection (push-down or push-up technique) but can also modify tip rotation by changing the axis at which the medial crura are fixed to the septum (**Fig. 13.17**). Cephalic rotation aids in shortening the nose. Shifting the medial cartilage cephalad will slightly increase the degree of tip rotation.[18] Other ideal candidates for this

technique are patients who have a hanging columella due to a long caudal septum and patients with a short upper lip, since fixing the medial crura to the caudal septum will usually produce slight extension of the upper lip.[2] Some patients consider the decreased mobility of the nasal tip to be a disadvantage (stiff feeling).

13.16 Push-Down Technique

If only moderate deprojection is needed and the septum is of adequate length, a push-down technique can be used. In this technique the medial crura are held down at the anterior border of the septum and are fixed in the desired position to the septum with fine nonabsorbable sutures. Changing the position of the medial crura can also affect rotation as in the tongue-in-groove technique (see **Fig. 13.17**). The shortening of the nose can be supported by an internal and external nose lift if there is excess skin that cannot shrink.[1]

13.17 Materials for Structural Grafts

The material of choice for grafting is septal cartilage, provided sufficient cartilage has been left from the previous operation. The stability of the septal framework must not be compromised. Another option is to use cartilage from the lower lateral cartilages that was removed in a cephalic trim. We also use conchal cartilage, tragal cartilage, and rib cartilage. Another commonly used material is autologous or allogeneic fascia. In very rare cases Medpor grafts (Stryker, Mahwah, NJ, USA) are used. We do not use silicone implants.[1]

13.18 Columellar Strut

Suturing the medial crura to a columellar strut can control projection and improve protection (tip support). The strut is placed in a pocket between the medial crura. In general, the medial crura are fixed to the strut with fine nonabsorbable sutures. The strut is usually fabricated from a straight piece of septal cartilage. If there is not enough septal cartilage left or if it is not straight enough, or if the anterior septum is to be reconstructed, the best solution is a double-layered sandwich graft made of conchal cartilage (**Fig. 13.18**). If the columellar strut is made of rib cartilage, the columella will be very stiff and susceptible to later deformation.

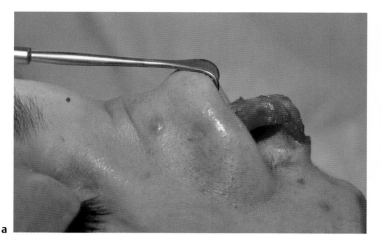
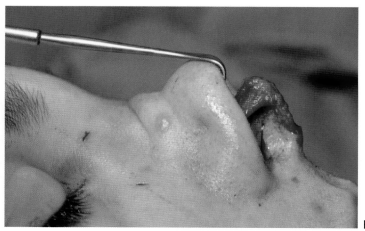

a b

Fig. 13.16 (**a**) The original domes occupy a low position. (**b**) The lateral steal technique reconstitutes the domes above the original position. This results in increased tip projection and cephalic rotation.

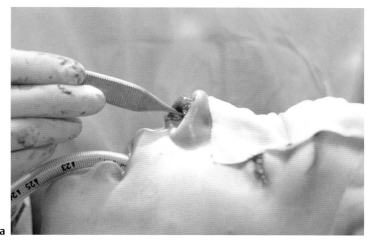
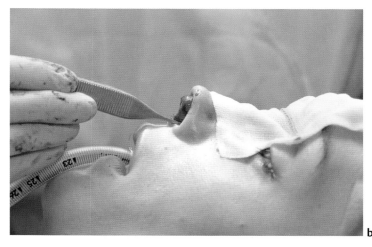

a

b

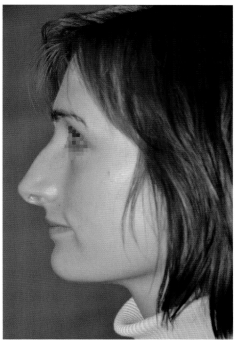
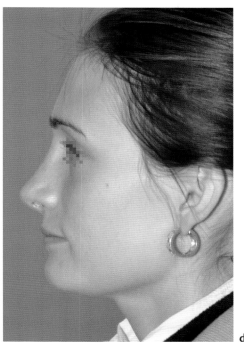

c

d

Fig. 13.17 (**a, b**) Both medial crura are pushed down and fixed to the anterior septal border temporarily with a needle and definitively with a 6–0 suture. In this case the septum was long enough to combine the push-down technique for deprojection with a tongue-in-groove tech- nique. The position of the medial crura is similarly changed, resulting in slight cephalic rotation of the tip. (**c, d**) Lateral views before and 3 months after rhinoplasty. A combined tongue-in-groove and push-down technique corrected the hanging columella and rotated the nasal tip.

13.19 Tip Graft

Tip grafts are used to contour the nasal tip, correct an underpro- jected nasal tip, and compensate for asymmetries. The grafts are fashioned from resected cephalic alar cartilage, septal cartilage (**Fig. 13.19**), or rib cartilage if necessary. To avoid visibility of the graft on the surface of the nose, the edges of the graft have to be flattened. In rare cases, especially in thin-skinned patients, tip grafts can also be made from one or more layers of fascia.

13.19.1 Shield Graft

Shield grafts are often used in secondary rhinoplasties (**Fig. 13.20**), for the correction of an underprojected nasal tip in thick-skinned patients, and for nose lengthening. They can also be used to imitate the "double break" of the nasal tip if desired (**Fig. 13.21**). Daniel distinguishes between "integrated" and "projected" grafts. The latter projects above the actual dome and is par- ticularly useful for tip contouring in patients with thicker skin (**Fig. 13.22**).[3] In these cases there is always a risk that the graft

edges will be visible beneath the skin. To prevent this, and to create smooth transitions, the edges can be recontoured with a small amount of soft, crushed cartilage or soft tissue.

13.19.2 CAP Graft

The contoured auricular projection (CAP) graft is placed directly over the domes to compensate for irregularities and increase tip projection[19] or to fill the dead space behind a projected shield graft over the domes (**Fig. 13.23**).

13.19.3 Batten Graft

Batten grafts are often used to stabilize very soft lateral alar car- tilages in primary rhinoplasties and prevent inspiratory alar col- lapse. They may also be used to correct a residual caudal defor- mity or reconstruct grossly overresected lower lateral cartilages (**Fig. 13.24**).[1,20] If the intermediate crura were not previously resected and are still stable, it is sufficient to restore the lateral crura with batten grafts (**Fig. 13.25**). The grafts can be made of

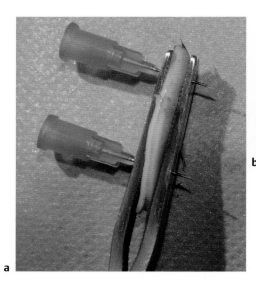

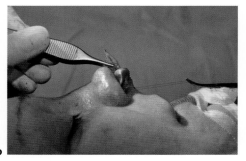

Fig. 13.18   (**a**) An Aiach-Gubisch clamp helps to hold the composite graft in an ideal position, making it easier to place the running suture for definitive graft fixation. (**b**) The sandwich graft is placed between the medial crura and then fixed to the residual septum and between the crura with nonabsorbable sutures.

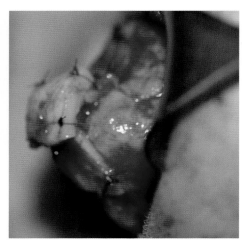

Fig. 13.19   Underprojection of the nasal tip is corrected with a tip graft made of septal cartilage.

septal cartilage. Extensive resection of cartilage, especially soft cartilage, leads to a collapse of the nostril, which can no longer maintain its shape during inspiration. It collapses along with the internal nasal valve, causing nasal airway obstruction. A collapse phenomenon may also occur in the cartilaginous lateral nasal wall during deep inspiration. This underscores the importance of a precise preoperative evaluation. Alar batten grafts or sidewall batten grafts are used to reinforce the weakened area. Conchal cartilage is excellent for this purpose, owing to its natural curvature.

Often we also see an inappropriate division of one or both sides of the lower lateral cartilages, usually not even at the same level. Also, a cartilage graft is needed to bridge the defect and restore the continuity of the crura. The domes are reestablished with suture techniques, relying mainly on intra- and transdomal sutures of nonabsorbable 6–0 material.

Extended batten grafts are used, for example, to support a less developed lower lateral cartilage or to correct a damaged and scarred lower lateral cartilage after previous surgery. Ideally these grafts are based on the piriform aperture.

13.19.4 Bending Technique

In many revisions we see an overresection or complete resection of the caudal cartilaginous framework even in thick-skinned patients. This was probably done with the intention of reducing and refining the nasal tip. As thick and heavy skin cannot shrink enough to match major changes in the cartilage framework, the

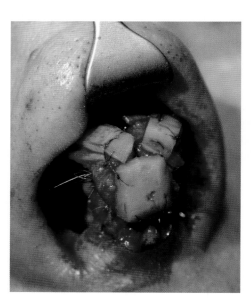

Fig. 13.20   A shield graft made of septal cartilage was used to extend the nose slightly in a secondary rhinoplasty. The edges of the graft were flattened to give an optimal shape.

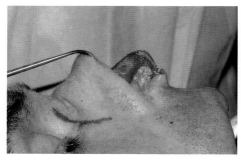

Fig. 13.21   The shield graft used to increase tip projection and extend the nose imitates the "double break" of the nasal tip.

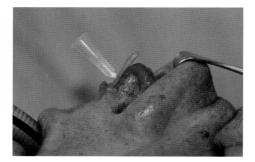

Fig. 13.22   The "projected" shield graft extends above the actual dome and is particularly useful for contouring thicker skin.

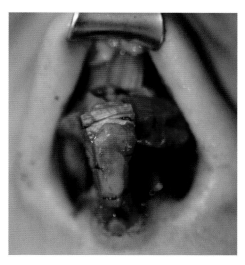

Fig. 13.23   The contoured auricular projection (CAP) graft made of allogeneic fascia lata is placed directly over the dome to fill the space behind the projected shield graft.

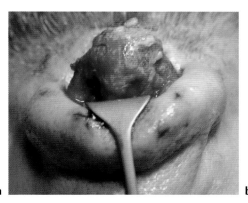

a

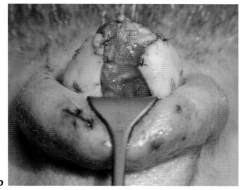

b

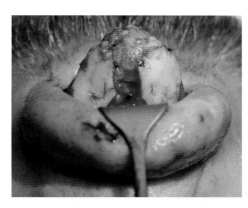

c

Fig. 13.24   (**a**) After eight previous operations elsewhere, both lower lateral cartilages were overresected and there was massive scar tissue with an absence of identifiable normal anatomic structures. (**b**) Both lower lateral cartilages were reconstructed with autologous tragal cartilage due to a lack of available septal and conchal cartilage. (**c**) A spanning suture was placed to control flaring of the reconstructed lower lateral cartilages.

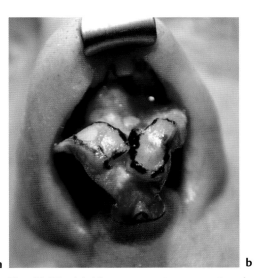

a

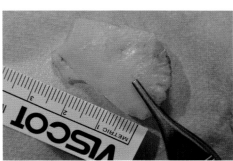

b

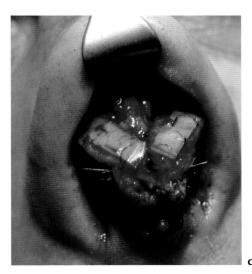

c

Fig. 13.25   (**a**) After one previous operation, both lower lateral cartilages are overresected and the medial crura are grossly deformed. (**b**) A piece of septal cartilage was harvested to recreate the internal valves with spreader grafts and reconstruct the lower lateral cartilages with batten grafts. (**c**) The deformity, excessive length and asymmetry of the medial crura were corrected by medial sliding. The batten grafts were fixed to the edges of the lower lateral cartilages medially and laterally to the vestibular skin.

nasal tip may become ptotic over the years due to a lack of cartilaginous support and the weight of the soft-tissue envelope. This leads to polly beak deformity with an underprojected nasal tip. In thin skin the overresection can cause a conspicuous asymmetry with visible and palpable cartilage ends and a pinching or retraction of the nostrils. The aesthetic effects in these cases may be accompanied by functional problems in the external nasal valve complex.[20]

All these cases require an anatomical reconstruction of the cartilaginous framework. In cases where intermediate crura were also resected or are unstable after prior reconstructive surgery, we prefer the bending technique (**Fig. 13.26**).[20]

Two long cartilage strips are harvested from the septum, provided there is enough septal cartilage remaining. A third strip is harvested to make a columellar strut. The strips are shaped with a burr to create the desired arch in the new dome area. They are then sutured medially to the stumps of the medial crura and laterally to the vestibular mucosa. The reconstructed cartilaginous framework is also fixed to the columellar strut. The domes are reconstituted with suture techniques, using mainly the intra- and transdomal techniques. A spanning suture controls alar flaring and a tip suspension suture fixes the nasal tip to the dorsal septal margin to prevent subsequent drooping of the tip. If there is not enough septal cartilage left to obtain a stable septal framework after the previous surgery, conchal or rib cartilage can be used and is basically treated the same way. Too much stiffness in the new dome can be corrected by dome division and cartilage reapproximation.[6,20]

The bending technique can also be used if tip projection needs to be increased but the caudal framework has insufficient length despite increasing the projection by suturing techniques, dome division, or an onlay graft. Another option in these cases is to extend the caudal cartilage framework by the bending technique.

13.19.5 Underbatten Graft

Underbatten grafts or lateral crural strut grafts can be used to reinforce unstable alar cartilages or flatten bulbous cartilages.[2] The supporting and stiffening grafts are positioned in a pocket carefully dissected between the undersurface of the lateral alar cartilages and the vestibular skin. The grafts are fixed with fine absorbable sutures (**Fig. 13.27**).

13.19.6 Interdomal Graft

Some patients complain about a "groove" between the domes. This can be rectified with an interdomal graft that fits between the domes and is secured with transdomal sutures (**Fig. 13.28**). This technique also ensures an adequate interdomal distance and can be used to add spacing for domes that are too close together.

13.19.7 Subdomal Graft

Subdomal grafts can also be used to increase the interdomal distance. Beyond this they can be used to correct a narrow domal angle, asymmetrical domes, and iatrogenic pinching of the lower lateral cartilages by transdomal sutures.[21] To increase the interdomal distance, the subdomal graft, preferably consisting of an 8- to 10-mm-long bar of septal cartilage 1.5–2 mm thick, is positioned under the dome and fixed with fine sutures (**Fig. 13.29**). Potential problems after graft insertion are cephalic rotation of the caudal end of the lower lateral cartilage and increased stiffness of the nasal tip.[21]

13.19.8 Alar Rim Grafts

Alar rim grafts are used to add volume to the concavity of the alar rim or relax and fill a collapsed nostril in cleft noses. They give the nostrils more support and prevent kinking. Alar rim grafts are soft, thin cartilage strips ~ 12–15 mm long and 2–3 mm wide. They are drawn into a previously dissected pocket that runs along the caudal border of the nostrils (**Fig. 13.30**). They are usually placed through an endonasal approach but may also be introduced through a stab incision in the alar fold.[1]

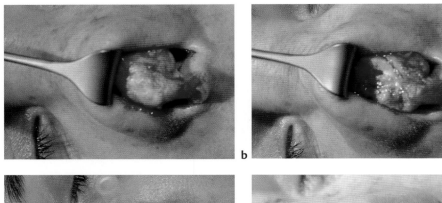
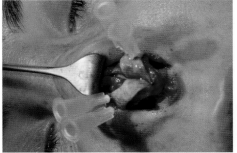
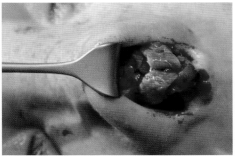
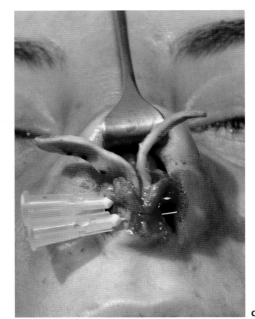

Fig. 13.26 (**a**) Intraoperative view shows massive scar tissue after two previous operations elsewhere. (**b**) Bilaterally resected lower lateral cartilages are seen after removal of the scar tissue. (**c**) Strips of conchal cartilage are fixed medially between the stumps of the medial crura. (**d**) The new lower lateral cartilages are temporarily fixed to the vestibular skin. (**e**) The strips are definitively fixed to the vestibular skin and joined medially, followed by the placement of a spanning suture and tip suspension suture.

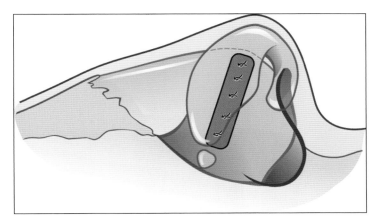

Fig. 13.27 The graft is positioned and sutured to the undersurface of the alar cartilages.

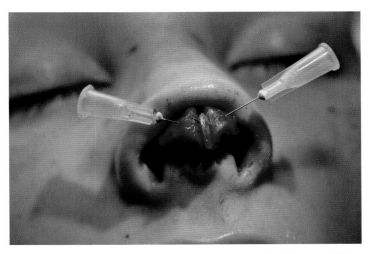

Fig. 13.28 An interdomal graft was fixed between the domes to fill the visible depression between the domes.

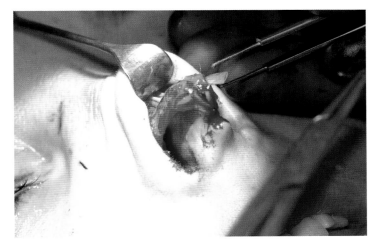

Fig. 13.29 A subdomal graft made of septal cartilage is positioned under the dome and fixed with fine sutures.

13.19.9 Caudal Septal Extension Graft

Overresection of the anterior septal border or anterior nasal spine often causes a decreased nasolabial angle or even a hidden columella. The loss of tip support leads to a caudal rotation that gives the nose the appearance of being too long. A caudal septal extension graft can add length to a too-short septum. The shape and orientation of the septal extension graft can be adjusted to make desired changes in the nasolabial angle, tip rotation, nasal length, and the relationship of the nostrils to the columella. Thus, for example, the lower portion of the graft can be made slightly longer to correct

a ptotic nasal tip with a sharp nasolabial angle. The medial cartilages are sutured up to the edge of the graft to support tip rotation. Choosing a graft with a longer extraction in the cranial part for an overrotated tip with a shorter nose, an extension of the nose can be achieved because the tip is moved more caudad.

The graft may be made of septal cartilage from the dorsal portions of the septum, or a double-layered sandwich graft can be fashioned from conchal cartilage. Alternatively, the reconstruction can be achieved by rotation of the entire septum.[22]

The graft is fixed to the septum with nonabsorbable sutures in an end-to-end or overlapping fashion. Additional fixation with a suture passed through a drill hole in the anterior nasal spine is also recommended. Thin cartilage splints called extended spreader grafts are also used to stabilize the septum and graft by bridging each other (**Fig. 13.31**).

13.20 Camouflage

Autologous soft tissue obtained during the dissection can be placed in the dome area to refine the tip contour and slightly increase projection (**Fig. 13.32**). Another option is the use of autologous or allogeneic fascia lata. Autologous soft tissue can also be used to line the occasionally retracted soft triangles at the end of an operation. Toriumi and Checcone also recommend perichondrium derived from conchal or rib cartilage to provide camouflage in the area of a shield graft.[2]

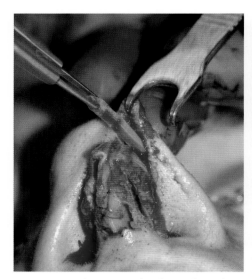 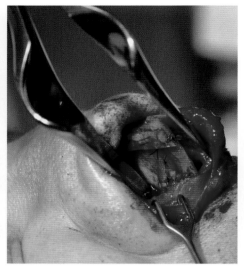 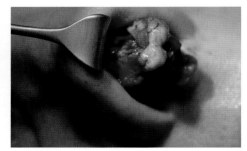

Fig. 13.30 Alar rim made of septal cartilage is drawn into a previously dissected pocket that runs along the caudal border of the nostril.

Fig. 13.31 Caudal septal extension graft made of septal cartilage overlaps the septum and is fixed with nonabsorbable sutures to the septum and anterior nasal spine. Extended spreader grafts additionally bridge the graft.

Fig. 13.32 The dome area is camouflaged with autologous scar tissue harvested during the dissection.

References

1. Eichhorn-Sens J, Gubisch W. Ästhetische Chirurgie der Nasenspitze. In: von Heimburg D, Lemperle G, eds. Ästhetische Chirurgie. Heidelberg, Germany: ecomed Medizin, Verlagsgruppe Hüthig Jehle Rehm GmbH; 2010

2. Toriumi DM, Checcone MA. New concepts in nasal tip contouring. Facial Plast Surg Clin North Am 2009;17(1):55–90, vi

3. Daniel RK. Rhinoplasty. An Atlas of Surgical Techniques. New York, NY: Springer; 2004

4. Gubisch W. Personal communication 2012. Publication in process

5. Gruber RP, Nahai F, Bogdan MA, Friedman GD. Changing the convexity and concavity of nasal cartilages and cartilage grafts with horizontal mattress sutures: part II. Clinical results. Plast Reconstr Surg 2005;115(2):595–606, discussion 607–608

6. Kridel RW, Yoon PJ, Koch RJ. Prevention and correction of nasal tip bossae in rhinoplasty. Arch Facial Plast Surg 2003;5(5):416–422

7. Papanastasiou S, Logan A. Management of the overprojecting nasal tip: a review. Aesthetic Plast Surg 2000;24(5):353–356

8. Rees TD. Rhinoplasty. In: Rees TD, ed. Aesthetic Plastic Surgery. Philadelphia, PA: WB Saunders; 1980

9. Simons RL. Vertical dome division in rhinoplasty. Otolaryngol Clin North Am 1987;20(4):785–796

10. Goldman IB. Surgical tips on the nasal tip. Eye Ear Nose Throat Mon 1954;33(10):583–586

11. Goldman IB. The importance of the mesial crura in nasal-tip reconstruction. AMA Arch Otolaryngol 1957;65(2):143–147

12. Davis AM, Simons RL, Rhee JS. Evaluation of the Goldman tip procedure in modern-day rhinoplasty. Arch Facial Plast Surg 2004;6(5):301–307

13. Anderson JR. The dynamics of rhinoplasty. In: Proceedings of the 9th International Congress of Otolaryngology, International Congress Series 206. Amsterdam, The Netherlands: Excerpta Medica; 1969

14. Eichhorn-Sens J, Gubisch W. [The sliding technique : a precise method for treating the overprojected nasal tip]. HNO 2009;57(12):1262–1272

15. Foda HM, Kridel RW. Lateral crural steal and lateral crural overlay: an objective evaluation. Arch Otolaryngol Head Neck Surg 1999;125(12):1365–1370

16. Kridel RW, Konior RJ. Controlled nasal tip rotation via the lateral crural overlay technique. Arch Otolaryngol Head Neck Surg 1991;117(4):411–415

17. Kridel RW, Konior RJ, Shumrick KA, Wright WK. Advances in nasal tip surgery. The lateral crural steal. Arch Otolaryngol Head Neck Surg 1989;115(10):1206–1212

18. Foda HM. Management of the droopy tip: a comparison of three alar cartilage-modifying techniques. Plast Reconstr Surg 2003;112(5):1408–1417, discussion 1418–1421

19. Porter JP, Tardy ME Jr, Cheng J. The contoured auricular projection graft for nasal tip projection. Arch Facial Plast Surg 1999;1(4):312–315

20. Gubisch W, Eichhorn-Sens J. Overresection of the lower lateral cartilages: a common conceptual mistake with functional and aesthetic consequences. Aesthetic Plast Surg 2009;33(1):6–13

21. Guyuron B, Poggi JT, Michelow BJ. The subdomal graft. Plast Reconstr Surg 2004;113(3):1037–1040, discussion 1041–1043

22. Gubisch W. Septumplastik durch extrakorporale Septumkorrektur. Stuttgart, Germany: Thieme; 1995

Section II

In the following, we present solutions to problems based on representative case reports drawn from our repertoire of reconstructive and revision surgery. Working from specific case details to general principles, we demonstrate why we have chosen a particular path—recognizing, of course, that many different paths can lead to the desired goal.

Our illustrative cases are arranged by anatomical regions. Another option would have been to divide them into minor and major revisions. But every surgeon knows that so-called minor revisions often take the brunt of patient dissatisfaction and attention. Similarly, the concept of a "simple" or "difficult" nose is problematic because rhinoplasty candidates often place very high expectations on the correction of simple or subtle flaws, while more serious deformities are easier to treat because any improvement in the patient's appearance is likely to be considered a success. The spectrum of illustrative case reports is drawn from the everyday case files of the contributing authors. Taken together, they paint a vivid picture of the many different problem situations that may arise in revision rhinoplasties.

14 Approaches to the Nasal Tip and Dorsum

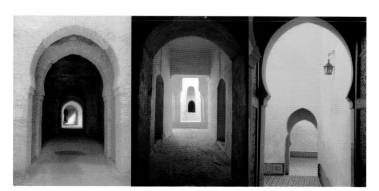

Fig. 14.1 How large should an approach be to open a hidden space?

14.1 Closed or Open Approach?

The first aesthetic rhinoplasty was performed by John Orlando Roe in 1887 using an endonasal approach.[1] Jacques Joseph performed the first reduction rhinoplasty through an external approach in 1898. Then, in 1904, Joseph was the first to report on the simultaneous intranasal correction of the anterior septum and a dorsal hump.[2] He continued to use the endonasal approach thereafter and systematically advanced it despite the staunch resistance of some leading contemporary surgeons such as Erich Lexer.[3–5] He passed his experience on to many later pioneers of rhinoplasty, such as Safian, Aufricht, and Maliniak, and thus laid the groundwork for the worldwide popularity of the closed technique. Proponents of the open approach, such as Rethi and Padovan, remained outsiders for many years.[6,7]

For decades the closed approach was used mainly for alar cartilage resections or reducing cartilage tension. These techniques relied on the "dynamics of rhinoplasty," or the cumulative effects of multiple surgical alterations.[8] For example, cephalic volume reduction of the alar cartilages combined with shortening and beveling of the dorsal septal border combine to produce a cephalic rotation of the nasal tip. Tip suture techniques were introduced only in recent decades. Although the proponents of the closed technique had long ago proven what could be accomplished through an endonasal approach, the booming and prospering field of facial plastic surgery, especially in the U.S., engendered a growing desire in the 1980s for a simple approach that would afford maximum visibility.[9] It was concluded that the open approach would shorten the learning curve for many surgeons inexperienced in rhinoplasties. Maximum exposure was seen as a rapid substitute for surgical experience. The open technique has evolved swiftly during the past 30 years and has prompted the development of new trends and techniques, giving rise to new suture techniques and many new and unexpected ways of applying and fixing cartilage grafts.[10,11] At present, ~ 88% of rhinoplasties in the U.S. are performed through an open approach.[12]

Meanwhile, the disadvantages of the open technique have become apparent and have sparked a critical discussion on the relative merits of the open and closed approaches (**Fig. 14.1**).[13–17] For example, controversy surrounds the fact that open rhinoplasties initially destabilize several structures that must later be repaired with grafts and sutures.[9] Typically, the surgeon must touch, dissect, repair, and reconstruct several structures for which the patient did not request treatment. The operating times are longer, and the larger wound area carries a greater risk of protracted wound healing and complications. The open approach itself may cause asymmetry due to edema, impaired nasal tip sensation, and problems with columellar closure. There is also a risk of unnatural nasal rigidity.[3]

For these reasons, a new version of the old closed rhinoplasty technique is experiencing a renaissance. This trend has benefited from the techniques devised for open approaches, which can also be applied and refined for endonasal use.

14.2 Endoscopic Approach

To avoid the problem of limited access and visibility in the closed approach, a fiberoptic Aufricht retractor and miniaturized instruments have been developed for endoscopic dissection of the nasal dorsum and nasal pyramid. This technique allows surgical maneuvers to be performed under optical control that were previously done blindly or controlled by audible feedback. This principle is illustrated by endoscopic dissection of the periosteum using specialized instruments.

The return to an advanced closed technique meets the desires of many of today's patients for a more efficient, goal-directed operation that is minimally invasive, takes less time, requires less down time, and eliminates external scars. Rhinoplasty is returning from an all-round operation in the mainstream of plastic surgery to a specialized field, and this should have positive effects. A good rule to follow in selecting an approach and operating technique is this: Preserve the functionality of the natural structure of the nose. You can rebuild form with grafts, but you cannot rebuild the natural functional elasticity of the nose.

14.3 Closed Approaches

14.3.1 Cartilage-Splitting Approach

The selection of an approach for revision rhinoplasty depends on the priorities of the patient, the degree of tissue scarring that has occurred in specific areas, and the patient's skin and connective-tissue type. The approach should be as invasive as necessary and as atraumatic as possible. The smaller the new raw surfaces, the better.

The cartilage-splitting approach is excellent for cephalic volume reduction of the alar cartilages in patients with a bulbous nasal tip.[3] It is less suitable for correcting asymmetries. It cannot alter the interdomal distance or the position of the tip defining points but can be used to harmonize the brow–tip aesthetic line, which is impaired by a bulbous tip and is significantly improved by smoothing the transition from the middle vault to the supratip area. Cephalic rotation follows the principles of rhinoplasty dynamics. Scar contracture will occur due to scarring between the caudal edge of the upper lateral cartilage and the intact alar cartilage. The level of the resection determines whether the tip defining points should be repositioned or preserved.

Cases 1–5 illustrate how specific approaches are chosen.

Case 1

Introduction

A 24-year-old woman presented 2 years after septal surgery with the concern of a drooping nasal tip that accentuated a preexisting hump (**Fig. 14.2**). She also complained of an intermittent whistling sound during nasal breathing. She desired a profile correction that would harmonize the junction of the nasal tip and dorsum in addition to repairing a septal perforation.

Findings

Frontal view (**Fig. 14.2a**) shows a broad, somewhat bulbous nasal tip with a disharmonious transition from the middle vault to the tip. Profile view (**Fig. 14.2b**) documents loss of tip protection and projection with a bony and cartilaginous hump. Basal view (**Fig. 14.2c**) shows a symmetrical, somewhat broad tip. Internal examination showed an ~ 1-cm septal perforation with residual deviation to the right.

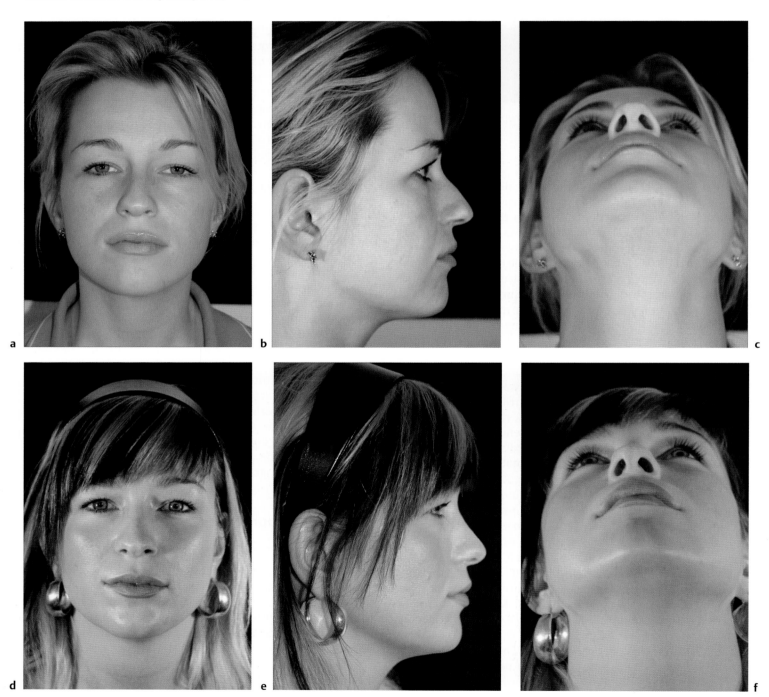

Fig. 14.2 (**a–c**) Appearance before revision rhinoplasty. (**d–f**) Appearance 2 years after revision rhinoplasty.

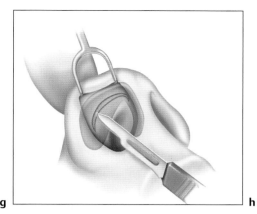
g

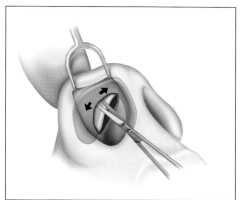
h

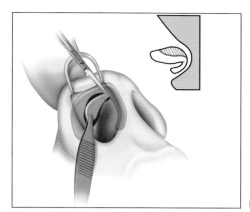
i

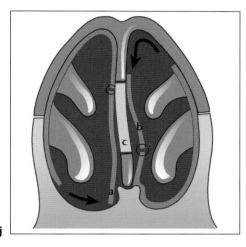
j

Fig. 14.2   (**g**) Cartilage-splitting approach to the nasal tip. Incision of the skin in the nasal vestibule. (**h**) Exposure of the cephalic portion of the lateral alar cartilage. (**i**) Cephalic volume reduction: the designated upper portion of the alar cartilage is resected. (**j**) Septal perforation repaired with the bridge flap technique; a, inferior mucosal flap; b, superior mucosal flap; c, cartilage.

Surgical Procedure

The septal perforation was closed with autologous tragal cartilage using the Schulz-Coulon bridge flap technique (**Fig. 14.2g**).[18]

For cephalic volume reduction of the alar cartilage, the dome was exposed and the dome area weakened by tailored compression with a broad, blunt Adson forceps. This was followed by *en bloc* resection of the bony and cartilaginous nasal hump plus medial and lateral curved osteotomies (**Fig. 14.2h–j**).

Psychology, Motivation, Personal Background

The patient, who worked as a hairdresser in Berlin, was bothered by her perforated septum. She sought consultation for that problem and also desired an aesthetic correction of her nasal tip and profile in the same sitting. Her motivation for the surgery was clear and understandable.

Discussion

A preoperative computer simulation was conducted with the patient to review possible profile adjustments, with and without a supratip break, and discuss how the nasal tip could be narrowed by reducing the interdomal distance with sutures. The patient elected to have the junction of the nasal dorsum and tip harmonized through a cartilage-splitting approach. An alternative would have been a suture technique with a delivery approach. The cartilage-splitting approach is effective for reducing tip volume but cannot be used to approximate the tip defining points or decrease the interdomal angle (**Fig. 14.3h–j**). Ultimately the choice depends on the wish of the patient, provided it is medically and aesthetically sound and technically feasible.

14.3.2 Delivery Approach

The delivery approach is an elegant endonasal technique that gives the practiced surgeon a variety of ways to correct and refine the nasal tip. A chondrocutaneous flap is raised from the alar cartilage and the skin of the nasal vestibule. Two incisions are used. First an intercartilaginous incision is made in the crease between the upper lateral cartilage and alar cartilage. Then the skin is incised along the caudal border of the alar cartilage. From there the alar skin is carefully undermined to the intercartilaginous incision, dissecting strictly along the contour of the cartilage. The alar cartilages can now be delivered through the incision and worked under vision while comparing each with the opposite side. Possible actions include cartilage resections, wedge or strip resections from the lateral alar cartilages, adjustment of cartilage tension by scoring or cross hatching, augmentation with autologous cartilage, and intra- or interdomal suture techniques. The approach is useful for correcting tip asymmetry and a bifid tip. Tip projection can be assessed and altered, and cephalic tip rotation can be produced. Domal suture techniques are particularly effective in candidates with a broad or boxy tip, thin skin, and scant subcutaneous fat and connective tissue. The alar cartilages themselves should be stable and elastic. Interdomal sutures are used to narrow the domes. Transdomal sutures can effectively approximate the tip defining point, usually after the removal of interdomal fat or connective tissue. In our experience both 5–0 PDS and 5–0 Prolene (undyed) can be used. Postoperative contraction of the overlying soft tissues will result in a stable tip shape after suture absorption. The knots should be placed internally, beneath the skin, and should not be placed on the cartilage surface.

Case 2

Introduction

A young woman wanted to have her nose reshaped by narrowing the nasal tip and changing the relationship of a narrow nasal pyramid, an even narrower middle vault, and the broad tip. Septal surgery 2 years earlier had already relieved nasal airway obstruction.

Findings

Internal examination revealed a straight, centered septum after previous septal surgery. Frontal view (**Fig. 14.3a**) shows a very thin middle vault, imparting an hourglass shape to the brow-tip aesthetic lines. This causes apparent thickening of the pyramid and ballooning of the tip. Profile view (**Fig. 14.3b**) shows a predominantly bony hump. Basal view (**Fig. 14.3c**) shows a boxy tip.

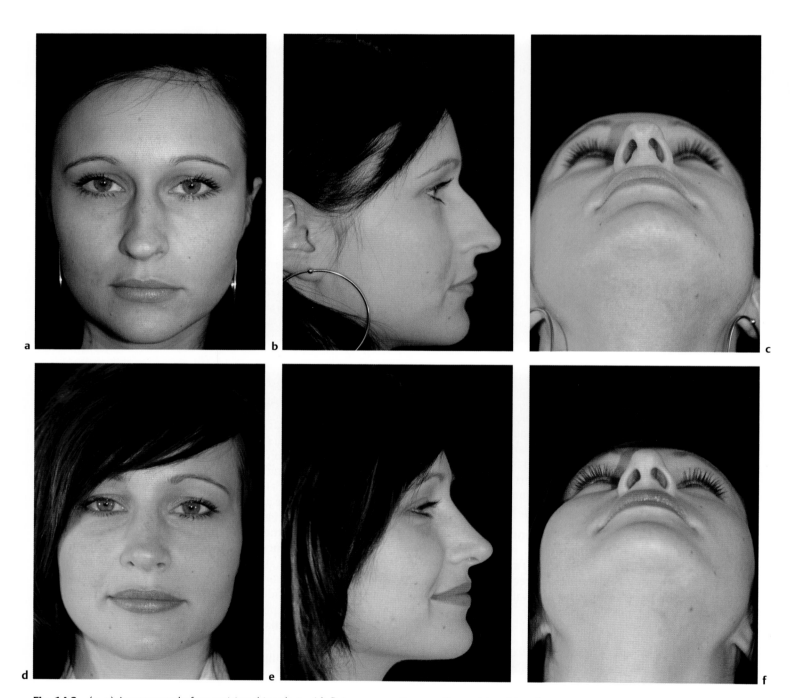

Fig. 14.3   (**a–c**) Appearance before revision rhinoplasty. (**d–f**) Appearance 2 years after revision rhinoplasty.

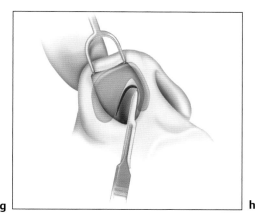
g

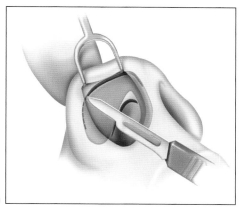
h

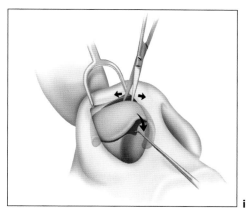
i

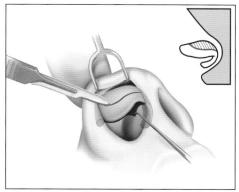
j

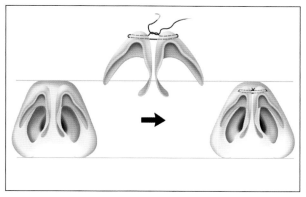
k

Fig. 14.3 (**g–j**) Delivery approach to the nasal tip using bilateral inter-cartilaginous and marginal incisions. The alar cartilage is delivered from the nose as a chondrocutaneous flap. (**g**) Intercartilaginous incision; (**h**) marginal incision; (**i, j**) exposure and delivery of the alar cartilage for cephalic volume reduction. (**k**) Transdomal sutures narrow the tip by reducing the interdomal angle and lateral flaring of the alar cartilages.

Surgical Procedure

Access was established with a posterior hemitransfixion incision and delivery approach, followed by the resection of a 3 × 10-mm cartilage strip from the septum (**Fig. 14.3g–k**). Cephalic volume reduction was performed, and a transdomal suture produced an inter- and intradomal effect on the nasal tip. 5–0 PDS mattress sutures were used. The dorsal hump was removed, followed by the endonasal placement of thin spreader grafts from the nasal septum.

Psychology, Motivation, Personal Background

The patient, who worked as a photographer, had a fine aesthetic sense and was intent on obtaining the desired aesthetic change. She had a clear motivation for the procedure. During preoperative computer simulation, the patient gained a clear understanding of the possibilities, risks, and expectations associated with the surgery.

Discussion

An open approach is unnecessary in a patient with good anatomic symmetry. The delivery approach enables the surgeon to correct the alar cartilages in any way desired. The dome area can be "weakened" by incomplete scoring or gentle crushing with a coarse, blunt Adson–Braun forceps. Volume reduction can also be obtained. The main challenge is to achieve a symmetrical suture placement (see **Fig. 14.3k**). By tightening the sutures, the surgeon can immediately assess the effect that is produced and can replace the sutures if asymmetry is noted. There is a diversity of opinion on whether absorbable or nonabsorbable sutures should be used. PDS sutures (5–0, undyed) are an acceptable compromise with a half-life greater than 100 days. Absorption is followed by stable scar fixation while the soft-tissue envelope contracts and molds to the nasal tip. The result of the delivery approach is illustrated in **Fig. 14.3d–f**.

14.4 Open Approach

The main indications for an open approach are asymmetries and deformities of the nasal tip, marked over- and underprojection, or deficient anatomic definition, which are frequent motivations for revision surgery. With a meticulous suture technique, the columellar incision will generally heal with an inconspicuous scar and should not be a factor in selecting the approach. The open approach gives excellent visibility and provides the surgeon with diagnostic information that is not available in closed approaches. Whether this visibility is necessary for the successful correction of a morphologic problem in a revision rhinoplasty will depend on the repertoire and experience of the surgeon. The technical advantages of the open approach in any given case should be weighed against the potential disadvantages, which have already been described.

The most common indications are as follows:

- Pronounced asymmetry of the nasal tip
- Marked over- or underprojection of the nasal tip
- Deformities of the nasal dorsum that require grafting
- Revisions (usually after multiple previous operations)
- Septal perforations larger than 8 mm
- Severe axial deviations
- Malformations such as cleft nose or Binder syndrome (maxillonasal dysplasia)
- Pronounced saddle nose deformities
- Nasal tumors (depending on location)

The steps involved in the open approach are illustrated in **Fig. 14.4**.

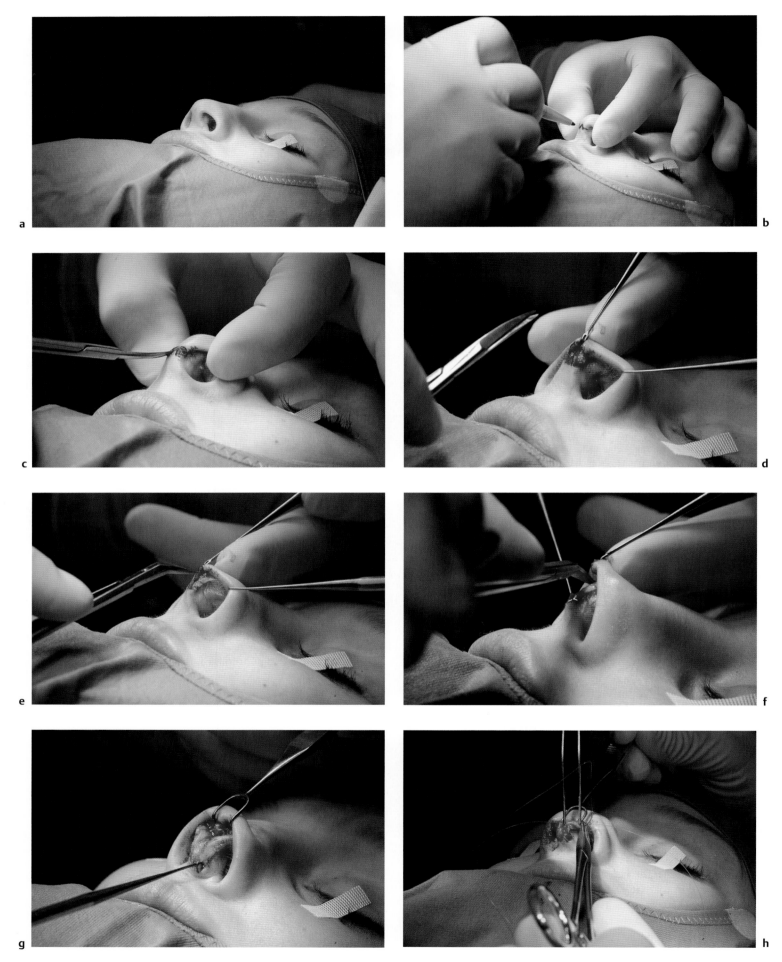

Fig. 14.4 Surgical approach. (**a**) Patient position. (**b**) The inverted-V incision line is marked at the center of the columella. (**c**) Precise incision with a no. 11 blade and further dissection with a pair of sharp, curved scissors. (**d, e**) Dissection along the medial crura of the alar cartilages. (**f**) Elevation of nasal tip soft tissues in the supraperichondrial plane. (**g**) Exposure of the alar cartilages. (**h**) The size, shape, and position of the alar cartilages are adjusted, here by means of interdomal sutures.

Case 3

Introduction

A 62-year-old woman had undergone two previous aesthetic rhinoplasties, which included septal surgery, and presented now with marked ptosis of the nasal tip caused by overresection of the anterior septal cartilage. The nasal tip showed decreased projection and protection with ptosis and deficient anterior septal cartilage (**Fig. 14.5**).

Findings

Internal examination showed a hidden columella with absence of an anterior cartilaginous septum. Frontal view (**Fig. 14.5a**) shows an inverted-V deformity, a short infratip triangle, and scar fixation of the thin skin after two previous operations. Profile view (**Fig. 14.5b**) shows a ptotic nasal tip. Basal view (**Fig. 14.5c**) shows a broad, deprojected tip.

Surgical Procedure

The septum was exposed through the very deep preexisting columellar scar. The duplicated mucosa of the anterior septum was carefully elevated, and conchal cartilage was implanted into the pocket. Tip protection was reinforced with a columellar strut. Additionally, the supratip area was augmented with an onlay graft made of conchal cartilage and connective tissue (**Fig. 14.5g**).

Psychology, Motivation, Personal Background

The patient had high aesthetic expectations of the procedure, a specific surgical goal, and a good understanding of the difficulties inherent in a third nasal operation.

Discussion

The open approach provided the best access and exposure for the definitive restoration of nasal tip protection and projection and for reconstructing the deficient anterior septum. The result is shown in **Fig. 14.5d–f**.

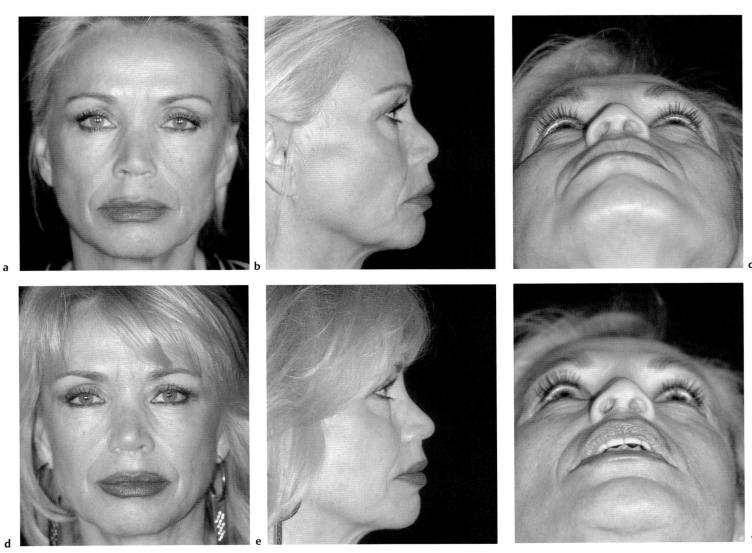

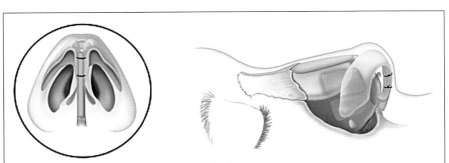

Fig. 14.5 (a–c) Appearance before revision rhinoplasty. (**d–f**) Appearance 2 years after revision rhinoplasty. (**g**) Diagram of the procedure.

Case 4

Introduction

A 17-year-old girl had undergone multiple previous operations for the repair of a cleft lip and palate. She sought now to optimize the aesthetic appearance of her nose (**Fig. 14.6**).

Findings

Frontal view (**Fig. 14.6a**) shows a broad nose at the level of the pyramid, middle vault and tip, a washed-out appearance of the bridge, and a slanted nasal base. Profile view (**Fig. 14.6b**) shows an underprojected nose with a flat profile and sharp nasolabial angle. Basal view (**Fig. 14.6c**) shows asymmetry of the nasal base and nostrils.

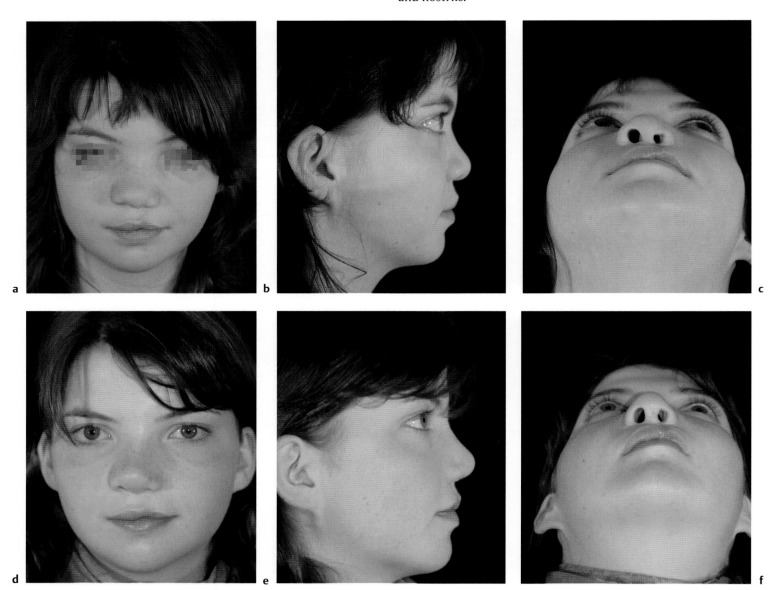

Fig. 14.6   (**a–c**) Appearance before revision rhinoplasty. (**d–f**) Appearance 2 years after revision rhinoplasty.

Surgical Procedure

The skin is incised for harvesting of rib cartilage (**Fig. 14.6g**). The perichondrium is elevated from the rib (**Fig. 14.6h**) and rib cartilage is harvested from the perichondrial sac (**Fig. 14.6i**). The graft is carved (**Fig. 14.6j**). Only a "balanced" graft taken from the central portion of the rib cartilage will retain a permanent, stable shape (**Fig. 14.6k**). Graft size is precisely determined with a Behrbohm surgical caliper (Karl Storz) (**Fig. 14.6l**). Supraperichondrial dissection of the nasal tip and dorsum is performed (**Fig. 14.6m**). A columellar pocket is developed to receive the supporting columellar strut (**Fig. 14.6n**). The columellar strut is sutured into place (**Fig. 14.6o, p**). The dorsal graft is fitted to the recipient site (**Fig. 14.6q**). The columellar strut and dorsal graft are connected to each other in "groove-and-tongue" fashion

(**Fig. 14.6r**). A tip graft is placed and attached (**Fig. 14.6s**). Skin sutures are placed (**Fig. 14.6t**). The right ala is adjusted to a lower position (**Fig. 14.6u**). Excess skin is excised, and the arch of the left nostril is formed (**Fig. 14.6v**).

Psychology, Motivation, Personal Background

The main priority was to achieve a clearly motivated aesthetic improvement of the underprojected nose.

Discussion

The open approach combined with the use of rib cartilage is usually the method of first choice for the correction of cleft nasal deformity (see also Case 52, Chapter 33). **Fig. 14.6d**, **Fig. 14.6e**, and **Fig. 14.6f** document a marked change relative to the initial findings in **Fig. 14.6a–c**.

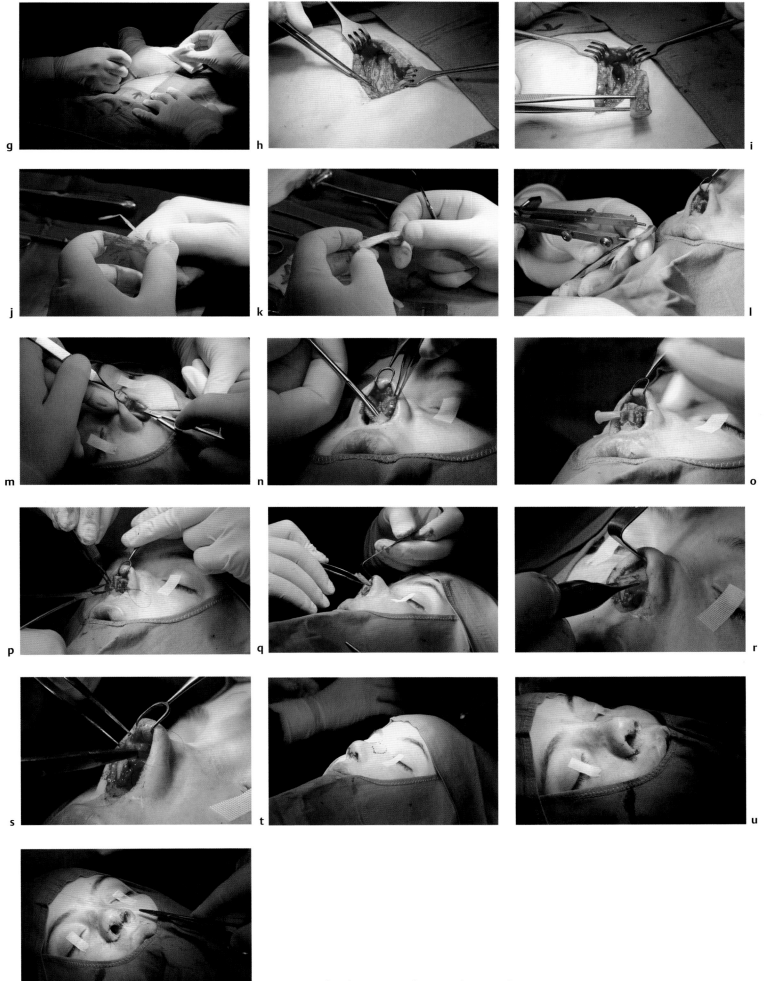

Fig. 14.6 (**g–v**) Sequence of steps in the operation.

Case 5

This case illustrates a disturbance of nasal growth following trauma and septorhinoplasty in childhood (operation by Jacqueline Eichhorn-Sens).

Introduction

The patient, a 24-year-old woman, had sustained nasal trauma in childhood and had undergone a septorhinoplasty elsewhere. She presented now with severe nasal airway obstruction and a disturbance of nasal growth.

Findings

Inspection revealed abnormal nasal growth with a saddle nose deformity and nasal deviation (**Fig. 14.7a–c**). The bony pyramid was wide and deviated. The brow-tip aesthetic lines were disharmonious. We found a droopy tip and a hidden columella. Internal examination showed a severe septal deviation with hypertrophy of both inferior turbinates.

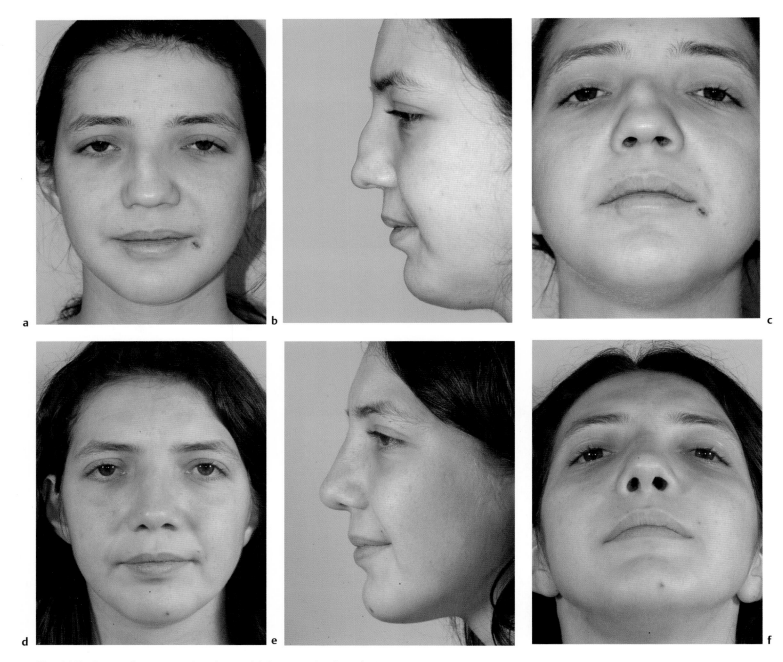

Fig. 14.7 Pre- and postoperative photos. (**a**) Preoperative frontal view shows a deviated nose with saddling of the cartilaginous dorsum and an undefined tip. (**b**) Basal view shows irregularities of the nasal dorsum, nasal deviation, and the undefined tip. (**c**) Lateral view shows a typical saddle nose deformity. The nasolabial angle is too short, and the tip is rotated downward. (**d–f**) At 1 year postoperatively the nose is straight and respiration is normal. (**d**) The nasal axis is straightened and the tip is well defined. (**e**) Basal view shows symmetrical nostrils and nasal tip with a straight columella. (**f**) Lateral view shows stable results for the dorsum and nasolabial angle.

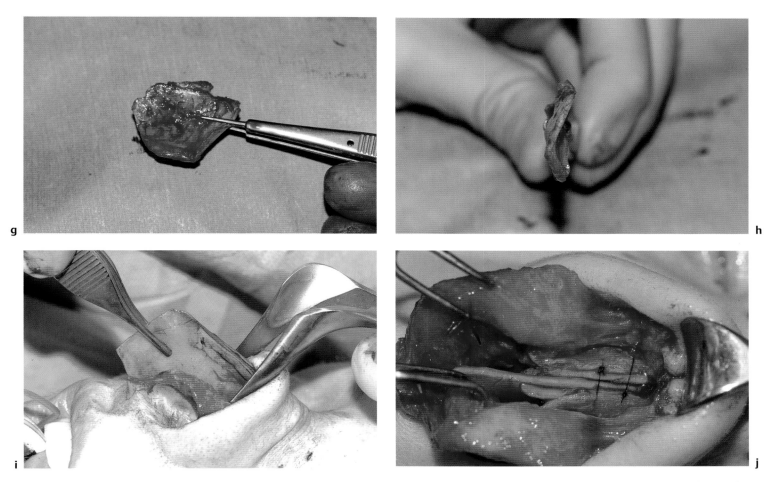

Fig. 14.7 (**g–j**) Intraoperative photos. (**g, h**) The severely deviated septum is shown. (**i**) The straightened nasal septum is repositioned. Spreader grafts are placed on the dorsal border. (**j**) The septum is suspended on the upper lateral cartilages.

Surgical Procedure

An open approach was used with a standard inverted-V mid-columellar incision. Analysis showed a severe septal deviation (**Fig. 14.7g, h**) with major loss of septal cartilage. The junction of the premaxilla and basal septum had been resected during previous surgery (growth zone). An extracorporeal septal reconstruction was performed that included the placement of bilateral spreader grafts (**Fig. 14.7i, j**). Conchal cartilage was harvested from one site. A double-layer conchal graft (sandwich graft) was placed for septal extension. A columellar strut graft was fabricated from septal cartilage and inserted.

The bony vault was straightened by lateral, transverse, and paramedian osteotomies. Submucous turbinectomy was performed on both sides. Nasal tip correction was achieved by cephalic volume reduction of the alar cartilages, dome division technique, and with transdomal sutures and a spanning suture. A one-layer fascia lata allograft was placed as an onlay graft to prevent postoperative irregularities of the nasal dorsum.

Psychology, Motivation, Personal Background

The patient had a history of childhood nasal trauma and a septorhinoplasty that had been performed elsewhere. Subsequent growth disturbance led to a typical saddle nose deformity with increasing nasal airway obstruction. The functional compromise and aesthetic deformity were both distressing for the patient. One year after revision rhinoplasty, the young woman was very satisfied with the functional and aesthetic outcome (**Fig. 14.7d–f**).

Discussion

Clinical evidence of the effects of nasal surgery in children, especially septal surgery, is still fragmentary. Verwoerd and Verwoerd-Verhoef[19] found a three-dimensional organization of the cartilaginous septum in children, noting that growth in the sphenodorsal zone of thick cartilage appears to be primarily responsible for the normal increase in the length and height of the nasal dorsum, while growth of the thickened basal rim in the sagittal plane is the driving force for the forward outgrowth of the (pre)maxillary region. The failure rate of septoplasties performed in children is ~ 20% worldwide. This failure rate may rise to 30% for septoplasties performed during the peak growth period of puberty.[20] In our practice we often see short noses and saddle nose deformities in patients who underwent nasal surgery in childhood.

References

1. Roe JO. The deformity termed "pug nose" and its correction by a simple operation. Med Rec 1887:621 (reprinted in Aesth Plast Surg 1986;10:89–91)

2. Joseph J. Intranasale Höckerabtragung. Berl Klin Wochenschr 1904;41:650

3. Behrbohm H, Tardy ME. Essentials of Septorhinoplasty. Approaches—Techniques—Philosophy. New York, NY: Thieme; 2003

4. Joseph J. Nasenplastik und sonstige Gesichtsplastik nebst einem Anhang über Mammaplastik. Leipzig, Germany: C Kabitzsch; 1931

5. Natvig P. Jacques Joseph–Surgical Sculptor. Philadelphia, PA: WB Saunders; 1982

6. Rethi A. Über die korrektiven Operationen der Nasendeformitäten. Chirurg 1929;1:1103

7. Padovan IF. External approach to rhinoplasty (decortication). Symp Otol Rhinol Laryngol Jug 1966;4:345–360

8. Tardy ME. Rhinoplasty: The Art and the Science. Philadelphia, PA: WB Saunders; 1997

9. Simons RL. A personal report: emphasizing the endonasal approach. Facial Plast Surg Clin North Am 2004;12(1):15–34

10. Gruber RP, Friedman GD. Suture algorithm for the broad or bulbous nasal tip. Plast Reconstr Surg 2002;110(7):1752–1764, discussion 1765–1768

11. Johnson CM, Toriumi DM. Open Structure Rhinoplasty. Philadelphia, PA: WB Saunders; 1990

12. Dayan S, Kanodia R. Has the pendulum swung too far?: trends in the teaching of endonasal rhinoplasty. Arch Facial Plast Surg 2009;11(6):414–416

13. Adamson PA, Galli SK. Rhinoplasty approaches: current state of the art. Arch Facial Plast Surg 2005;7(1):32–37

14. Berghaus A. Rhinoplastik: Offene oder geschlossene Technik? HNO 2010;58(9):878–881

15. Foda HM. External rhinoplasty: a critical analysis of 500 cases. J Laryngol Otol 2003;117(6):473–477

16. Fritz K. "Open approach"—der "Fortschritt" zurück an den Beginn der Septorhinoplastik. HNO 2000;48(8):562–567

17. Rohrich RJ, Muzaffar A. A Plastic Surgeon's Perspective. Course Manual Rhinoplasty. Chicago; 2001:491–524

18. Schultz-Coulon HJ. Three-layer repair of nasoseptal defects. Otolaryngol Head Neck Surg 2005;132(2):213–218

19. Verwoerd CDA, Verwoerd-Verhoef HL. Rhinosurgery in children: basic concepts. Facial Plast Surg 2007;23(4):219–230

20. Pirsig W. Rhinoplasty and the airway in children. Facial Plast Surg 1986;3:225–241

15 Revision Septoplasty

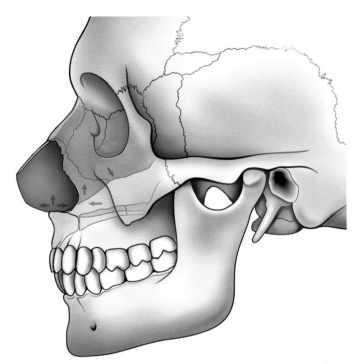

Fig. 15.1 Anatomy of the medial nasal wall. Blue, light blue: quadrangular cartilage; yellow: vomer; purple: perpendicular plate. The arrows represent the vectors of the most common "tectonic shifts."

The nasal septum is part of the medial nasal wall. It is composed anatomically of various bony and cartilaginous structures: the perpendicular plate of the ethmoid bone, the vomer, the posterior nasal spine, the transverse palatine suture, the maxilla with the anterior nasal spine, the incisive bone, the caudal rim of the anterior piriform aperture, and the quadrangular cartilage. It is common for these elements to move and shift relative to one another during cranial growth. Multiple components are always involved in bowing of the medial nasal wall.[1] The septal cartilage functions as a kind of "crumple zone" for absorbing unphysiologic stresses (**Fig. 15.1**).

Septal deviation may occur during periods of special "tectonic unrest" in cranial growth (e.g., during puberty) or may result from trauma relating to nasal, septal, or midfacial fractures. Postoperative septal deviation may develop because the original surgeon ignored this problem during the primary rhinoplasty, or may result from inadequate fixation, scar traction, or incomplete relaxation of the cartilage. Besides bowing, the septum may also be too long or too high for the nasal cavity in certain of its dimensions, resulting in septal subluxation or a tension septum. The nasal septum is attached to the bony nasal pyramid in the keystone area. It also has firm attachments to the upper lateral cartilages and alar cartilages. The septal cartilage and upper lateral cartilages form an anatomic unit. The cartilaginous septum joins with the anterior edge of the upper lateral cartilages to form the "internal nasal valve," which is the narrowest part of the nasal airway.

The nasal septum is important in revision septorhinoplasties for several reasons:

- Its functional importance for nasal breathing
- Its function as a "pillar" to support the nasal dorsum
- Its role in shaping the nasal tip (tip support mechanism)
- Its role in maintaining the position of the nasal tip
- The attachment of the cartilaginous septum to the midface in the keystone area
- Its involvement in axial deviations and crooked noses

15.1 Functional Importance of the Nasal Septum

15.1.1 Functional Importance for Nasal Breathing in Revision Surgery

Since ~ 20 to 30% of patients complain of impaired nasal breathing or dry membranes after functional rhinoplastic surgery, the concept of septal surgery should be continually reviewed.[2] What should functional surgery look like? A curved septum in itself will not necessarily cause breathing problems. The goal of septal surgery should be a centrally positioned septum that divides the vestibule and nasal cavity into two airways of approximately equal size.

15.1.2 Supportive Function

Slight bowing, especially in the thin, fragile cartilage of the nasal septum, may generate intrinsic forces that contribute significantly to the overall supportive function of the cartilaginous nose.[3] If the cartilage is weakened at one site or a gentle curve is straightened, this may cause the cartilage to give way and produce dorsal saddling. The mechanical strength of the septal cartilage may be evident preoperatively and can be assessed by internal and external palpation, but often its supportive properties can be fully appreciated only during the operation.

15.1.3 Shape and Position of the Nasal Tip

The tip support mechanisms critically influence the shape and position of the nasal tip. For example, the attachment of the medial crural footplates to the anterior edge of the caudal septum significantly affects the projection and protection of the nasal tip and the configuration of the three septal angles. The rhinosurgeon should understand the various ways in which the projection, shape, position, and rotation of the nasal tip can be modified by septal surgery.[4–7] The major and minor tip support mechanisms described by Tardy are still of crucial importance and are outlined below.[7]

Major tip support:

- Size, shape, thickness, and resilience of the alar cartilages
- Attachment of the upper lateral cartilages to the cephalic margin of the alar cartilages

■ Wrap-around attachment of the medial crural footplates to the caudal septum

Minor tip support (may contribute major support in some anatomic variants):

■ Anterior septal angle

■ Skin of the nasal tip

■ Membranous septum

■ Caudal septum

■ Nasal spine

■ Ligamentous sling spanning the paired domes of the alar cartilages

■ Sesamoid cartilage complex extending the support of the lateral crura to the piriform margin

The area of the rhinion is rightly called the keystone area because, like the architectural keystone in a gothic arch, it supports the entire nasal dome and attaches it to the piriform aperture. If that attachment is released and is not repaired, an inverted-V deformity will result due to separation of the cartilaginous nose from the piriform aperture.

15.1.4 Axial Deviations and the Crooked Nose

Gustave Aufricht summarized the role of the nasal septum by noting that "Where the septum goes, there goes the nose." While it is true that a septoplasty cannot correct all deformities, nothing can be accomplished without it. This applies equally to the functional tension nose, the reconstruction of saddle deformities, and the correction of a cartilaginous crooked nose. In all these cases, the selective release of tension or a stable reconstruction of the septum is the key to a successful outcome.

15.1.5 The Vomeronasal Organ—the Seventh Sense?

The term "pheromones" was coined by A. Butenandt for molecules that are produced by a species and evoke certain reactions in animals of that species. The vomeronasal organ (Jacobson's organ) is essential for the social and mating behaviors of all mammals.[8] Many observations and studies have shown that pheromones also transmit signals in humans.

The vomeronasal organ has been identified as a pair of tiny, blind-terminating canals located in the anterior nasal septum. Morphologic findings suggest that the vomeronasal organ consists of functioning sensory epithelium (**Fig. 15.2**). Further studies are needed to identify its central projections to the hypothalamus and determine its functional importance.

15.2 Brief History of Septoplasty

In 1867, Leinhardt described the first submucous resections of the nasal septum for correction of the anterior septum. Hartmann and Petersen expanded the method, also applying it to deviations of the posterior septum.[9,10] Gustav Killian (1860–1920) injected a cocaine–epinephrine solution beneath the two mucosal layers to separate the mucosa from the cartilage on both sides and developed the technique of the submucous septal resection.[11] The overresection of healthy cartilage from the anterior septum led to late complications such as depression of the cartilaginous nasal dorsum and retraction of the columella, with the functional and aesthetic problems of a saddle nose and hidden columella. Mucosal lesions related to the overresection or poor vascularity of the scarred mucosal layers predisposed patients to perforations. As an alternative to the Killian resection, therefore, Maurice Cottle (1896–1981) introduced his cartilage-conserving technique, which was better able to preserve the supportive function of the septal cartilage.[12] In modern parlance the Cottle septoplasty is considered to be synonymous with cartilage-conserving septal surgery. Today the classic "maxilla–premaxilla approach for extensive septal surgery" no longer has this connotation and is no longer practiced in the classic manner. Some authors advocate a conservative approach while others report good results with an extracorporeal septoplasty in which the septum is removed from the nose, straightened externally, and reimplanted.

15.3 Preoperative and Intraoperative Analysis

A functional and morphologic analysis provides an important basis for developing an individual surgical plan.[6,7,13,14] Special rules apply to surgery of the pediatric nasal septum (see Chapter 6, Section 6.1).[15] It is important in revision surgery to evaluate the extent of cartilage defects, residual or recurrent deviations, and scarring and hydration of the mucosa. Because deviations are so varied in their morphology and relevance, a variety of surgical techniques should be available. There is no such thing as a standard septal operation. The less traumatizing the procedure, the fewer problems will arise in wound healing. For this reason, the reorientation and trimming of deviated segments should always be considered as an initial option before proceeding with an external septoplasty.

15.4 Swinging-Door and Swinging Double-Door Techniques

Mobilizing the septal cartilage in a swinging-door fashion after a horizontal and vertical chondrotomy is the standard technique for the correction of anterior deviations. Mucosal tunnels are developed, and the anterior nasal spine is exposed. The quadrangular cartilage is then released from the bony nasal floor, perpendicular plate, and vomer by vertical and horizontal incisions (**Fig. 15.3**).

Often the septum can be straightened in this approach by resecting slivers of cartilage to achieve shortening and relaxation and by the removal of ridges and spurs. It should be noted that permanently straightening a deviated cartilage by making scoring incisions on the concave side is rarely successful in revision settings. Preexisting and new scar contractures tend to redeflect the cartilage toward the deviated side. Transseptal mattress sutures can be placed to counteract this tendency during postoperative healing. Scoring also weakens the biostatic properties of the cartilage and compromises its mechanical stability.

Fig. 15.4 shows the main intraoperative details for a septal correction through a hemitransfixion incision, which is perhaps the most widely used rhinosurgical approach in general.

Vertical division of the deviated cartilage at the apex of the curve is an effective technique that yields good long-term results. It allows the fragmented cartilage to be repositioned in the midline without tension. The swinging-door technique is suitable for this procedure.

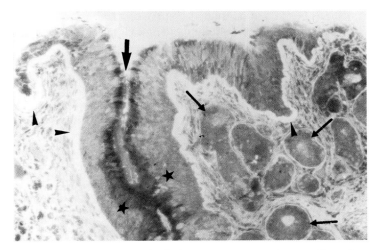

Fig. 15.2 Photomicrograph of a human vomeronasal organ. The orifice (*large arrow*) opens into a duct lined by a thickening epithelium (*). The superficial epithelium is backed by a thick basement membrane (*arrowheads*), which becomes thinner at deeper levels. *Small arrows:* convoluted glandular fragments. (Figure courtesy of Prof. Dr. V. Jahnke, Berlin.)

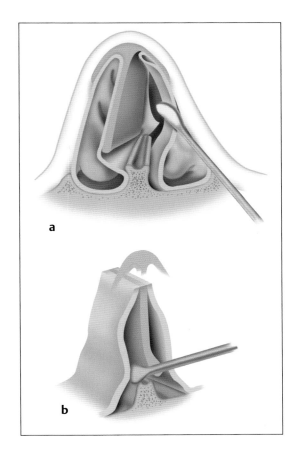

Fig. 15.3 (**a**) Principle of the swinging-door technique in a submucous septoplasty. The right mucosal flap remains attached to the septal cartilage, here in the area of the middle and posterior septum. (**b**) In a revision septoplasty, it may be best to separate the entire mucoperichondrium from the septal cartilage. The figure shows the anterior half of the "double door."

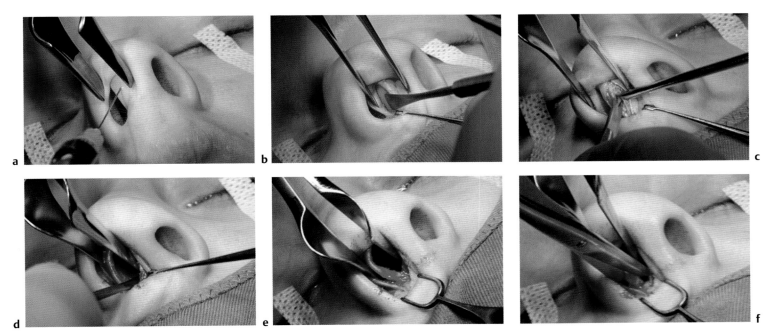

Fig. 15.4 Details of surgical dissection in a septoplasty. (**a**) Hydrodissection of the mucoperichondrium accounts for almost half the operation. Targeted fluid injection already separates the mucosa from the cartilage. (**b**) The surgical plane between the mucoperichondrium and septal cartilage can be identified by the bluish-gray color of the cartilage. (**c**) Connective tissue fibers on the floor of the inferior tunnel are sharply divided. (**d**) The anterior septal border and "septal table" are exposed. (**e**) An inferior tunnel is developed. (**f**) The basal septum is shortened.

15.5 Dynamics of Septoplasty

The principle of the step-by-step rhinoplasty technique described by M. E. Tardy applies equally well to septoplasty. After each step, the surgeon pauses to assess the effect that the step has produced and its implications for the next step.[7] In the revision of a previously operated crooked nose deformity, it may be necessary to detach the upper lateral cartilage from the septal cartilage, shorten it on one side if needed, and reattach it to the septum or neoseptum, with or without the placement of spreader grafts. The surgeon can also judge whether symmetry of the external nose can be achieved by correction of the septum and upper lateral cartilages alone, or whether perichondrium or fascia should also be added to camouflage slight residual asymmetries. Spreader grafts are excellent for straightening a deviated, previously operated septum. They are placed parallel to the dorsal border of the septum on one or both sides.

15.6 Cartilage Grafts

The replacement of missing septal cartilage is of major importance in revision septoplasties. Different cartilage tissues vary markedly in their mechanical stability and resilience. Auricular cartilage is more prone to rapid fraying. Septal cartilage should never be crushed because this creates a pulped material that has unpredictable properties during wound healing and will usually undergo complete or partial resorption. Controlled compression of the cartilage with a squeezer (Karl Storz) can selectively modify the cartilage alignment. This technique is particularly effective on septal cartilage. The quality of cartilage grafts can be ranked as follows: septal cartilage (first choice), conchal cartilage (second choice), and rib cartilage (third choice).

15.7 Cartilage Transfers

Cartilage transfers are suitable in patients with severe anterior septal deformities, cartilage defects, lack of nasal tip protection, or saddling of the supratip area, usually after trauma, prior surgery, or rhinitis sicca. Access is gained through a hemitransfixion incision. The mucoperichondrium is completely elevated by developing superior and inferior tunnels to expose the septal cartilage, bony vomer, and perpendicular plate. Ideally the anterior cartilage is replaced with portions of the posterior septal cartilage. If there is not enough posterior septal cartilage available, autologous cartilage can be harvested from the conchal bowl or tragus, or, less commonly, from a rib.

15.8 Splinted Septal Reconstruction

Bönisch described a mosaic-like reconstruction of the nasal septum in which the individual fragments are aligned and stabilized by suturing to a PDS Flexible Plate (MentorWorldwide LLC, Santa Barbara, CA).[16] This technique has yielded good results. The use of a thin plate avoids having to place too much absorbable material into the nose during the septoplasty.

15.9 Extracorporeal Septal Reconstruction
Jacqueline Eichhorn-Sens

A key issue in secondary rhinoplasties is whether or not the septum has residual deformity. Does at least a straight L-shaped framework exist, or is the outer framework deformed? Is the anterior part of the septum deviated or absent?

A straight septal framework is a prerequisite for a straight nose and physiologic nasal breathing. Standard septoplasty techniques are often unsuccessful on severely deviated septal cartilages, and in such cases a straight septal framework can be obtained only by an extracorporeal septal reconstruction (**Fig. 15.6**).

If the anterior septal border has been resected, possible effects are drooping of the tip, a pseudohump deformity, or an acute nasolabial angle (**Fig. 15.7**). As an alternative to the techniques described in the preceding chapters, the whole septum can be removed to reconstruct a straight framework and then reimplanted in a more anterior position so that the anterior septum is also restored.

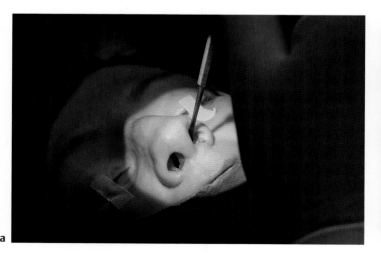
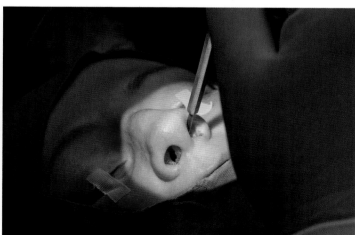

a   b

Fig. 15.5 (**a, b**) The "Freer test" at the end of the septoplasty confirms successful elimination of all morphologic obstructions

The extracorporeal septoplasty or extracorporeal septal reconstruction as described by Wolfgang Gubisch provides an option for correcting these difficult cases.[17] The reconstruction of a straight septum requires removing the whole septum in one piece, meaning that both the cartilaginous and bony part of the septum are harvested.

15.9.1 Operative Technique

In extracorporeal septal reconstructions we always use an open approach with a standard inverted-V midcolumellar incision. Before separating the upper lateral cartilages from the septum, we do an extramucosal dissection at the junction of the dorsal septal border and upper lateral cartilages so that an intact mucosal wall can be preserved.

On reaching the subperichondrial plane, both superior tunnels are dissected to the junction of the premaxilla and vomerine groove. Then the inferior tunnels are developed. When dissection of the superior and inferior tunnels is completed, they are interconnected by cutting the adhesive fibers between them. The complete cartilaginous and bony septum is then removed in one piece.

The required lengths of the septal dorsum and anterior border are measured. The next step is to reconstruct a straight septal plate (**Fig. 15.6e, f**) or at least a straight L-shaped strut of the necessary dimensions. First, all irregularities are smoothed out, particularly addressing the thickened junction of the bony and cartilaginous septum. Irregularities in the bony part are best thinned with a cylindrical bur. All spurs and deformities are removed.

It may be possible to straighten the deviated cartilaginous septum by scoring. To prevent recurrence, another straight cartilage strip or a thinned, perforated piece of bony septum should be fixed to the scarified cartilage to straighten it permanently (**Fig. 15.8**). Sometimes the straightened portion can be stabilized with quilting sutures. Another option is to suture a curved cartilage graft to the convex side of the remaining septum, enabling the curve to act as a "counterspring" to prevent redeviation.[18]

In some cases the straight portions of the septum can be rotated to obtain a residual septum that is intrinsically straight and can provide the dimensions necessary for a successful reconstruction.

Reconstruction is more difficult in cases with multiple fracture sites and cartilage fragments that have healed in a dislocated position. One solution is to create a neoseptum by cutting out small, straight pieces of cartilage, assembling them like a jigsaw puzzle, and suturing them to a thinned perpendicular plate or PDS Flexible Plate to construct a template for suturing and stabilizing the cartilage fragments. Fixation can be aided by drilling holes in the perpendicular plate (**Fig. 15.7**). Later the septum is stabilized by placing multiple mattress sutures through the septal mucosa, passing them blindly through the holes. The holes also provide sites for connective tissue ingrowth that will further enhance stability.

If a PDS plate is used for septal reconstruction, it is important to avoid tearing of the mucosa. Otherwise there will be a substantial risk of septal necrosis and perforation.[19]

The use of spreader grafts or extended spreader grafts is recommended in every septal reconstruction.[20] They are fixed to the dorsum of the reconstructed septum to restore the integrity of the internal nasal valves, restore the dorsal aesthetic lines, and augment the stability of the septal framework.[20]

Once a straight neoseptum of the necessary size has been created, stable fixation of the reimplanted septum is essential for a good aesthetic and functional outcome. Two fixation points are needed to eliminate the risk of graft slippage,[17] so the septum should be fixed to the anterior spine and to the upper lateral cartilages. If the upper lateral cartilages are too short, the reconstructed septum can be fixed to the nasal bone.

In patients with short nasal bones and long upper lateral cartilages, the neoseptum can be attached to the upper lateral cartilages with multiple back-and-forth sutures. In the opposite case, where the nasal bones are long and the upper lateral cartilages are short, holes should be drilled into the nasal bones to fix the reimplanted septum to the bones and securely bridge the keystone area. The neoseptum is also fixed to the anterior spine with multiple sutures passed through a hole drilled with a Lindemann bur to eliminate the risk of slippage. Fixation to the periosteum alone is not secure enough.

Before fixing the neoseptum to the anterior spine, check to make sure that the spine is precisely on the midline. If the spine is very wide and is only minimally displaced from the midline, bone can be removed from one side of the spine to establish an overall centered position. A hole is then drilled through the anterior spine, the length of the anterior septum is tailored as needed, and the anterior septum is approximated and fixed to the bone.

If the anterior spine has been displaced from the midline by more than 3–4 mm, the spine must be fractured and recentered. The spine can be detached with a Lindemann bur, which should cut through both the spine and the premaxilla. The whole structure is then returned to the midline and secured there with a microplate and microscrew.

If there is insufficient septal cartilage remaining, especially in cases where extensive cartilage was removed in a previous operation, the bony portions of the septum can be used along with conchal or rib cartilage to construct a straight columellar strut and/or a straight L-shaped septum. Thin Medpor (Stryker Craniomaxillofacial, Kalamazoo, MI) sheets can also be used in rare cases.

If bony portions of the septum must be used, the bone is ground very thin with a cylindrical bur. The bone should also be perforated with multiple drill holes for the reasons noted above. Anteriorly, an auricular sandwich graft is placed as a columellar strut to provide support without creating a stiff columella (**Fig. 15.7**).

In multiple revision cases, often there is not enough straight cartilaginous or bony material left to construct an L-shaped framework. The first option to consider in these cases is to harvest conchal cartilage, usually from both ears, and use it to create a double-layer L-shaped sandwich graft[20] for constructing a straight anterior septal border. The sandwich graft will be fixed to the anterior spine, and the graft should additionally be fixed to the dorsal frame of the septum to create a more stable construct.

Following the septal reconstruction, transseptal mattress sutures and intranasal septal silicone splints are placed to protect the surgical result. The splints remain in place for 2 weeks. A nasal cast is applied and remains in place for a total of 2 weeks.

The functional and aesthetic outcome of an extracorporeal septoplasty is permanent and can be accurately predicted. In a retrospective study of 2,301 patients who had an extracorporeal septoplasty between 1981 and 2004 with a 1- to 6-year follow-up in 404 patients, Gubisch found that the septum was straight and centered in 92% of the patients, and 96% rated their nasal breathing as good or excellent.[17]

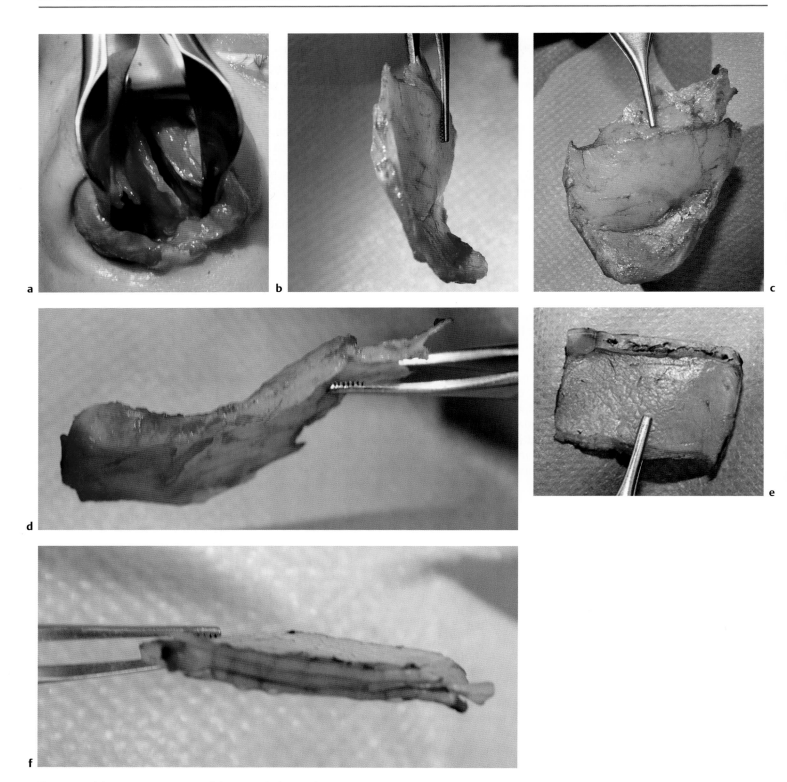

Fig. 15.6 (**a**) Intraoperative view of the severely deviated septum in situ. (**b–d**) The septum is removed from the nose in one piece. It is severely deviated in all dimensions, so there is no point in trying to correct it in an endonasal position. (**e, f**) A straight new septum with the necessary dimensions has been constructed. The spreader grafts have already been placed.

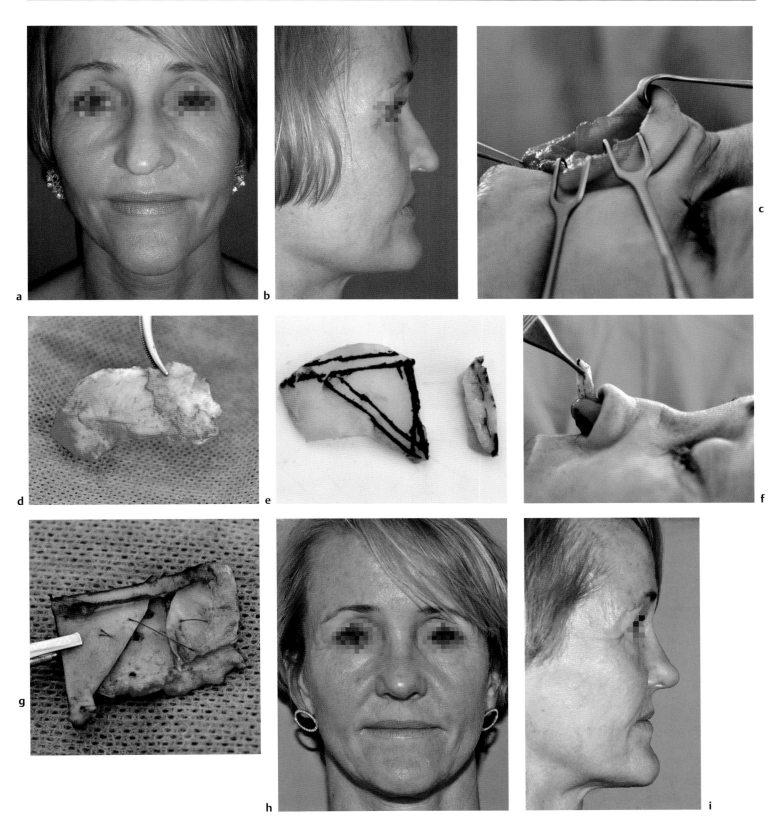

Fig. 15.7 (**a, b**) After a previous operation elsewhere, the patient still suffered from functional problems. The remaining septum was still grossly deviated, resulting in a crooked nose. Additionally, the anterior septal border had been removed in the previous operation, resulting in a retracted columella, a drooping nasal tip, and a long nose. (**c**) Intraoperative view shows absence of the anterior septal border due to overresection in the previous operation. (**d**) The remaining septum was removed in one piece. It was still deviated and contained many scars.

(**e**) Graft planning. Conchal cartilage was also harvested to fashion a straight, double-layer sandwich graft. (**f**) The conchal double-layer graft was used to reconstruct the anterior septal border. (**g**) The remaining straight pieces of septal cartilage were fixed to a thinned perpendicular plate with nonabsorbable sutures. (**h, i**) Eight months later the patient is free of functional complaints. The nasal axis is straight, and the nasolabial angle, nasal length, and tip projection and protection are improved.

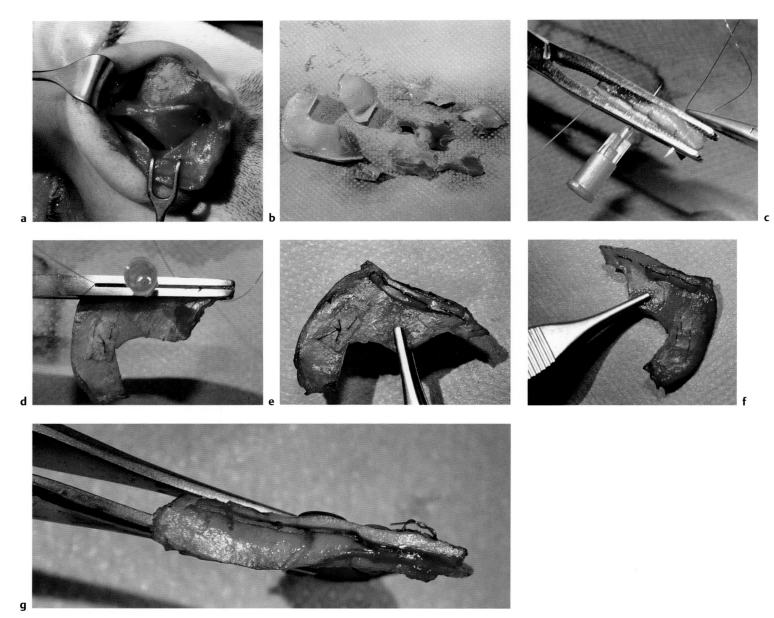

Fig. 15.8 (a) Intraoperative view shows the severely deformed septum in situ following trauma and previous surgery. (b) These are all the remaining pieces of the septum. (c, d) The Aiach–Gubisch clamp helps in fixing the spreader grafts to the dorsal side of the new septum. (e, f) The cartilage was badly deformed, so this part had to be additionally straightened by fixing a thinned, straight piece of septal bone to the cartilage. The new septum is constructed as a stable, straight L-shaped framework of the necessary dimensions. (g) There was not enough septal cartilage left to make a second whole spreader graft, but the missing part could be replaced by the "natural" kinking of the new septum.

The extracorporeal septoplasty is an important technique for correcting the difficult septum after previous surgery in cases where the remaining framework is still deviated and/or large portions of the septum have been harvested. All rhinosurgeons should therefore become proficient in this technique.

15.10 Endoscopic Surgery of the Medial Nasal Wall

Endoscopic septoplasty was initially performed only as an adjunct to endoscopic surgery of the paranasal sinuses (**Fig. 15.9**).[1]

The main indications for endoscopic septoplasty are:

- Obstruction of the middle meatus by a high deviated septum

- Submucous exposure and removal of the posterior septal cartilage along with portions of the perpendicular plate. External straightening by cross-hatching, careful morselization, or cartilage scoring

- Cartilage reimplantation

- Straightened nasal septum with decompression of the middle meatus

The tremendous advantages of endoscopy in the intraoperative visualization and analysis of findings and dissections have made it an operating technique of the future.[21] The application of video technology has opened up whole new worlds of microsurgery tailored to individual findings (**Fig. 14.6**).

The approaches shown in **Fig. 15.11** may be used alone or may be combined with the familiar hemitransfixion incision (**Fig. 15.10a–d**).[22]

15.10.1 Posterior Endoscopic Hemitransfixion Incision and Intercartilaginous Incision

The mucoperichondrium is elevated on both sides of the cartilage, perpendicular plate, and vomer with special dissectors (e.g., Behrbohm) or a Freer elevator. The mucosa is much easier to undermine on the posterior septum than anteriorly. Note: Mucosal

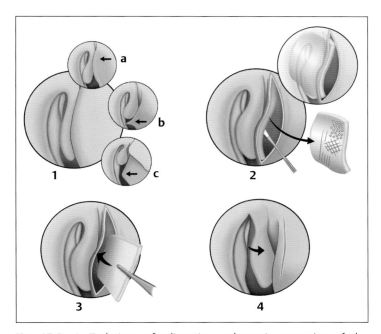

Fig. 15.9 1, Technique of adjunctive endoscopic correction of the posterior nasal septum. (**a**) Posterior deviation. (**b**) Vomer spur. (**c**) Vomer ridge. 2, Removal of the deviated posterior septum, external straightening by cross hatching, morselization or incomplete cartilage incisions. 3, Reimplantation of the cartilage. 4, Straightening of the septum with the decompression of the middle turbinate.

perforations at this stage should be scrupulously repaired. There is a considerable risk of posterior perforations, which can be avoided only by a meticulous operating technique preceded by careful hydrodissection. Deviated portions of the cartilaginous and bony septum are excised basally and dorsally with septal scissors. The excised tissue is deburred, straightened with a cartilage crusher, and reimplanted. The mucosa must be precisely approximated. The septum should be approached anterior to a septal tubercle, if present. A small blood vessel is often encountered in the upper part of the incision and may cause significant epistaxis in the days after the surgery. The bleeding should be controlled by electrocautery. The intercartilaginous incision provides wide exposure of the entire septal cartilage.

15.10.2 Hemitransfixion Incision and Endoscopic Dissection

Endoscopic dissection via a hemitransfixion incision offers several advantages:

- Precise analysis of the pathogenesis and morphology of a deviation
- Optically guided dissection at each stage of the procedure
- Better visibility in the posterior mucosal tunnels
- Minimal surgical trauma
- Magnification effect with a constant depth of focus
- Endoscopic dissection technique

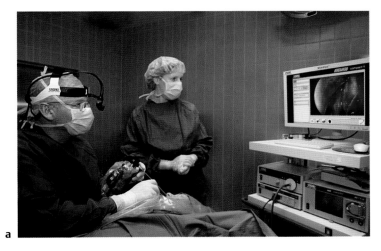

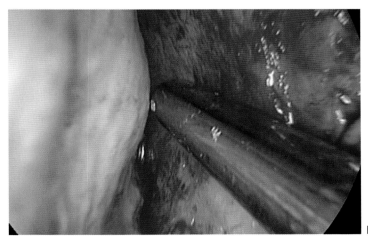

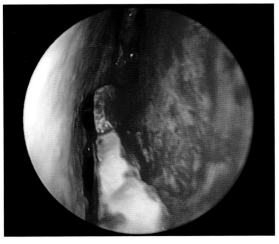

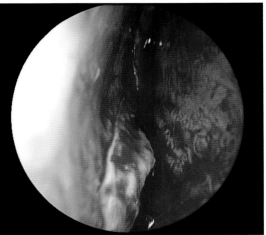

Fig. 15.10 Endoscopic septoplasty. (**a**) Operating room setup with video tower. (**b**) Endoscopic dissection of a superior tunnel. (**c, d**) Removal of a basal ridge.

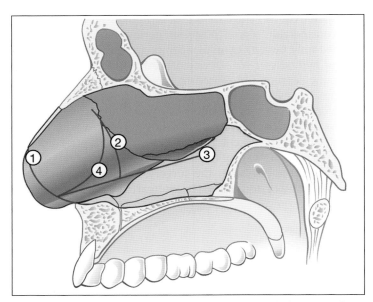

Fig. 15.11 Approaches for endoscopic septal surgery: 1, hemitransfixion incision; 2, posterior hemitransfixion incision; 3, horizontal incision; 4, intercartilaginous incision.

References

1. Behrbohm H. Septal surgery with functional and aesthetic goals. In: Behrbohm H, Tardy ME, eds. Essentials of Septorhinoplasty. New York, NY: Thieme; 2003:9–11

2. Mlynski G. Impaired function of the upper respiratory tract. Restorative procedures for upper airway dysfunction, nasal breathing [in German]. Laryngorhinootologie 2005;84(Suppl 1):S101–S117

3. Hildebrandt T. Principles of modern septoplasty. In: Behrbohm H, Tardy ME, eds. Essentials of Septorhinoplasty. New York, NY: Thieme; 2003:108–115

4. Heppt W, Gubisch W. Septal surgery in rhinoplasty. Facial Plast Surg 2011;27(2):167–178

5. Hildebrandt T, Behrbohm H. The influence of the septum on the aesthetics of the nasal tip. Mediaservice 2000. Interactive CD, KS 533

6. Mattias C. Surgery of the nasal septum and turbinates. GMS Curr Top Otorhinolaryngol Head Neck Surg 2007;6:Doc10. Epub 2008 Mar 14

7. Tardy ME. Rhinoplasty. The Art and the Science. 2 vols. Philadelphia, PA: WB Saunders; 1997

8. Behrbohm H, Kaschke O. Pathophysiologie, Differentialdiagnostik und Therapie von Störungen des Geruchsinns. 5 Weissensee HNO Fortbildung. HNO aktuell 1999;7:21–27

9. Hartmann A. Partielle Resektion der Nasenscheidewand bei hochgradiger Verkrümmung derselben. Dtsch Med Wochenschr 1882;8:691–692

10. Petersen F. Über subperichondrale Resektion der knorpeligen Nasenscheidewand. Berl Klin Wschr 1883;20:329–330

11. Killian G. Die submuköse Fensterresektion der Nasenscheidewand. Arch Laryngo Rhinol (Berl) 1904;16:362–387

12. Cottle MH, Loring RM, Fischer GG, Gaynon IE. The maxilla-premaxilla approach to extensive nasal septum surgery. AMA Arch Otolaryngol 1958;68(3):301–313

13. Baumann I. [Septoplasty update]. Laryngorhinootologie 2010;89(6):373–384

14. Keefe MA, Cupp CL. The septum in rhinoplasty. Otolaryngol Clin North Am 1999;32(1):15–36

15. Schultz-Coulon H-J. Die Korrektur ausgeprägter Deformitäten des ventro-kaudalen Septumabschnitts beim Kind. HNO 1983;31(1):6–9

16. Bönisch M, Mink A. Heilungsprozess des Knorpels in Verbindung mit PDS-Folie. HNO 2000;48(10):743–746

17. Gubisch W. Twenty-five years experience with extracorporeal septoplasty. Facial Plast Surg 2006;22(4):230–239

18. Gorney M. The septum in rhinoplasty: "form follows function". In: Gruber RP, Peck GC, eds. Rhinoplasty. State of the Art. St. Louis, MO: Mosby-Year Book; 1993:301–313

19. Fuchshuber GF. Komplikationen bei der Nasenseptumrekonstruktion mit Polydioxanfolie [inaugural dissertation]. Heidelberg, Germany: Ruprecht-Karls-Universität; 2003

20. Eichhorn-Sens J, Gubisch W. Sekundäre Rhinoplastik. In: von Heimburg D, Lemperle G, eds. Ästhetische Chirurgie. Heidelberg, Germany: ecomed Medizin; 2010

21. Wormald P-J. Endoscopic Sinus Surgery. Anatomy, Three-Dimensional Reconstruction, and Surgical Technique. Endoscopic Septoplasty. New York, NY: Thieme; 2007:23–26

22. Behrbohm H, Birke H, Dalchow C. Von der Septumplastik zur "swinging-double-door"-Technik. HNO-Nachrichten 2009;2:32–37

16 Complexity of Events

The nose is a complex of anatomic structural elements invested by a fibroaponeurotic sheath (the superficial musculoaponeurotic system, SMAS), which binds the elements together and maintains a tension that is important for function and aesthetics. Our case report of a primary and revision septoplasty will illustrate the potentially complex effects of nasal surgery that divides the fibrous attachments between the structural elements of the nasal tip without altering the tip shape itself. Shortening the anterior septum can lead to a loss of nasal tip projection with lateral flaring of the alar cartilages.[1] Weakening or dividing the fibrous attachments between the domes of the alar cartilages leads to a generalized loss of tension in the tip and supratip area. This

is true despite histologic studies showing that a long-postulated interdomal ligament per se does not exist. The framework of the nasal tip, normally held in tension by the soft-tissue envelope of connective tissue, subcutaneous tissue, and skin, may lose its shape in an unpredictable way. The results are lateral flaring of the alar cartilages, depression of the supratip area, and drooping of the nasal tip with cephalic or caudal rotation.

The case report also illustrates the reconstructive steps that are always necessary when this system is destabilized by approaches such as hemitransfixion incisions, the creation of large columellar pockets, nasal tip approaches, etc.[2]

Case 1

Introduction

A 40-year-old woman underwent septoplasty and noticed a marked, complex change in the appearance of her nose just a few weeks after the operation. She desired a prompt restoration of the old shape, especially with regard to straightening and narrowing of the tip and the correction of dorsal saddling.

Findings

Frontal view (**Fig. 16.1a**) shows a cartilaginous broad nose and nasal tip asymmetry, which creates the impression of a crooked nose deviated to the right. Profile view (**Fig. 16.1b**) shows saddling of the supratip area. Basal view (**Fig. 16.1c**) shows that the supratip saddling does not affect the shape of the nasal tip viewed from below. **Fig. 16.1d**, **Fig. 16.1e**, and **Fig. 16.1f** were taken 6 months after revision septoplasty. At this time you see a gentle overcorrection in the supratip area, which will go away in the next few months.

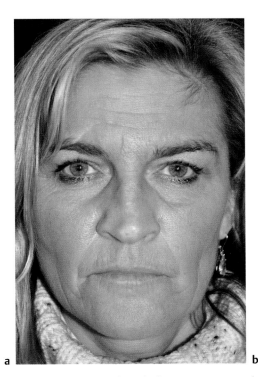
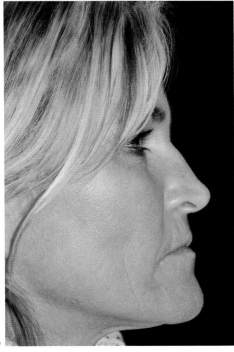
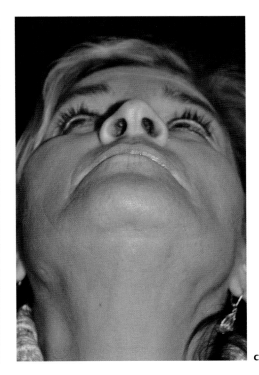

a b c

Fig. 16.1 (**a–c**) Findings before revision septoplasty. (*Continued on next page*)

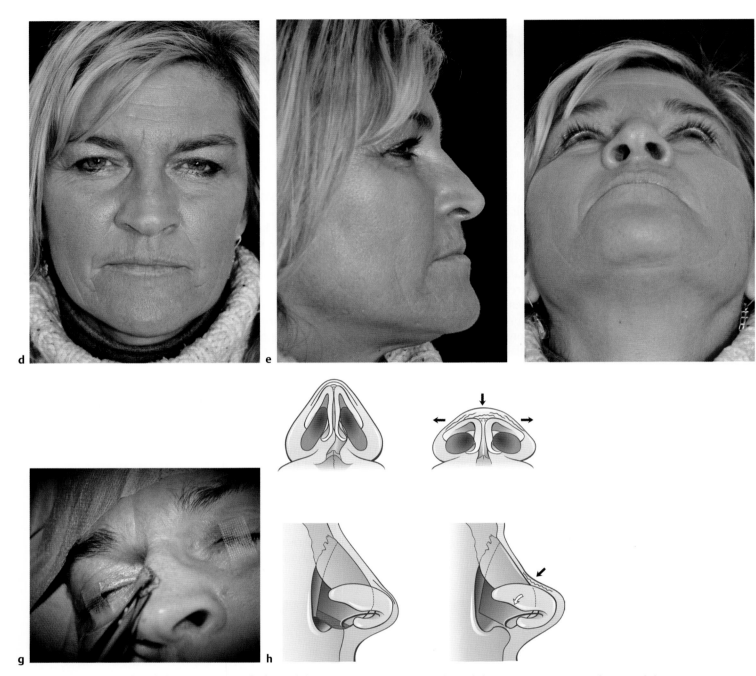

Fig. 16.1 (*Continued*) (**d–f**) Postoperative findings. (**g**) Intraoperative view: augmentation of the supratip area. (**h**) The alar and septal cartilages, superficial musculoaponeurotic system, skin, subcutaneous and connective tissues combine to give support and shape to the nasal tip. Any settling of the anterior septum or division of the connective-tissue fibers between the domes may cause widening of the nasal tip (after Rettinger, 2007).

Surgical Procedure

A graft was harvested from the conchal cavity. The supratip area was exposed directly through a medial intercartilaginous approach. A narrow pocket was developed, and the implant was inserted, followed by closure (**Fig. 16.1g**).

Psychology, Motivation, Personal Background

Immediately after the primary septoplasty, the patient felt that the postoperative change in her nose was too drastic and wanted it returned to the "old shape" as soon as possible. Since it was unlikely that the findings would improve over time, her desire for an immediate revision was reasonable and a revision septoplasty was scheduled.

Discussion

To restore permanent tension to the connective tissue system in the supratip area, the graft should be fitted into a tight pocket and should be slightly oversized. This enables the implant to function as a kind of "keystone" for the supratip region. Resorption will integrate the graft into the profile while preserving its function.

References

1. Hildebrandt T, Behrbohm H. Functional and Aesthetic Surgery of the Nose. The Influence of the Septum on the Aesthetic Lines of the Nasal Tip. Tuttlingen, Germany: Endo-Press; 2004

2. Rettinger G. Risks and complications in rhinoplasty. An update on functional and aesthetic surgery of the nose and ear. GMS Curr Top in Otorhinolaryngol Head Neck Surg 2007;6:73—88

17 Polly Beak Deformity

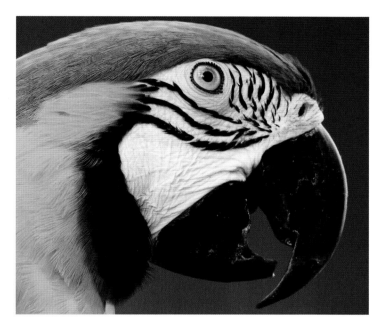

Fig. 17.1 The polly beak.

"Polly" is derived from the name "Molly." In the Cockney rhyming slang once spoken by sailors and pirates, "pretty Polly" meant money. Using the term "Polly" for "parrot" alludes to the profit that was to be made from selling parrots brought back from distant shores. Today it is still common for parrots to be named "Polly," and "Polly want a cracker" is often the first phrase that parrots are taught to speak.[1]

A polly beak (**Fig. 17.1**) is present when the supratip area projects higher than the tip defining point. This condition is marked by a convex transition from the cartilaginous nasal dorsum to the nasal tip, which resembles a parrot's beak in profile view. Risk factors for a postoperative polly beak are a deep nasal root, a high cartilaginous dorsum, and a low nasal tip.[2] A polly beak deformity may arise by various mechanisms, which call for different corrective measures. It is important, therefore, to determine the specific cause of a polly beak deformity in each patient before proceeding with revision surgery. **Fig. 17.2** shows the pathogenic mechanisms of polly beak deformity and possible ways of preventing them.

17.1 Soft-Tissue Polly Beak

Overvigorous dissection or leaving rough edges or cartilage fragments at the surgical site may evoke an intense connective-tissue reaction and scarring in the supratip area. This is particularly common in thick-skinned patients.[3] Since postoperative swelling can mimic a soft-tissue polly beak, unnecessary revisions can be avoided by always waiting until the swelling has completely subsided.[4]

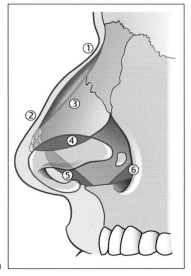

a

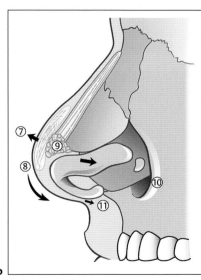

b

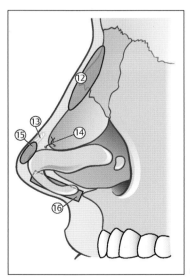

c

Fig. 17.2 Pathogenic mechanisms and possible solutions for preventing polly beak deformity. (**a**) The risk of polly beak deformity is increased by a deep nasofrontal angle (1), a high cartilaginous nasal dorsum, and an underprojected nasal tip. Thick skin in the supratip area (2) is also predisposing. The most common steps in the surgical correction of a humped nose: removal of a bony and cartilaginous hump (3), cephalic volume reduction of the alar cartilages (4), reduction of the anterior septal border, here by releasing the attachments of the medial crural footplates to the anterior septal border (5), and shortening the basal septal cartilage produce the desired profile change (6). (**b**) Principal causes of polly beak deformity. A granulating inflammation in the supratip area (7), often caused by rough cartilage edges (9), subcutaneous swelling and scarring, loss of projection (8) and protection due to collapse of the domes and medial crura (11) and a shortened septum (10). (**c**) Ways to prevent polly beak deformity: raising the nasal dorsum and increasing the nasofrontal angle (12), circumscribed thinning of the subcutaneous tissue beneath thick skin (13), possible fixation with a loose suture (14), lifting the nasal tip with a tip graft (15), or improving projection and protection with a columellar strut (16).

Case 2

Introduction
A 34-year-old woman had undergone two septorhinoplasties elsewhere 4 and 6 years previously. An active jogger, she still had difficulty breathing through the nose and also wanted a better aesthetic outcome. The result after two operations failed to meet her expectations. Moreover, her occupation as a bartender in a Berlin hotel placed her constantly in the public eye, and this increased her desire to have an attractive nose.

Findings
Frontal view (**Fig. 17.3a**) shows a crooked nose with a slight inverted-V deformity on the left side, subluxation of the septum on the right side, and a long infratip triangle. Profile view (**Fig. 17.3b**) shows thick skin, an overprojected tip, absence of a double break, poor tip definition, and a polly beak deformity. Basal view (**Fig. 17.3c**) shows septal subluxation with nostril asymmetry. **Fig. 17.3d**, **Fig. 17.3e**, and **Fig. 17.3f** show her appearance 2 years after revision surgery.

Surgical Procedure
The anterior septum was exposed through a hemitransfixion incision, and the basal septum was shortened. Other intraoperative details: spinal suture, intercartilaginous incision, elevation of the soft-tissue envelope, removal of thick scars over rough edges on the dorsal septum at the level of the anterior septal angle, reosteotomy on both sides, and spreader graft placement on the left side (**Fig. 17.3g, h**).

Psychology, Motivation, Personal Background
The patient viewed the previous operations as total failures. Her decision to have another rhinoplasty was not an easy one, but she placed high expectations on the result. During preoperative visits she gained a realistic level of expectation and an understanding of the problems associated with her skin type.

Discussion
This case illustrates a typical soft-tissue polly beak deformity. The patient's skin type predisposed her to this complication (**Fig. 17.2b**).

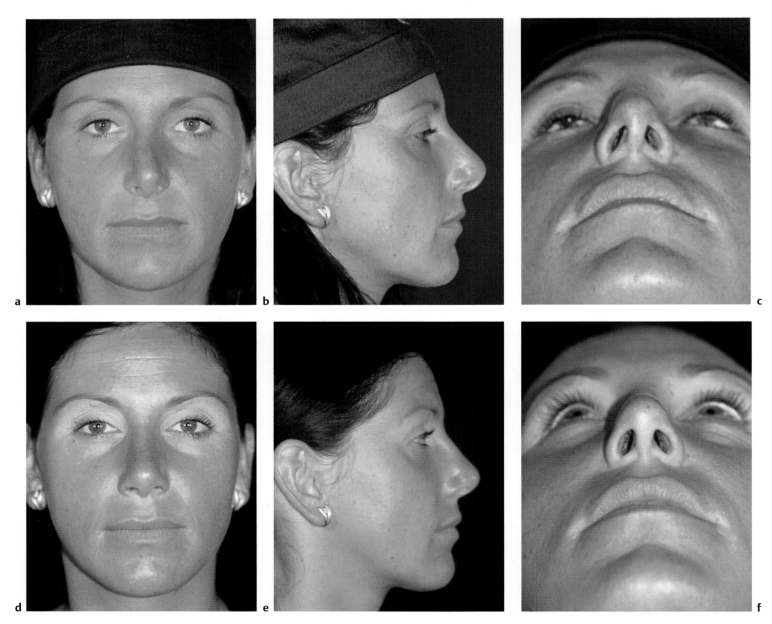

Fig. 17.3 (**a–c**) Findings before revision surgery. (**d–f**) Findings 2 years after revision surgery.

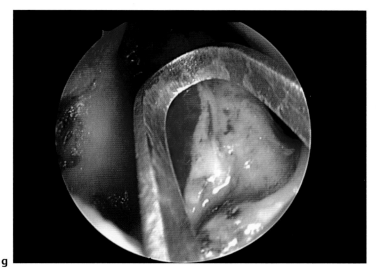

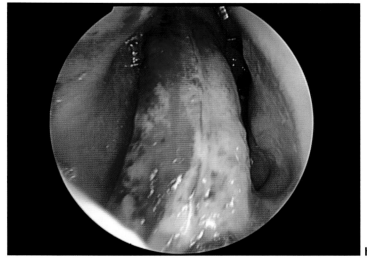

g

h

Fig. 17.3 (**g, h**) Intraoperative views. Resection and smoothing in the supratip area with microcurette (after Behrbohm, Karl Storz, Tuttlingen) (see **Fig. 18.4**).

Case 3

Introduction
A 72-year-old woman had undergone a previous rhinoplasty in her youth. She related stories about her life in Hamburg, and I asked her to write an account of her nasal surgery. This is what she wrote:

"How I came to have two nasal operations: Actually I had no problem with my looks (see photos in **Fig. 17.4a, b**) until my boyfriend, a dermatologist who specialized in cosmetic surgery, convinced me that I had a wide nose that looked 'Eastern Prussian.'

"Fashion models in the 1970s mostly had small, thin noses that were usually the result of cosmetic surgery. Since I wanted to be as photogenic as possible—even though I worked in the natural sciences—I agreed to have a rhinoplasty. My new nose was well received in my social circles and no one criticized the result. As time passed, however, a moderate 'polly beak' started to develop on my nose. I also suffered repeated sinus infections during that time, and I was supposed to have sinus surgery before getting a dental implant. It took me several years to decide. I also had corrective nasal surgery at the same time. I see now that the first operation did not yield an optimum result. Looking back, I like my natural nose and my current nose better. I lived for over 30 years with a nose that did not fit my facial proportions very well. What if I had just kept my original nose? You can't go with every passing fad of what constitutes beauty."

Findings
Frontal view (**Fig. 17.4c**) shows a slender nasal dorsum with a pinched tip and inspiratory alar collapse. Profile view (**Fig. 17.4d**) shows a polly beak deformity due to overresection of the bony nasal dorsum. Basal view (**Fig. 17.4e**) shows slight nostril asymmetry. **Fig. 17.4f**, **Fig. 17.4g**, and **Fig. 17.4h** show the corresponding views 2 years after revision surgery.

Surgical Procedure
Endoscopic sinus surgery was performed to improve sinus drainage. A hemitransfixion incision was made on the right side, and two mucosal tunnels and a swinging door were created, followed by basal shortening of the septal cartilage and incisions to straighten the anterior septum. The soft-tissue envelope was elevated from the nasal dorsum, and hyperplastic scars were removed from the supratip area. The nasal dorsum was augmented with crushed septal cartilage.

Discussion
The goal of the revision surgery was to remove the cartilaginous polly beak and raise the upper dorsum. The bone-cartilage junction was smoothed by augmentation.

17.2 Cartilaginous Polly Beak

Loss of nasal tip projection and protection is the main cause of postoperative polly beak deformity. M. E. Tardy, Jr. divided cartilaginous polly beaks into three categories: those compromising tip support and tip projection, those causing a false tip projection, and those tending to accentuate or mask a prominent cartilaginous dorsum.[5] Transitional forms may also occur. Thus, in our own experience as well, understanding the tip support mechanisms is the key to the prevention of polly beak. If there is concern about postoperative drooping of the nasal tip, this risk should be considered at operation and measures should be taken to prevent it.[6,7] A postoperative polly beak may also result from inadequate shortening of the dorsal septal and upper lateral cartilages as well as overresection of the nasal dorsum.[8] In patients with a deep nasal root, any resection of the bony dorsum should be done sparingly, and augmentation of the nasofrontal angle should be considered.[4]

The tip support mechanisms play a major role in the correction of polly beak deformity.

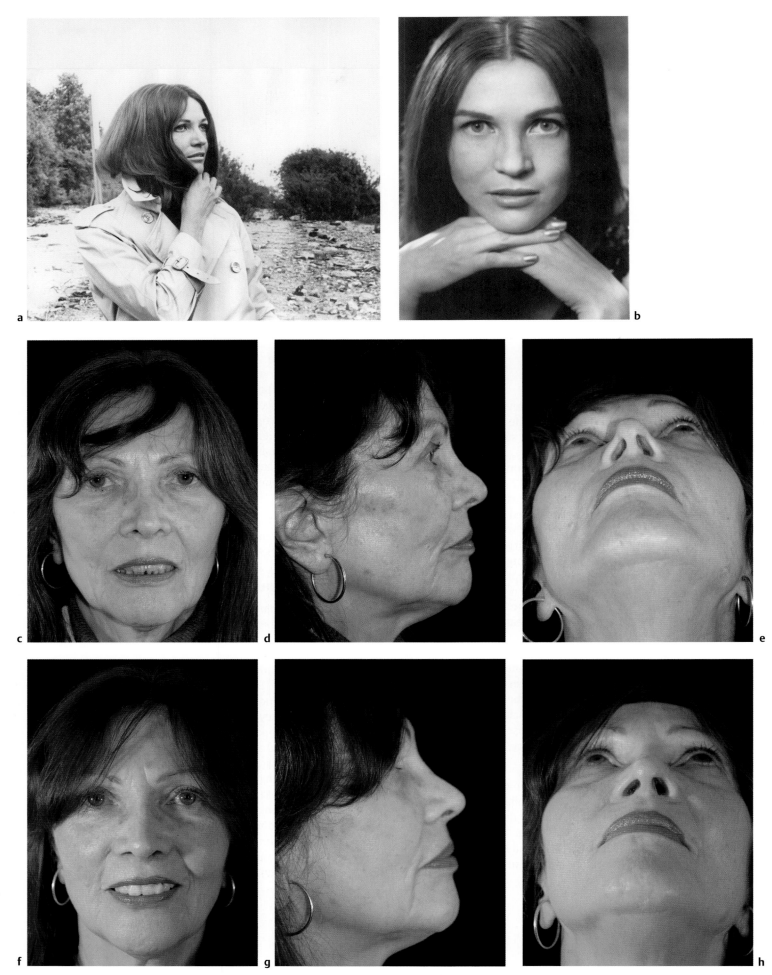

Fig. 17.4 (**a, b**) Photographs of the patient as a young woman before her first rhinoplasty. (**c–e**) Findings before revision surgery. (**f–h**) Findings 2 years after revision surgery.

Case 4

Introduction
A 25-year-old woman presented 2 years after a rhinoplasty in her home town, which involved the removal of a nasal hump. She was generally unhappy with the deformity of the nasal dorsum and sought aesthetic improvement.

Findings
Frontal view (**Fig. 17.5a**) shows deformity of the nasal dorsum, supratip area, and nasal tip. Profile view (**Fig. 17.5b**) shows a cartilaginous polly beak and hanging tip. Basal view (**Fig. 17.5c**) shows a broad, slightly asymmetrical nasal base. **Fig. 17.5d**, **Fig. 17.5e**, and **Fig. 17.5f** show the corresponding views 1 year after revision surgery.

Surgical Procedure
Delivery approach with cephalic reduction of the alar cartilages and elevation of the soft-tissue envelope. The upper lateral car- tilages were detached from the dorsal septal margin. The dorsal septum and superior borders of the upper lateral cartilages were shortened. Spreader grafts were fixed to the septum and upper lateral cartilages with 5–0 Prolene sutures (**Fig. 17.5g–j**).

Psychology, Motivation, Personal Background
A psychologically stable woman was firmly resolved to have the previous outcome improved by a revision procedure.

Discussion
The main goals of revision surgery were to reduce the height of the cartilaginous nasal dorsum and stabilize the shortened superior borders of the upper lateral cartilages. This was accomplished with spreader grafts sutured to the upper lateral cartilages at the dorsal septal margin. The nasal tip was well defined and did not require lifting or stabilization.

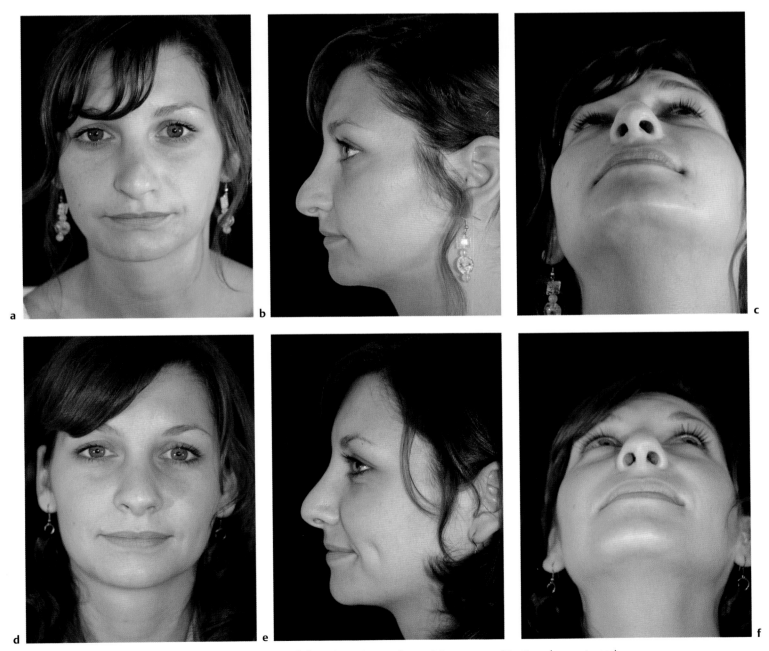

Fig. 17.5 (**a–c**) Findings before revision rhinoplasty. (**d–f**) Findings 1 year after revision surgery. (*Continued on next page*)

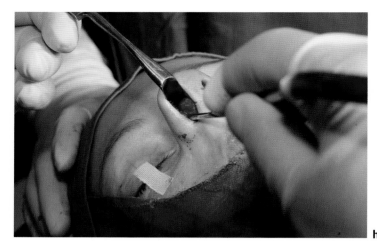

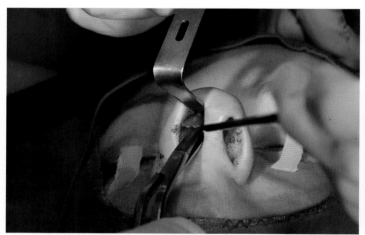

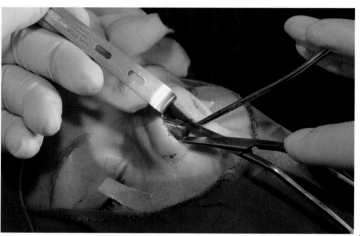

Fig. 17.5 (*Continued*)   (**g**) Sharp removal of the cartilaginous polly beak. (**h**) Intranasal approach to the nasal dorsum and supratip area. (**i**) Sharp removal of the cartilaginous polly beak. (**j**) Positioning of the dorsal septal border and the higher cartilages before suturing with PDS 5–0.

References

1. Behrbohm H. Septorhinoplastik in verschiedenen Lebensabschnitten. Part 2b: Das mittlere Lebensalter. HNO aktuell 2004;12:59–68

2. Rettinger G. Risks and complications in rhinoplasty. An update on functional and aesthetic surgery of the nose and ear. GMS Curr Top Otorhinolaryngol Head Neck Surg 2008;6:73–90

3. Hanasono MM, Kridel RW, Pastorek NJ, Glasgold MJ, Koch RJ. Correction of the soft tissue pollybeak using triamcinolone injection. Arch Facial Plast Surg 2002;4(1):26–30, discussion 31

4. Kim DW, Toriumi DM. Open structure rhinoplasty. In: Behrbohm H, Tardy ME, eds. Essentials of Septorhinoplasty. New York, NY: Thieme; 2003:118–136

5. Tardy ME Jr, Kron TK, Younger R, Key M. The cartilaginous pollybeak: etiology, prevention, and treatment. Facial Plast Surg 1989;6(2):113–120

6. Guyuron B, DeLuca L, Lash R. Supratip deformity: a closer look. Plast Reconstr Surg 2000;105(3):1140–1151, discussion 1152–1153

7. Jung D-H, Lin RY, Jang HJ, Claravall HJ, Lam SM. Correction of pollybeak and dimpling deformities of the nasal tip in the contracted, short nose by the use of a supratip transposition flap. Arch Facial Plast Surg 2009;11(5): 311–319

8. Bagal AA, Adamson PA. Revision rhinoplasty. Facial Plast Surg 2002; 18(4):233–244

18 Problems with the Nasal Dorsum

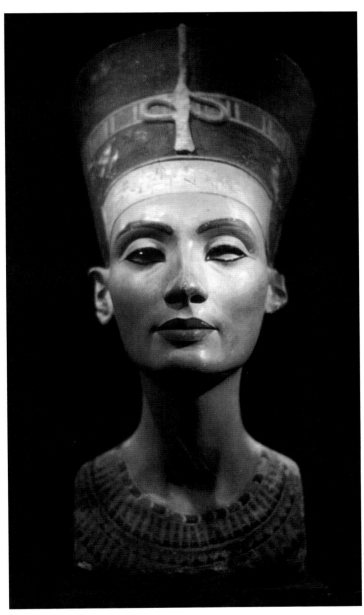

Fig. 18.1 Nefertiti in the New Museum in Berlin.

The name Nefertiti (**Fig. 18.1**) means "The beautiful one has arrived." The favorite wife of the pharaoh Akhenaten, she lived in the 14th century BC. She was immortalized by the familiar bust made of limestone and plaster, currently on display at the Neues Museum in Berlin. She is considered an icon of feminine beauty and charisma. Anyone who gazes into her eyes will never forget the impression.

The problems that may involve the nasal dorsum are numerous and diverse, ranging from an inverted-V deformity, open roof, and displaced osteotomy fragments to cysts and irregularities of the nasal dorsum. A correspondingly large range of solutions have been recommended for addressing these problems.[1-5]

18.1 Inverted-V Deformity

The inverted-V deformity is an aesthetically and functionally troublesome complication of rhinoplasty that is particularly common after the removal of large dorsal humps. It appears as a groove running along the piriform aperture between the bony nasal pyramid and the flexible cartilaginous part of the nose. It produces a fairly conspicuous and characteristic shadow shaped like an inverted V, which the patient may perceive as unsightly. The inverted-V deformity may appear shortly after the resolution of postoperative swelling or may develop as a late complication. Early appearance of the deformity suggests that the cause relates to displacement, loosening or detachment of the upper lateral cartilage from the nasal pyramid during the operation. Excessive rasping creates the greatest risk of intraoperative trauma. For this reason, rasping should be done as sparingly as possible and, when necessary, should be directed at an oblique angle to the piriform aperture. In our experience, standard 4-cm rasps have become obsolete for aesthetic rhinoplasty. Alternatives have been developed that minimize the risk of upper lateral cartilage trauma through the use of smaller, flatter instruments. In addition, diamond files should always be used in preference to coarse rasps. Short nasal bones, long upper lateral cartilages, and a large nasal hump are a triad that predisposes to the inverted-V deformity. Even with technically correct lateral osteotomies, scar contraction occurs in the late healing phase that tends to medialize the osteotomy fragments. As a result, the nasal dorsum sags below the pyramid, causing stenosis of the nasal cavity or internal nasal valve. The best way to prevent this problem is by the placement of spreader grafts or extended spreader grafts.[6]

Case 5

Case elements: inverted-V deformity, undefined nasal tip, over-projected dorsum, extracorporeal septoplasty (operation by Jacqueline Eichhorn-Sens).

Introduction

The patient was unhappy with the functional and aesthetic results of a previous rhinoplasty performed elsewhere. Functional problems were caused by residual septal deviation, internal valve stenosis, and inferior turbinate hypertrophy.

Findings

Frontal inspection showed disharmony of the brow-tip aesthetic lines and a conspicuous inverted-V deformity (**Fig. 18.2a**), suggesting that the upper lateral cartilages had been separated from the bone in the previous rhinoplasty. The bony pyramid was wide and asymmetrical. A deep nasal root and bony hump were noted in the profile view (**Fig. 18.2b**). The nasal tip was wide and bulky, asymmetrical, and not well defined (**Fig. 18.2a, b**). Endo-

nasal inspection revealed a deviated septum, especially at the anterior nasal border; the rest was deviated and round bodied (**Fig. 18.2g, h**). On examination with a glass probe, manual expansion of the anterior nasal valve produced an immediate sensation of improved breathing, confirming that the internal valve was stenotic and required reconstruction.

Surgical Procedure

An open approach was performed through a standard inverted-V midcolumellar incision. Analysis showed that the anterior septal border was deviated and the whole septal cartilage was under tension. Therefore, we decided to remove the septum (**Fig. 18.2g, h**) and perform an extracorporeal septal reconstruction. We smoothed out all irregularities, particularly addressing the thickened area at the junction of the bony and the cartilaginous septum.

The rest of the septum was then rotated 180 degrees to obtain a straight residual septum. A thinned perpendicular plane was sutured to the new anterior septal border to support the

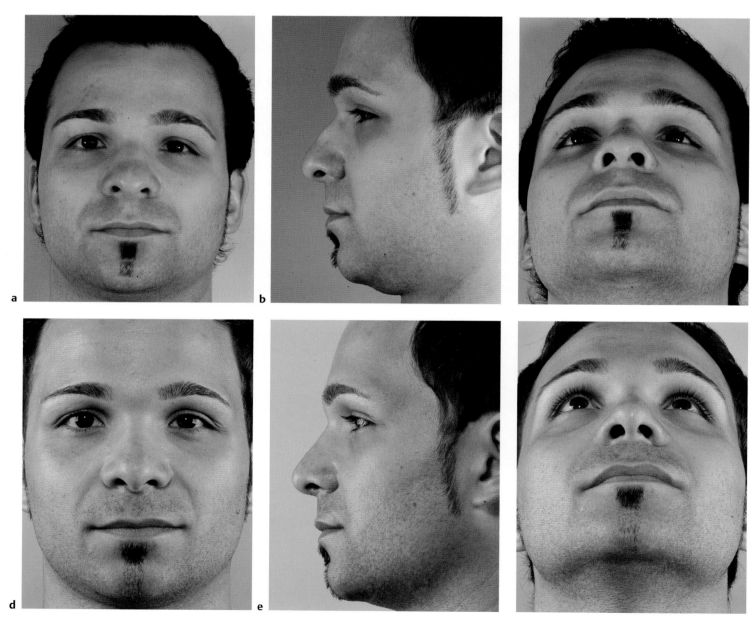

Fig. 18.2 (**a**) Preoperative frontal view shows disharmony of the brow-tip aesthetic lines, a conspicuous inverted-V deformity, deviation of the nose, and a wide, undefined nasal tip. (**b**) Profile view shows a bony hook and overprojected cartilaginous dorsum. (**c**) The asymmetrical, undefined tip is conspicuous in the basal view. (**d–f**) Follow-up views at 18

months. Nasal breathing is normal. (**d**) Frontal view. The brow-tip aesthetic lines are symmetrical, the nasal axis is straight, and the tip is well defined. (**e**) Basal view displays a symmetrical and well-defined tip. (**f**) Profile view shows a more pleasing appearance of the dorsum with stable correction of the nasolabial angle.

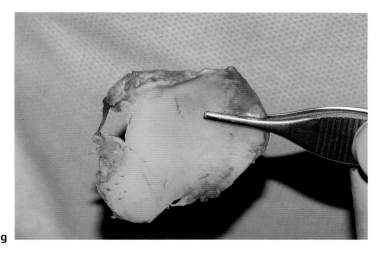

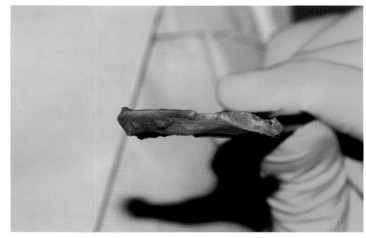

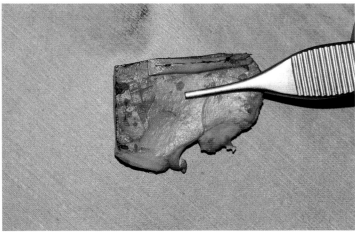

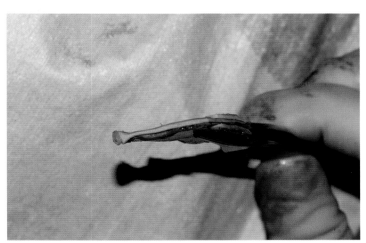

Fig. 18.2 (**g, h**) The anterior septal border was deviated, and all of the septal cartilage was under tension. (**i, j**) A thin piece of perpendicular plate was sutured to the new anterior septal border to straighten it per-manently and give it support. At this point the new anterior border is fully straightened. Spreader grafts have been placed in the dorsum.

cartilage piece (**Fig. 18.2i**). We sutured spreader grafts made of septal cartilage to the dorsal part of the new septum to restore the integrity of the internal nasal valves, reestablish the dorsal aesthetic lines, and increase the stability of the framework (**Fig. 18.2i, j**). Lateral, paramedian, and transverse osteotomies were performed on both sides following reduction of the bony hump. The new straight septum was repositioned and anchored to the upper lateral cartilages with multiple back-and-forth sutures. Anterior fixation was achieved with several sutures passed through a small drill hole in the anterior spine. A cartilage graft was placed on the nasal root. The dorsum was additionally covered with a layer of homologous fascia lata. For correction of the nasal tip, the cephalic portions of the lower lateral cartilages were resected and the dome area was reconstituted with trans-domal sutures. A spanning suture was placed to control flaring, and a tip suspension suture stabilized the nasal tip in the ideal position.

Psychology, Motivation, Personal Background

The previous operation had been done elsewhere to correct functional problems, but the septum was still deviated. Additionally, the upper lateral cartilages had been separated from the bone in the previous operation, narrowing the internal valves and exacerbating the airway problems. The patient also suffered from aesthetic deformities including a conspicuous inverted V, a hooked nose, and a broad, undefined nasal tip. Thus, the patient could reasonably expect functional and aesthetic improvements from the revision surgery. When seen 18 months postopera-tively, the patient was satisfied with the aesthetic and functional outcome (**Fig. 18.2d–f**).

Discussion

It is reasonable to ask whether the septal cartilage could have been straightened without removing the entire septum. The most important issue involves the outer framework of the septum: Is at least a straight L-shaped framework present, or is the outer framework deformed? In this case the framework, especially the anterior septal border, was not straight. A straight septal frame-work is essential for a straight nose. Therefore, every effort was made to straighten the septum.

Case 6

Introduction
A 32-year-old woman presented 10 years and 8 months after undergoing a septorhinoplasty at another hospital. She worked as a waitress at a popular resort on the Baltic Sea and desired a rapid and permanent improvement of the primary outcome.

Findings
Frontal view (**Fig. 18.3a**) shows an inverted-V deformity with undercorrection of the cartilaginous nasal dorsum. Oblique (**Fig. 18.3b**) and profile views (**Fig. 18.3c**) show a residual hump, irregularities all along the nasal dorsum, and incomplete removal of a nasal hump with a cartilaginous polly beak.

Follow-up views after revision rhinoplasty show the findings at 2 years (**Fig. 18.3d–f**) and at 10 years (**Fig. 18.3g, h**).

Psychology, Motivation, Personal Background
The patient felt that the result of the primary operation was worse than her original nose. She was highly motivated to seek a maximal degree of improvement.

Surgical Procedure
A 4 × 12-mm cartilage strip was harvested from the lower septum through an open approach. Cartilage remnants were removed from the septum, the upper lateral cartilages were detached, the dorsal septal margin was shortened, bilateral spreader grafts were placed, and medial and lateral curved osteotomies were performed on both sides. The entire nasal dorsum was camouflaged with allogeneic human fascia lata.

Discussion
The nasal dorsum was augmented with allogeneic, devitalized, freeze-dried fascia lata. Fascia is a useful material for dorsal nasal camouflage, although its tendency to expand in vivo leads to protracted swelling that may last for months. It should be decided on a case-by-case basis whether autologous tissue would be a better option than allografts.

18.2 Residual Hump

There are several typical problems that may arise after the surgical correction of a humped nose. Besides an inverted-V deformity, rocker deformity, or open roof, a postoperative residual hump is particularly distressful because patients equate it with a failed operation. The main decision to be made in these cases is whether to take a wait-and-see approach or proceed at once to revision surgery. Residual humps may be predominantly bony or cartilaginous. They may result from the faulty placement of an osteotomy line during removal, persistent periosteal swelling, appositional bone growth, granulating inflammation, or organized hematomas. Atraumatic handling of the periosteum at surgery is the best way to promote rapid and uneventful healing of the nasal dorsum.

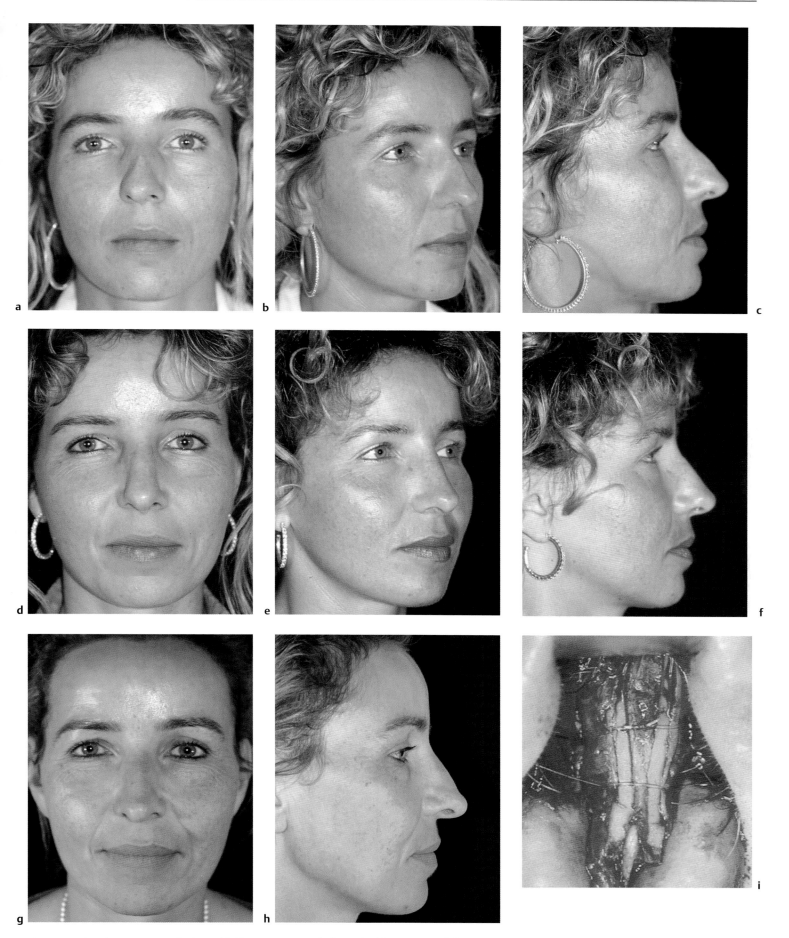

Fig. 18.3 (**a–c**) Preoperative findings. (**d–f**) Postoperative findings. (**g, h**) Long-term follow-up 10 years after revision surgery. (**i**) Intraoperative view. Spreader grafts have been placed on both sides.

Case 7 (Late Revision)

Introduction
The patient presented at 41 years of age with nasal airway obstruction and aesthetic complaints. She sought correction of the nasal dorsum, correction of the dorsum-tip junction, and narrowing of the tip.

Findings before Primary Rhinoplasty
Frontal view (**Fig. 18.4a**) shows a prominent nasal dorsum with a plateau in the supratip area and a broad nasal tip. Profile view (**Fig. 18.4b**) shows a bony and cartilaginous hump with overprojection and a small nasofrontal angle. Oblique view is shown in **Fig. 18.4c**.

Findings before Revision Rhinoplasty
Frontal view (**Fig. 18.4d**) and profile view (**Fig. 18.4e**) show a residual hump. **Fig. 18.4f–h** show the corresponding views after revision surgery.

Surgical Procedure
The soft-tissue envelope was elevated from the nasal dorsum through a medial intercartilaginous incision. Scars and granulations were removed with a nasal dorsal curette and mini-scraper.

Psychology, Motivation, Personal Background
The doctor and patient had been hopeful that the prominence over the bony nasal pyramid would resolve with time. A wait-and-see approach is usually justified in patients with residual swelling of this magnitude. But if the residual hump does not resolve because of periosteal new bone formation or other causes, revision surgery is the only remaining option.

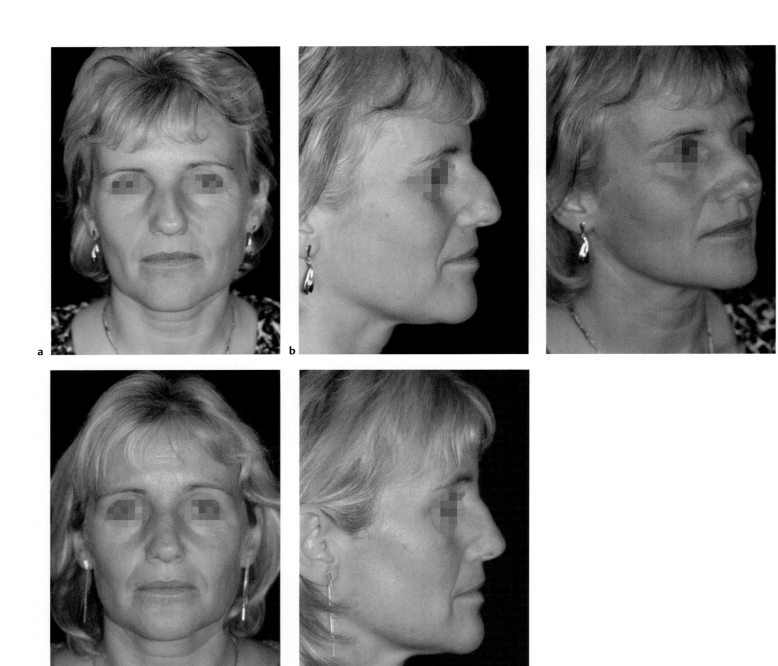

a   b   c   d   e

Fig. 18.4   (**a–c**) Findings before the primary rhinoplasty. (**d, e**) Findings before revision rhinoplasty.

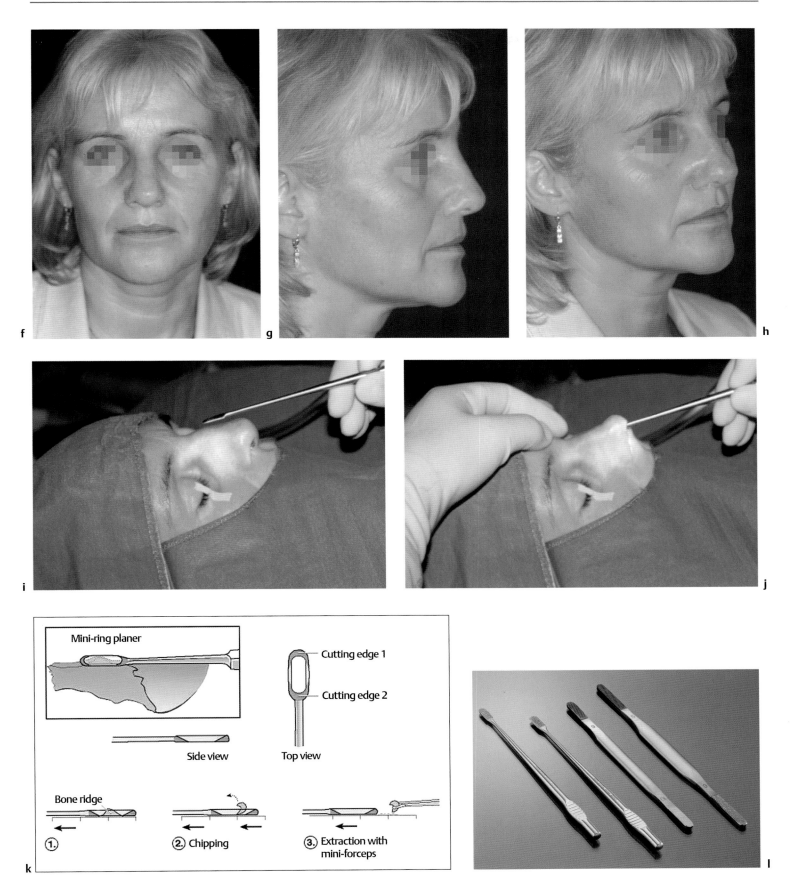

Fig. 18.4   (**f–h**) Findings after revision rhinoplasty. (**i**) Intraoperative view. (**i**) Use of a miniature rasp combined with a microcurette. (**j**) Positioning the microcurette through a small intranasal incision. (**k**) Cutting and smoothing action of the microcurette. (**l**) Small and mini-rasps and diamond files. (Karl Storz, Tuttlingen.)

Case 8 (Early Revision)

Introduction
The patient presented 3 months after a primary rhinoplasty for the removal of a nasal hump.

Findings
Frontal view (**Fig. 18.5a**) shows a broad nasal pyramid. Profile view (**Fig. 18.5b**) shows a residual hump with a hard consistency. Basal view is shown in **Fig. 18.5c**, **Fig. 18.5d**, **Fig. 18.5e**, and **Fig. 18.5f** show the follow-up views 1 year after revision surgery.

Surgical Procedure
The residual hump was removed (**Fig. 18.5g**).

Psychology, Motivation, Personal Background
If the dorsum is not adequately reduced, leaving a residual hump, more is required than reassuring the patient and engendering false hopes. The surgeon should take the initiative in recommending an early revision and spare the patient an unnecessary and frustrating wait for an illusory goal.

Discussion
The surgeon should wait until the nose has fully healed and is stable before proceeding with a revision rhinoplasty. Generally this will take at least 8 months, and even longer in some cases. The problem of a premature revision is that it adds a new period of destabilization to the existing variables of incomplete stabilization, scarring, and graft integration, creating a situation that is difficult to manage and predict. There are exceptions, however, in which it is appropriate to proceed with an early revision. These cases would include technically flawed osteotomies with displaced fragments, displaced implants, a residual hump, septal deviation, septal hematoma, suture fistulas, and wound infections. These complications are considered valid indications for an early revision procedure.

In cases where such an indication exists, the doctor should take the initiative, offer the patient a revision, and determine the timing. Surgeons should never ignore an obvious problem such as displaced grafts or implants, causing their patients to "wander around" and seek help from other doctors.

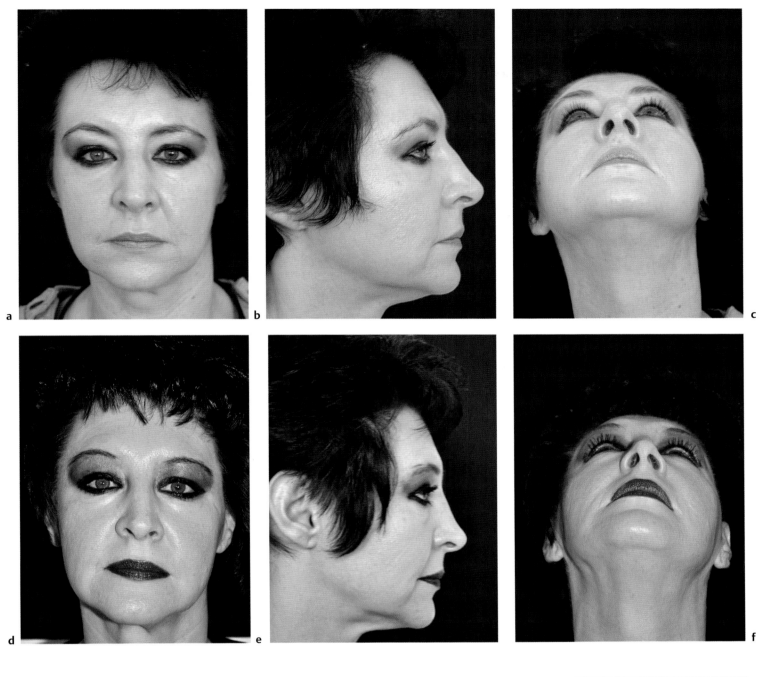

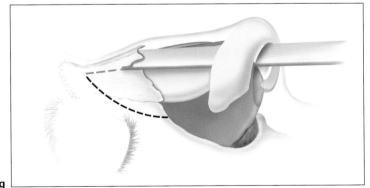

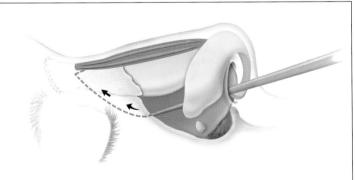

Fig. 18.5 (a–c) Findings before revision rhinoplasty. (d–f) Findings 1 year after revision rhinoplasty. (g) Residual hump is removed with a guarded Rubin osteotome. (h) Curved low lateral osteotomy, beginning higher on the ascending process at the level of the inferior concha, coursing lower onto the ascending, and finally curving upward toward the medial-oblique oseotomy site.

18.3 Open-Roof Deformity

Open-roof deformity is manifested by a broadening of the bony nasal dorsum. It occurs when the nasal bones are left separated after the removal of a bony hump. This may result from incomplete or technically flawed lateral osteotomies, greenstick fractures, or residual bony bridges left between the septal and nasal bones due to inadequate paramedian osteotomies.[1] This gap in the bony nasal pyramid may allow the soft tissues to sag, causing palpable and sometimes visible irregularities in the nasal dorsum. Direct contact is established between the outer skin and endonasal mucosa, often leading to neuralgia, headaches, sensory disturbances, and a cold sensation. In most cases these symptoms will disappear after revision surgery.

A wide nose with an open-roof deformity may also result from nasal trauma. Injuries to the nasal bones may cause lateralization of the bones or may avulse portions of the maxillary frontal process, creating an open roof.[3]

The open roof should definitely be closed to prevent scar contractures and unpredictable deformities of both the bony and cartilaginous dorsum. These tissue reactions may also affect the upper lateral cartilages and internal nasal valve, leading to stenosis. The underlying pathogenic mechanisms are similar to those in an inverted-V deformity. The open roof is closed by means of medial and lateral curved osteotomies.

Case 9

Introduction

A 24-year-old woman presented 1 year after undergoing a septorhinoplasty with hump removal. The young cosmetician complained of a wide bony nasal pyramid, crooked nose, and asymmetry in the supratip area.

Findings

Frontal view (**Fig. 18.6a**) shows a wide nose with an open-roof deformity and slight asymmetry caused by scar induration in the left supratip area. Profile view (**Fig. 18.6b**) shows a residual hump and polly beak deformity. Basal view is shown in **Fig. 18.6c**. **Fig. 18.6g**, **Fig. 18.6h**, and **Fig. 18.6i** were taken 1 year after the second revision.

Surgical Procedures

Two revision rhinoplasties were performed:

1. First revision in 2010: hemitransfixion incision, intercartilaginous incision, elevation of the soft-tissue envelope, scar tissue excised from the supratip area. Reosteotomy of a residual hump, medial and lateral curved osteotomies. The upper lateral cartilages were detached from the dorsal septal border and fixed with 5–0 PDS sutures.

2. Second revision in 2011: reosteotomy on the right side and excision of scar tissue, especially in the left supratip area (**Fig. 18.6g–l**). Adjunct: 0.4 mg triamcinolone was injected into the area after surgery.

Psychology, Motivation, Personal Background

The patient perceived the postoperative asymmetry as cosmetically objectionable, and this motivated her to seek improvement.

Discussion

The osteotomies and mobilization in a primary rhinoplasty are often too high or incomplete. The osteotomy fragments in the present case had not been completely mobilized, especially on the right side, and so the revision focused on reosteotomies.

18.4 Tissue Memory

If the nasal bones are too short or lateral osteotomies are placed too high, incomplete closure may result. Postoperative scar tissue may contract medially toward the defect, or the osteotomy fragments may tend to move laterally in patients with small, mobile, floating nasal bones. Because this tendency is often difficult to control, it is called tissue memory. Greenstick fractures have a springlike tendency causing the bony pyramid to return to its original configuration after surgery.

18.5 Rocker Deformity

Rocker deformity occurs when osteotomies are placed too high above the nasofrontal suture or extend into the thick frontal bone. The thick upper portion of the osteotomized nasal bone tends to "rock" laterally while the thin lower portion moves medially, producing a lateral rocker deformity. Treatment consists of backfracturing, that is, making new osteotomies at a lower level through the thinner nasal bones to create a lower point for mobilizing the bone fragments. A 2-mm osteotome can be used percutaneously to create more appropriate transverse osteotomies.

18.6 Dorsal Nasal Cyst

Dorsal nasal cyst formation results from the entrapment or displacement of endonasal respiratory epithelium into the nasal dorsum. This may occur through an osteotomy site or may develop when the anatomic boundary between the two compartments is breached in an open-roof deformity. Ciliated epithelium becomes trapped beneath the skin of the nasal dorsum during postoperative scarring. Goblet cells and seromucous glands continue to produce secretions, causing a cyst to form. The treatment of choice is complete extirpation.[7]

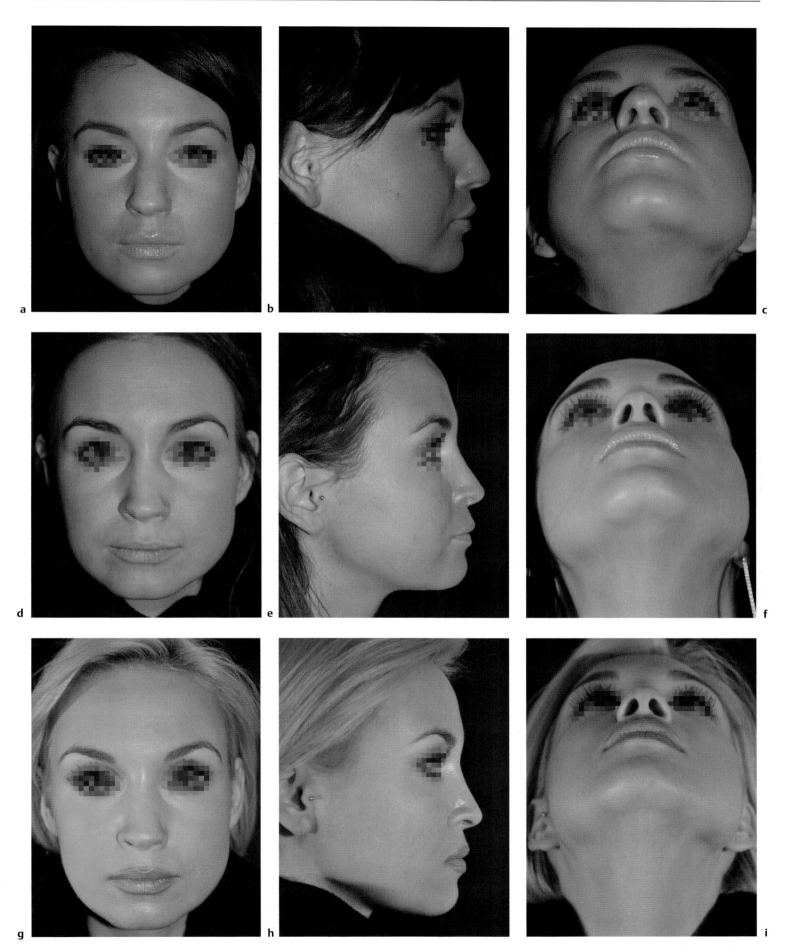

Fig. 18.6 (**a–c**) Findings before revision rhinoplasty. (**d–f**) Findings 1 year after revision rhinoplasty. (**g–i**) Findings 1 year after second revision rhinoplasty. (*Continued on next page*)

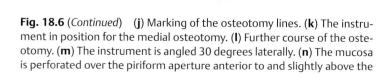

Fig. 18.6 (*Continued*)   (**j**) Marking of the osteotomy lines. (**k**) The instrument in position for the medial osteotomy. (**l**) Further course of the osteotomy. (**m**) The instrument is angled 30 degrees laterally. (**n**) The mucosa is perforated over the piriform aperture anterior to and slightly above the head of the inferior turbinate. (**o–p**) Continuation of the lateral curved osteotomy. (**p**) Changing the direction of the lateral osteotomy. (**q**) Osteotome is advanced 30 degrees medially.

Case 10

Case elements: inverted-V deformity, undefined nasal tip, over-projected dorsum, extracorporeal septoplasty (operation by Wolfgang Gubisch).

Introduction

A 35-year-old woman presented after a previous septorhino-plasty with hump removal. Her nose appeared to be too long because the tip had been neglected in the previous operation. The nasal dorsum showed irregularities, the nostrils were asymmetrical, and the right ala had a kinked appearance. The anterior septal border was mobile after the septoplasty and produced a "click" when moved over the anterior spine.

Diagnosis

Inspection revealed a long nose following hump removal in a previous rhinoplasty (**Fig. 18.7a, b**). The tip looked wide, undefined, and asymmetrical. The right ala showed kinking (**Fig. 18.7c**). The tip was rotated caudally and the nasolabial angle was too small (**Fig. 18.7b**). Visible irregularities were noted on the nasal dorsum. On palpation of the columella, the anterior septal border could be moved over the anterior spine with a clicking sound. Endonasal inspection showed residual septal deviation.

Surgical Procedure

The revision was performed through an open approach. After dissection of the tip, it was found that dome area had been asymmetrically resected on both sides and the right lower lateral cartilage had been overresected in the previous surgery (**Fig. 18.7g**). The caudal end of the septum had lost contact with the anterior nasal spine, and the anterior septum had been overresected (**Fig. 18.7h**). We corrected the residual septal deviation. Conchal cartilage was harvested from one site, and a double-layer conchal sandwich graft was fashioned as a columellar strut to improve tip support (**Fig. 18.7i**). The sandwich graft was sutured to the anterior nasal spine and to the anterior septal border. The right lower lateral cartilage was corrected with a batten graft. Rim grafts of septal cartilage stabilized the nasal vestibule. Tip con-

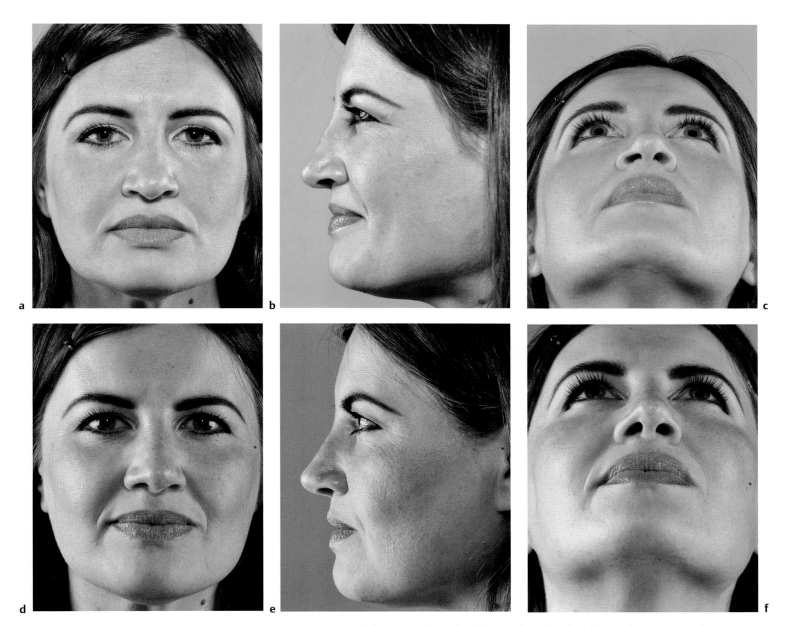

Fig. 18.7 (**a**) Preoperative frontal view: the nose is too long and the tip is asymmetrical, wide, and poorly defined. The bony dorsum is asymmetrical, and dorsal irregularities are visible. (**b**) Profile view: the nose appears too long and the nasolabial angle is too small. The tip is rotated caudally. (**c**) Basal view shows nostril asymmetry and deviation of the col-umella with kinking of the right ala. (**d**) Frontal view 1 year after revision rhinoplasty. The tip is well defined. (**e**) Profile view shows good correction of tip rotation and the nasolabial angle. The nose is shortened, and nasal length is in harmony with the rest of the face. (**f**) Basal view shows stabilization of the left ala and a well-defined nasal tip. (*Continued on next page*)

figuration was corrected bilaterally by a modified dome division technique, taking advantage of the preexisting incisions in the dome area (**Fig. 18.7j**). To prevent a sharp, narrowed tip in the years after the dome division, the dome area was covered with a double-layer homologous fascia lata graft. A spanning suture was placed. A shield graft of septal cartilage was used to configure the infratip break point. The nasal dorsum was contoured with diced conchal cartilage wrapped in homologous fascia lata (diced cartilage in fascia, DCF).

Psychology, Motivation, Personal Background

The young woman still had breathing issues after her previous operation. She was also unhappy with the appearance of her nose. One year after revision surgery she was pleased with the aesthetic and functional outcome (**Fig. 18.7d–f**).

Discussion

Our graft material of first choice is septal cartilage, when it is available. But a sandwich graft made of conchal cartilage is more suitable for improving tip support in the columella, as in the present case.

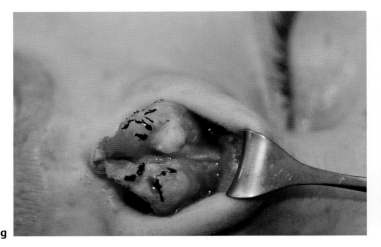

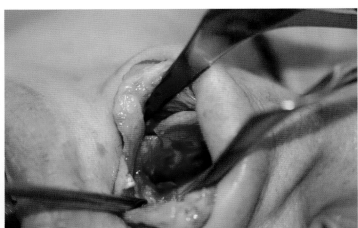

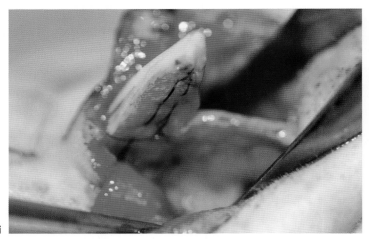

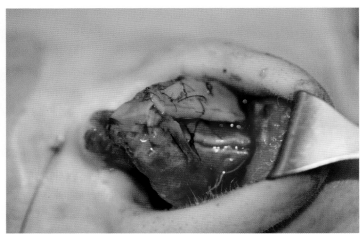

Fig. 18.7 (*Continued*)   (**g**) Bilateral incisions in the dome area and asymmetrical cartilage resection. (**h**) Intraoperative view of the overresected anterior septum. The caudal end of the septum is not in contact with the anterior nasal spine. (**i**) A double-layer sandwich graft of conchal cartilage was used to reconstruct the anterior septum and provide tip support. (**j**) The right lower lateral cartilage was covered with a batten graft of septal cartilage. The spanning suture and shield graft are also shown.

18.7 Tip Ptosis and Residual Hump

Case 11

The goal in this case was to correct a persistent dorsal hump while preserving ethnic identity (operation by Holger Gassner).

Introduction

A 26-year-old woman presented after previous open-structure rhinoplasty with a persistent dorsal hump, ptotic nasal tip, and left-sided nasal obstruction. She requested minor cosmetic changes that would preserve her ethnic identity.

Diagnosis

Frontal view (**Fig. 18.8a**) shows a narrow middle vault with an inverted-V deformity. Profile view (**Fig. 18.8b, c**) shows a persistent bony hump. The nasal tip is ptotic and derotated. The oblique view (**Fig. 18.8d**) accentuates the droopy tip, which makes the nose appear too long.

Surgical Procedure

The previous open approach was revised. The dorsal hump was removed using a No. 11 scalpel and a 14-mm Rubin osteotome (**Fig. 18.8e, f**), which resulted in an open roof (see **Fig. 18.8g**). The narrow middle vault was reconstructed with conventional spreader grafts, which were fashioned from split septal cartilage (**Fig. 18.8h**). The tip was rotated and projected with a modified tongue-in-groove technique, partially preserving the membranous septum to prevent a rigid nasal tip. These maneuvers resulted in conservative hump reduction, moderate tip rotation, adequate middle vault width, and preservation of the natural softness of her nasal tip (**Fig. 18.8i–l**).

Psychology, Motivation, Personal Background

Patients with a non-Caucasian ethnic background must be very carefully evaluated with regard to their expectations. This patient requested preservation of her ethnic identity. Overzealous rotation of the nasal tip in this case would have resulted in an unnaturally short nasal appearance.

Discussion

We strive to preserve septal cartilage, which contributes to nasal function and may be valuable in the event of future revision surgery. In the majority of cases, we detach the upper lateral cartilage from the septum and fashion auto-spreader grafts. In cases where the height of the upper lateral cartilages is insufficient, split septal cartilage provides a cartilage-sparing alternative for reconstruction of the middle vault.

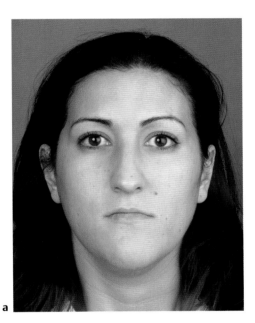

a

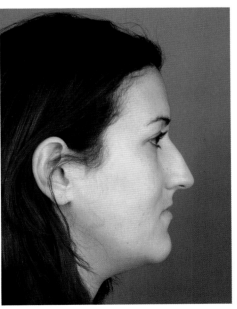

b

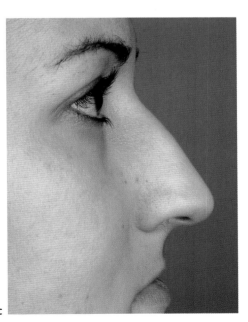

c

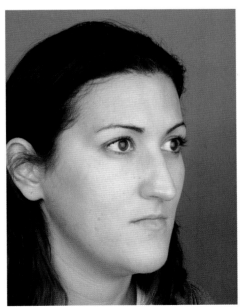

d

Fig. 18.8   (a–d) Preoperative views show an elongated nose with a ptotic and underprojected tip, a mild dorsal hump, and C-shaped deviation of the nose. (*Continued on next page*)

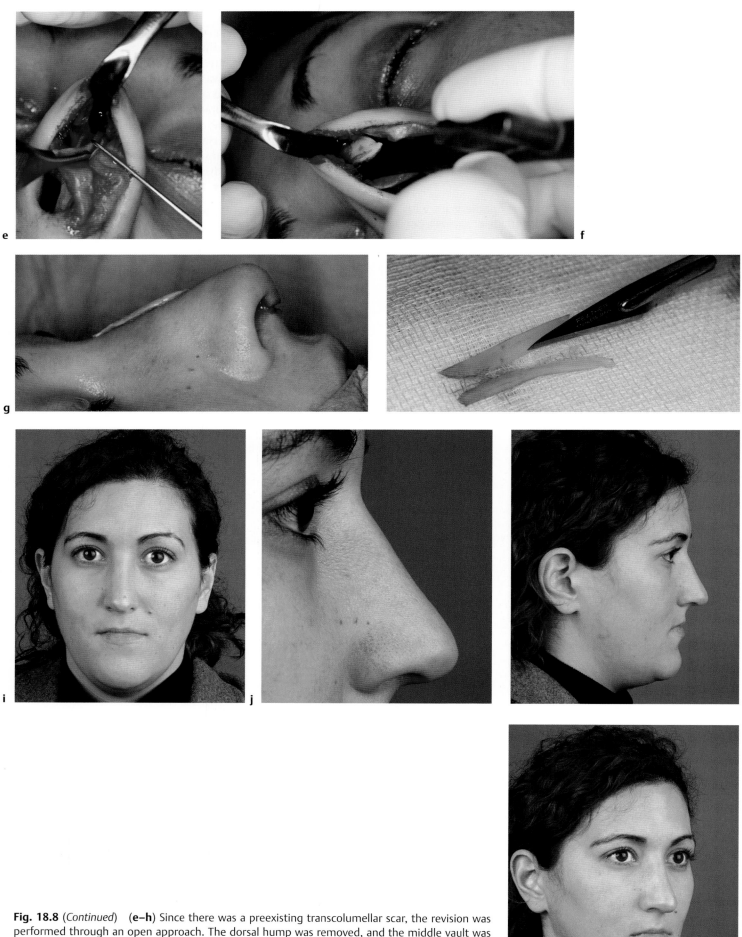

Fig. 18.8 (*Continued*)   (**e–h**) Since there was a preexisting transcolumellar scar, the revision was performed through an open approach. The dorsal hump was removed, and the middle vault was reconstructed with split septal cartilage spreader grafts. (**i–l**) Any appearance of a scooped dorsum or visible supratip break was to be avoided in this patient. A straight dorsal line was created, and the tip was left less rotated than would be the case in a nonethnic rhinoplasty. A smooth transition was created from the supratip area to the tip.

Case 12

This case involved dorsal irregularities secondary to posttraumatic atrophic scarring of the dorsal skin (operation by Holger Gassner).

Introduction

A 28-year-old woman presented after three previous rhinoplasties for the revision of dorsal irregularities. She was not bothered by the amorphous and rounded appearance of her nasal tip, but requested improvement of visible and palpable irregularities in the dorsal skin.

Diagnosis

The profile views (**Figs. 18.9a–c**) show irregularities and depressions over the upper and middle thirds. On palpation, the skin is paper-thin and some of the bony irregularities are speculated and tender on palpation. The skylight view (**Fig. 18.9d**) shows marked hypopigmentation of the atrophic dorsal skin scar. The amorphous appearance of the nasal tip and the mild polly beak deformity did not concern the patient and were not to be addressed.

Surgical Procedure

Elevation of the dorsal skin through bilateral intercartilaginous incisions was tedious and difficult due to scar adhesions and a very thick soft-tissue envelope. Gentle hydrodissection with local anesthetic solution and dissection under microscopic control allowed the dorsal skin to be elevated without additional trauma. The skeletal irregularities were corrected by careful smoothing with a fine rasp, dissection with a No. 15 blade, the placement of thinly shaved auricular cartilage grafts, and camouflage with deep temporal fascia. Fascia and cartilage were harvested though a common retroauricular incision (**Fig. 18.9e**). The fascia was then placed on the nasal dorsum as a single-layer graft (**Fig. 18.9f**). **Figs. 18.9g–j** show a markedly smoother dorsal profile, which also became notably less tender to palpation during the first postoperative year.

Psychology, Motivation, Personal Background

Additional correction of the patient's nasal tip deformity seemed intuitive in this case. The author only touched very lightly on this aspect of her nose, but did in no way stress the issue. The patient was merely concerned about her dorsum.

Careful assessment of the patient's desires and expectations is of paramount importance during the preoperative discussion. The patient was very happy with the outcome, which was the result of a patient-oriented "please fix this one problem" approach rather than a surgeon-oriented "let me do your nose" approach.

Discussion

Atrophic changes in the dorsal skin are among the most difficult problems to correct in rhinoplasty. Adequate preventive strategies include meticulous microscopic dissection in the supraperichondrial and subperiosteal plane. We favor sharp dissection and recommend minimal use of blunt dissection techniques such as spreading movements with a scissors.

The placement of stacked, soft, and thin autologous material is excellent for camouflaging visible and palpable irregularities. The author prefers autologous grafts over allogeneic or synthetic material.

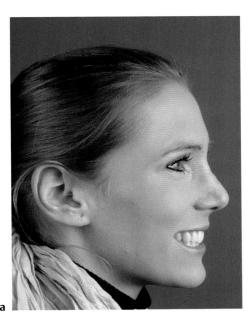

a

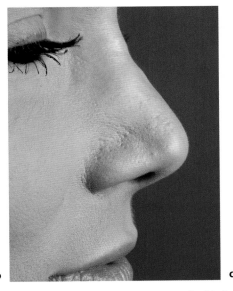

b

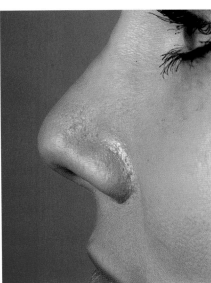

c

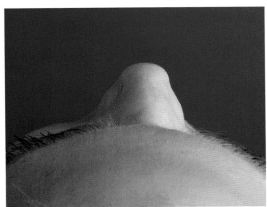

d

Fig. 18.9 (**a–d**) Preoperative views highlight the atrophy of the dorsal skin. The underlying irregularities are accentuated by the paper-thin skin and soft-tissue envelope. The skin is smooth, glistening, and hypopigmented. (*Continued on next page*)

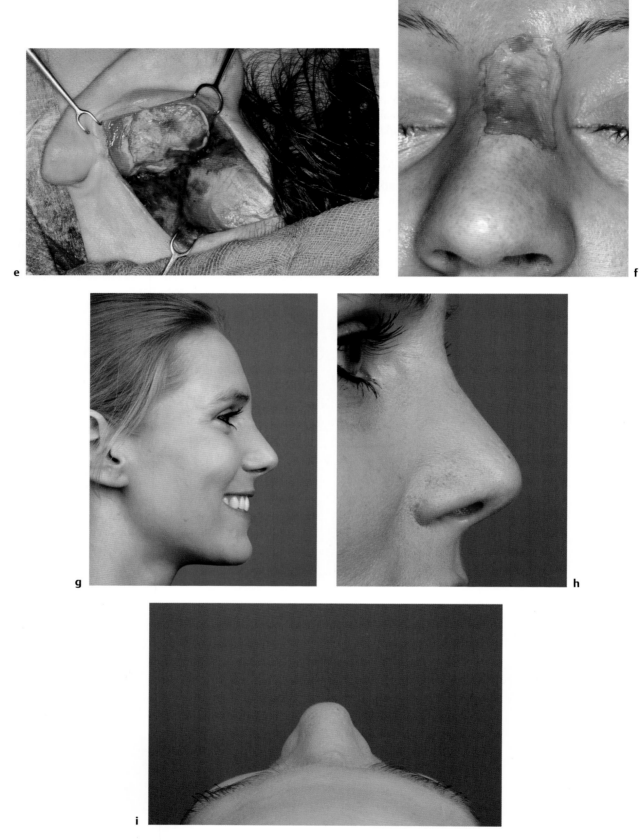

Fig. 18.9 (*Continued*) (**e**) Retroauricular harvest of deep temporal fascia. The fascia is approached in an avascular plane deep to the temporoparietal fascia. The temporalis muscle is located below this fascia. (**f**) Deep temporal fascia provides additional soft-tissue coverage to augment the thickness of the atrophic skin over the visible irregularities. (**g–i**) Postoperative views show gentle augmentation of the previously depressed proximal nasal dorsum. Visible and palpable irregularities have been smoothed by the fascial graft.

Case 13

Introduction

A 36-year-old woman presented with the concern of a hard, visible irregularity on the nasal dorsum 8 years after a rhinoplasty with hump removal in her Spanish homeland.

Findings

Frontal view (**Fig. 18.10a**) shows a bony irregularity on the right side of the nasal dorsum. Profile view (**Fig. 18.10b**) shows a residual hump with an irregularity. Oblique view (**Fig. 18.10c**) localizes the irregularity to the level of the rhinion at the bone-cartilage junction. Appearance 2 years after revision rhinoplasty can be seen in **Fig. 18.10d** and **Fig. 18.10e**.

Palpation

The palpable irregularity had a bony consistency and was adherent to the overlying skin.

Surgical Procedure

The soft-tissue envelope was carefully elevated from the dorsum, exposing a scar-tissue plaque several millimeters thick, which was removed in small pieces. A bony excrescence was removed from the undersurface of the skin with a small scraper blade, with all scraping movements directed toward the dorsum (**Fig. 18.10f**).

Psychology, Motivation, Personal Background

Dissatisfaction with the result of the initial operation in this case was a strong motivator for a secondary rhinoplasty. This type of situation provides a good foundation for revision surgery.

Discussion

Sites at which the periosteum is stripped, elevated, or even touched always determine the risk of granulating inflammations or late osseous reactions. Hence the surgeon should always proceed very cautiously in these areas. Visual control is very helpful in this setting.

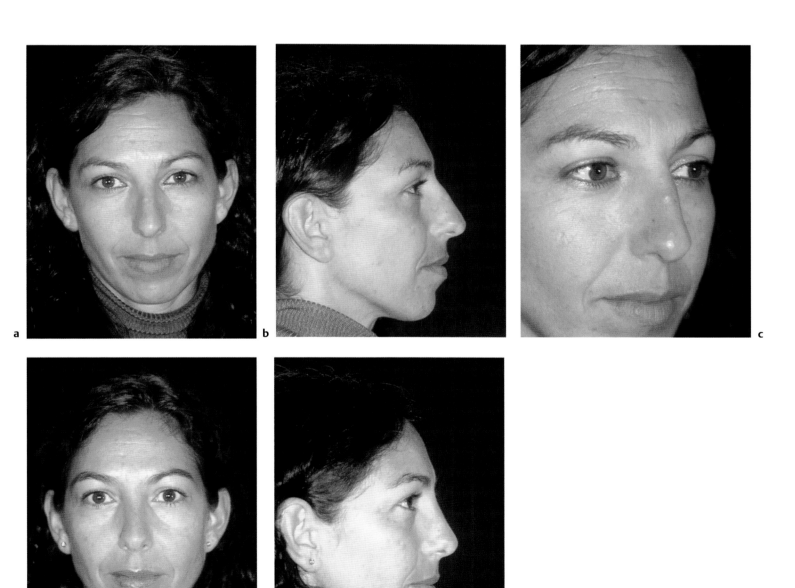

Fig. 18.10 (**a–c**) Findings 8 years after rhinoplasty. (**d, e**) Findings 2 years after revision rhinoplasty. (*Continued on next page*)

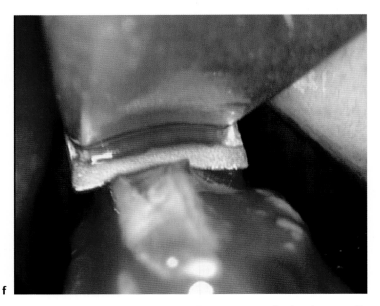

f

Fig. 18.10 (*Continued*)   (**f**) The nasal dorsum is smoothed endoscopically with specially designed miniature instruments. (Karl Storz, Tuttlingen.)

References

1. Cobo R. Correction of dorsal abnormalities in revision rhinoplasty. Facial Plast Surg 2008;24(3):327–338

2. Sykes JM. Management of the middle nasal third in revision rhinoplasty. Facial Plast Surg 2008;24(3):339–347

3. Sykes JM, Tapias V, Kim J-E. Management of the nasal dorsum. Facial Plast Surg 2011;27(2):192–202

4. Toriumi DM. Management of the middle nasal vault. Oper Tech Plast Reconstr Surg 1995;2:16–30

5. Zoumalan RA, Carron MA, Tajudeen BA, Miller PJ. Treatment of dorsal deviation. Otolaryngol Clin North Am 2009;42(3):579–586

6. Sheen JH. Spreader graft: a method of reconstructing the roof of the middle nasal vault following rhinoplasty. Plast Reconstr Surg 1984;73(2): 230–239

7. Zijlker TD, Vuyk HD. Nasal dorsal cyst after rhinoplasty. Rhinology 1993;31(2):89–91

19 Deviation of the Nasal Dorsum

"Don't you think my nose is crooked?" This question should prompt the surgeon to make a detailed search for the underlying cause. A crooked appearance of the nose may have various causes ranging from asymmetrical swelling, inadequate osteotomies, graft displacement, or residual septal deviation to less-than-optimum suture techniques.[1–4] Key factors to be considered are the time elapsed since the last operation, the choice of surgical approach, and the technique that will be used. Palpation is a reasonably accurate method of distinguishing between tissue swelling and displacement.

A deviated nasal dorsum always creates the impression of a crooked, asymmetric nose. Correction of the deviation should always be based on the anatomic problem. Deviations can be classified in simple terms as a bony or cartilaginous deviation, a C- or S-shaped deviation, or a pseudo-crooked nose due, for example, to asymmetric brow-tip aesthetic lines. It is helpful to draw an imaginary horizontal line between the pupils, then drop a straight vertical line from the center of the glabella through the nasal dorsum, tip, columella, philtrum, and menton.[5,6] This simple method can quickly distinguish between axial deviation

and asymmetry of the dorsum while also assessing the degree of facial asymmetry.

Osteotomies are the most important tool for correcting deviations of the nasal pyramid. It is important to clarify the role of residual septal deviations. In the middle third of a deviated dorsum, much can be accomplished with contouring onlay grafts that are placed in tight pockets. In patients with significant cartilaginous deviation, it should be determined whether the upper lateral cartilages are symmetrical or whether side-to-side differences have caused abnormal tension or overlaps with the alar cartilages. This will aid the surgeon in deciding among various options: detachment of the upper lateral cartilages from the septum, shortening, the placement of spreader grafts, or the use of positioning sutures. Experience has shown that osteotomies are the treatment of choice if even the slightest residual tension exists at the bone-cartilage junction. Spreader grafts have become the "workhorse" for straightening of the middle third.[7,8] They can be placed through an endonasal or open approach or may be used in an extracorporeal septoplasty.

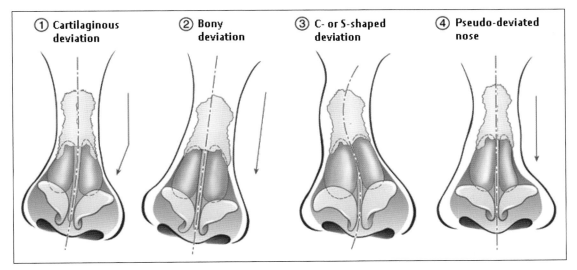

① Cartilaginous deviation **② Bony deviation** **③ C- or S-shaped deviation** **④ Pseudo-deviated nose**

Fig. 19.1 Different types of nasal deviation.

Case 14

Introduction

An 18-year-old male presented 2 years after a previous septoplasty with a desire to have his nose straightened and "shortened."

Findings

Frontal view (**Fig. 19.2a**) shows a bony deviation of the nose to the left. Profile view (**Fig. 19.2b**) shows an overprojected nasal tip. Basal view (**Fig. 19.2c**) shows elliptical nostrils with narrowing of the valve area. **Fig. 19.2d**, **Fig. 19.2e**, and **Fig. 19.2f** are follow-up views taken 2 years after revision surgery.

Surgical Procedure

Operative details: closed approach, resection of the medial crural footplates, submucous septoplasty, and dislocation of the alar cartilages with lateral sliding. Medial and lateral curved osteotomies were performed on both sides, with a double osteotomy and wedge resection on the right side and a single osteotomy on the left side (**Fig. 19.2g, h**).

Psychology, Motivation, Personal Background

The patient was highly motivated to have his overprojected nose straightened and deprojected.

Discussion

The decision for a closed approach was based on the symmetrical nasal tip and the anticipated effects of the endonasal manipulations.

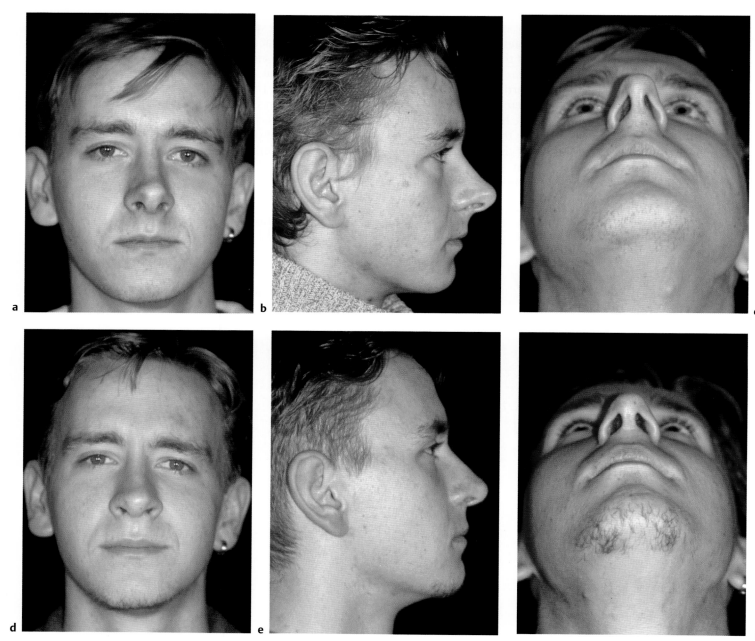

Fig. 19.2 (**a–c**) Preoperative findings. (**d–f**) Findings 2 years after revision rhinoplasty.

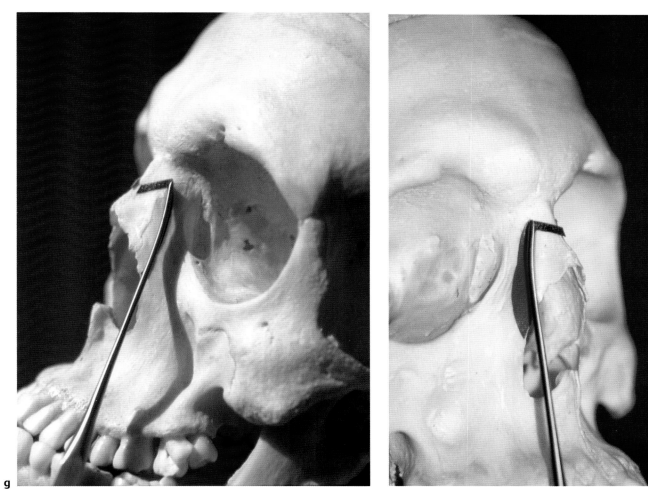

g   h

Fig. 19.2 (**g, h**) Principle of a lateral curved osteotomy and a double curved osteotomy with a wedge excision on the right side, demonstrated in a model skull.

Case 15

Introduction

A 25-year-old woman presented with the desire to have her nose straightened. She also wanted a nasal hump removed to harmonize her profile. She had breathing issues as well, particularly on the left side. One year after primary rhinoplasty she presented again with the concern of an asymmetrical nasal dorsum.

Initial Findings

Frontal view before primary rhinoplasty (**Fig. 19.3a**) shows asymmetry of the nasal dorsum with convexity on the right side and concavity on the left side in the supratip area. Profile view (**Fig. 19.3b**) shows overcorrection of the dorsum with a scooped appearance. Basal view (**Fig. 19.3c**) shows slight widening of the nasal tip. **Fig. 19.3g**, **Fig. 19.3h**, **Fig. 19.3i**, and **Fig. 19.3j** were taken 2 years after revision surgery.

Surgical Procedure

Primary rhinoplasty: hemitransfixion incision, submucous septoplasty, splitting approach, en bloc resection of the bony and cartilaginous hump, medial and lateral curved osteotomies with a double osteotomy on the left side.

Revision rhinoplasty: lysis of dorsal scars and adhesions, additional cephalic alar cartilage reduction, and augmentation of the opposite side with the removed cartilage. Augmentation of the supratip area.

Psychology, Motivation, Personal Background

The patient had positive and realistic expectations and self-image. Her understandable desire for a symmetrical nose was the goal of the revision rhinoplasty.

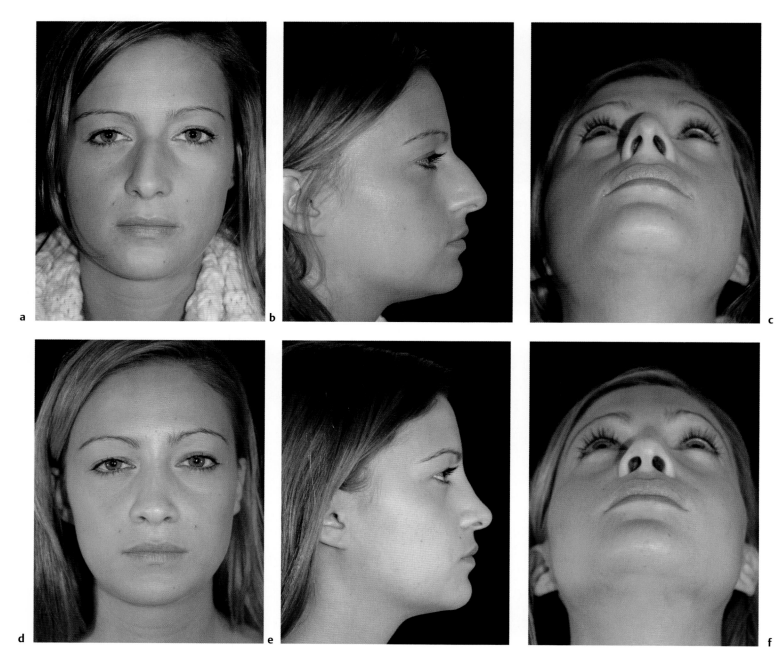

Fig. 19.3 (**a–c**) Findings before the primary rhinoplasty. (**d–f**) Findings before revision rhinoplasty.

Discussion

This case illustrates the risk of dorsal deviation due to the asymmetrical resection of structural elements as well as the unpredictable postoperative change that may occur in the supportive function of the anterior septal cartilage, with an associated risk of unintended collapse.

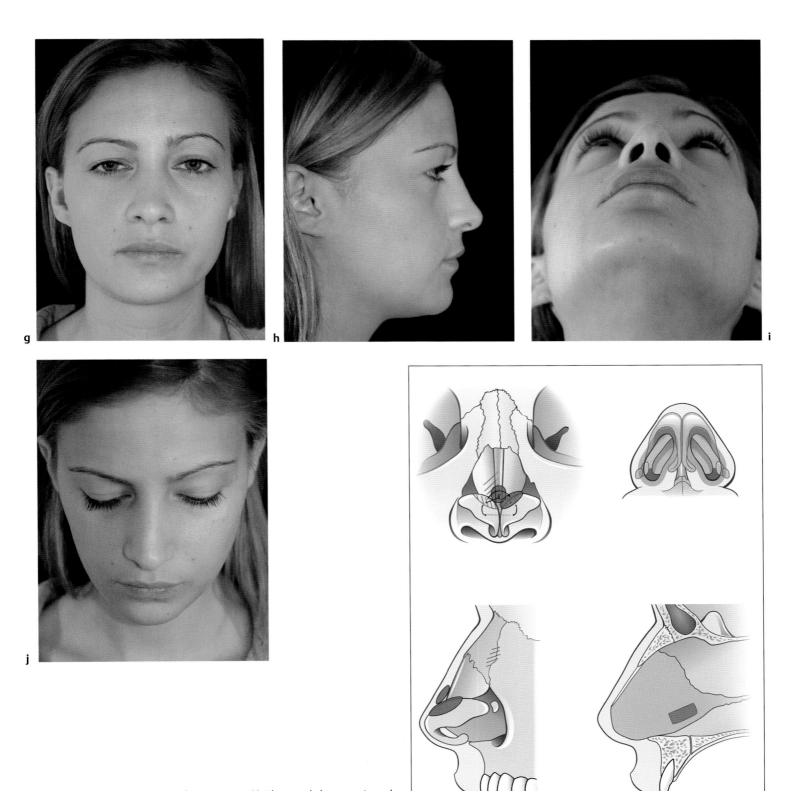

Fig. 19.3 (**g–i**) Two years after revision. (**j**) The nasal dorsum viewed from above. (**k**) Steps involved in the primary and secondary rhinoplasties (red, resections; blue, grafts).

Case 16

This case illustrates the postoperative deviation of an L-shaped rib graft (operation by Wolfgang Gubisch).

Introduction

After sustaining nasal trauma in childhood and undergoing one previous operation 37 years ago, the patient presented at age 58 with severe functional problems. The L-shaped rib graft was extremely deviated and also fractured.

Findings

On inspection, the patient had a severely twisted nose 37 years after undergoing nasal reconstruction with an autologous rib graft. The costal cartilage had become deviated over the years (**Fig. 19.4a**). The skin over the dorsum was altered and showed telangiectasias (**Figs. 19.4a, b**). In basal view the columella was off the midline and the entire vestibule was deviated (**Fig. 19.4c**). The nasal pyramid was very wide and asymmetrical (**Fig. 19.4a**). Viewed in profile, the root of the nose appears too deep (**Fig. 19.4b**). The vestibular mucosa was very dry on endonasal inspection.

Surgical Procedure

The revision employed an open approach through the old columellar scar using a standard inverted-V incision. Analysis revealed a deviated L-shaped rib graft in the columella, the upper portion of which had been fractured (**Fig. 19.4g**). Conchal cartilage was harvested from the left ear to customize a double-layer sandwich graft for reconstructing the columella and anterior septal border (**Fig. 19.4h**). Though the anterior nasal spine was rudimentary, it was possible to drill a hole through it for fixation of the sandwich graft. The wide bony pyramid was corrected with a lateral low-to-low osteotomy, paramedian osteotomy, and

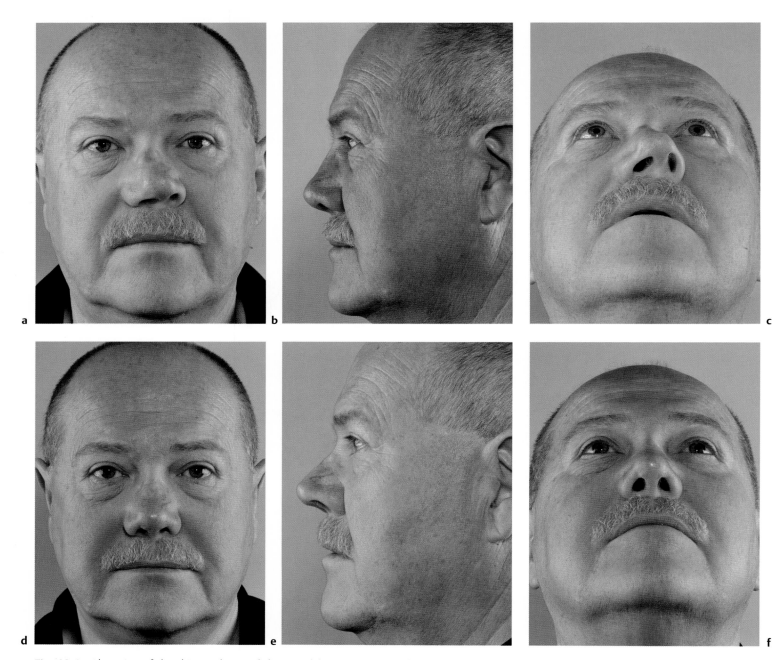

Fig. 19.4 Alteration of the skin on the nasal dorsum. (**a**) Preoperative frontal view shows a severely twisted nose and an extremely deviated nasal tip. (**b**) Profile view. The nose is too short, the columella is retracted, the tip is overprojected, and the dorsum is too low over the nasal root. (**c**) Basal view shows displacement and deviation of the columella and nostril asymmetry. (**d**) Postoperative frontal view shows a stable result 1 year after revision septorhinoplasty. (**e**) Profile view after revision. (**f**) Basal view shows symmetrical nostrils and a straight columella.

transverse osteotomy performed on both sides. The nasal dorsum was reconstructed with diced cartilage wrapped in autologous deep temporal fascia (**Fig. 19.4i, j**), followed by the placement of a shield graft and rim grafts made of costal cartilage.

Psychology, Motivation, Personal Background

The patient suffered from nasal airway obstruction and from the aesthetic appearance of his twisted nose. The skin over the dorsum was very thin, altered, and showed telangiectasias. The patient told us that 37 years ago the skin in that area had undergone second-intention healing. One year after revision rhinoplasty, he is happy with the functional and aesthetic outcome (**Fig. 19.4d–f**).

Discussion

Instead of DCF (diced cartilage in fascia), onlay grafts made from conchal cartilage or auricle cartilage had to be used. Sometimes these grafts become displaced and palpable, however. Grafts made of costal cartilage have the disadvantage of becoming deviated over the years.

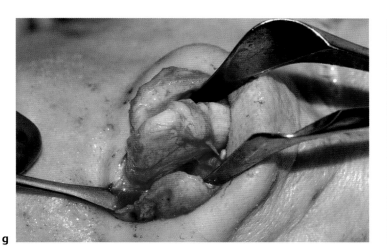

g

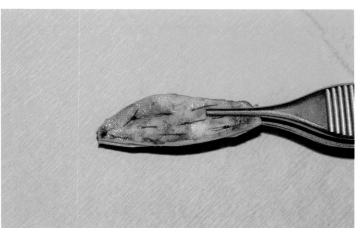

h

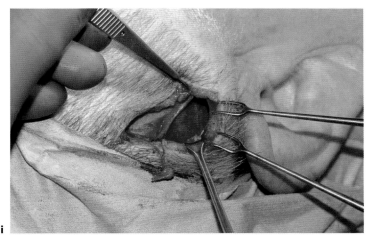

i

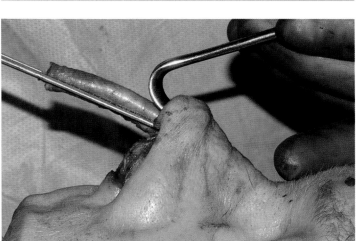

j

Fig. 19.4 (**g**) The L-strut (rib graft) is extremely deviated, behind the midline, and fractured in its upper portion. (**h**) A double-layer conchal sandwich graft is tailored for use as a septal extension graft and for reconstructing the anterior septal border. (**i**) Deep temporal fascia is harvested. (**j**) The nasal dorsum is reconstructed with diced cartilage wrapped in autologous temporal muscle fascia.

Case 17

This case illustrates the severe deviation of a rib graft with complete obstruction of the left vestibule (operation by Jacqueline Eichhorn-Sens).

Introduction

A 63-year-old man presented 40 years after nasal trauma followed by multiple previous nasal operations. Twenty-seven years after the last revision surgery and nasal reconstruction with an L-shaped rib graft, the patient presented with an extreme deviation of the graft and complete obstruction of the left vestibule.

Findings

The left vestibule was completely obstructed by an extremely deviated and broken rib graft (**Fig. 19.5c**). The patient was unable to breath through the left nostril. The skin on the nasal dorsum was altered after multiple previous operations (**Fig. 19.5a, b**).

Palpation revealed an unnaturally rigid tip and a thick columella that "clicked" when moved across the midline.

Surgical Procedure

Conchal cartilage was harvested (**Fig. 19.5g**) and used to fabricate a double-layer sandwich graft (**Fig. 19.5h, i**). The nose was exposed through an open approach, and the deviated rib graft was found at the columella. The rib graft was also found to be broken into three pieces. The caudal piece was securely fixed by scar tissue in the area of the anterior nasal spine. The original anterior nasal spine could not be found, so a hole was drilled through the caudal piece of the rib graft. This appeared to be the best way to fix the conchal cartilage sandwich graft, which was used as a septal extension graft and columellar strut (**Fig. 19.5j**). The conchal sandwich graft was fixed to the drill hole with nonabsorbable sutures. The caudal end of the double-layer conchal sandwich graft was joined in tongue-in-groove fashion to the old

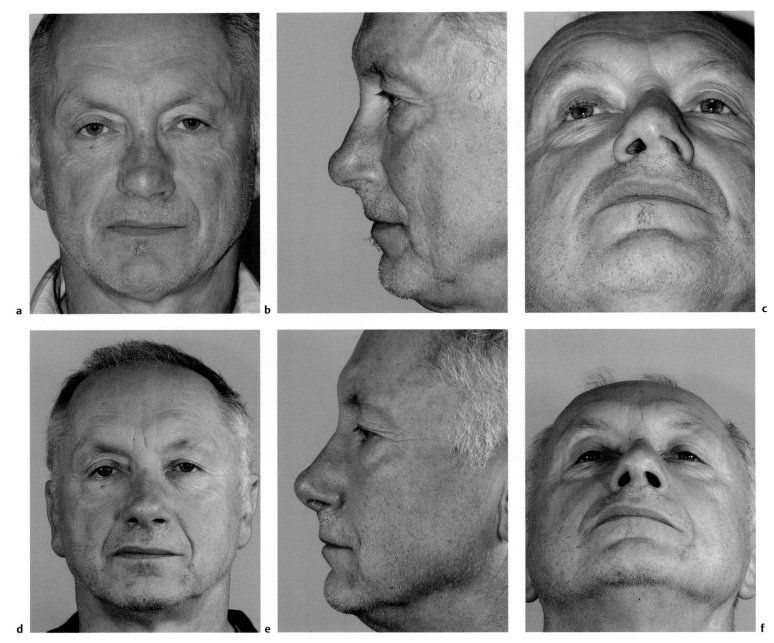

Fig. 19.5 (**a**) Preoperative frontal view shows alteration of the dorsal nasal skin after multiple previous operations. The tip is not well defined. The brow-tip aesthetic lines are interrupted bilaterally in the supratip area. (**b**) Profile view. The tip has a protuberant appearance. (**c**) Basal view shows extreme deviation of the columella and obstruction of the left vestibule. (**d**) Postoperative frontal view 7 months after revision rhinoplasty. (**e**) Profile view after revision shows an harmonious nasal dorsum and tip. (**f**) Basal view documents correction of the nasal vestibule.

piece of rib cartilage. The other pieces of rib cartilage were found to be extremely deviated and had to be removed. Transdomal sutures and a spanning suture were placed for tip correction.

Psychology, Motivation, Personal Background

This patient had sustained severe nasal trauma 40 years ago and underwent several operations thereafter. It had been 27 years since the last operation. The rib graft that had been used to reconstruct the anterior septum became more and more deviated over the years. Now the left vestibule was completely obstructed by the deviated rib graft in the columella. The patient complained

that he had to periodically remove foul-smelling material from the left nostril because the deviated splint obstructed normal drainage. The main goal of the revision, then, was to correct the functional problems. One year after revision surgery the patient was very satisfied with the result (**Fig. 19.5d–f**).

Discussion

We prefer to use an auricular sandwich graft as a columellar strut so that the columella itself is not stiff. This is one advantage over using rib cartilage or perpendicular plate in the area of the anterior septal border.

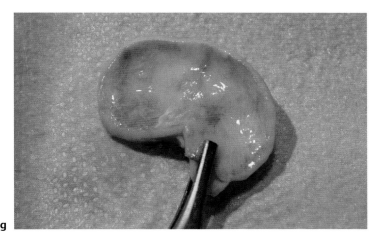
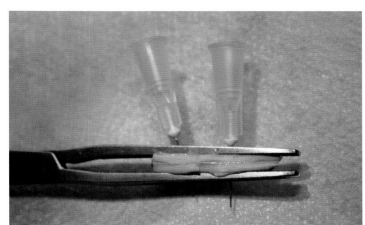
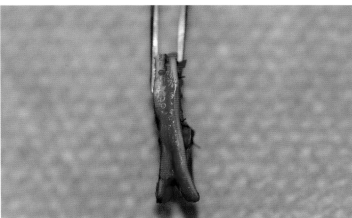
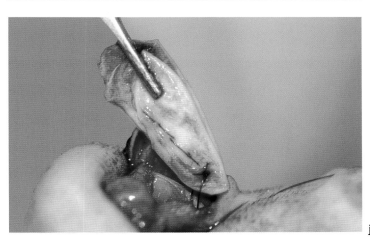

Fig. 19.5 (**g**) Conchal cartilage is harvested. (**h**) An Aiach–Gubisch forceps helps to hold the graft together in an ideal position. A running suture provides definitive fixation. (**i**) The graft is straight. The "feet" of the graft ride upon the remaining straight rib cartilage. (**j**) The sandwich graft is placed between the medial crura and fixed to the rib cartilage, septum, and between the medial crura with nonabsorbable sutures.

Case 18

Introduction

A 54-year-old woman presented with photographs that had been taken at age 25 (**Fig. 19.6a, b**). Years later she was involved in a severe traffic accident, sustaining midfacial fractures that destroyed the bony and cartilaginous nasal skeleton. Afterward she underwent three septorhinoplasties elsewhere using autologous rib cartilage, the most recent performed 6 years ago. She presented now with marked deviation of the nasal dorsum.

Findings

Frontal view (**Fig. 19.6c**) shows deviation of the cartilaginous nasal dorsum by a displaced and warped rib graft. Profile view (**Fig. 19.6d**) shows a short nose, a large nasolabial angle, and a cartilaginous hump. Basal view (**Fig. 19.6e**) shows nostril asymmetry. Endonasal inspection revealed a 5-mm septal perforation. Bilateral otapostasis was also present.

Findings 3 years after the last revision rhinoplasty

Fig. 19.6f, **Fig. 19.6g**, and **Fig. 19.6h** were taken after the first revision. **Fig. 19.6i**, **Fig. 19.6j**, and **Fig. 19.6k** were taken after the second revision.

Surgical Procedures

One revision rhinoplasty was performed, followed by a finesse rhinoplasty to correct minor imperfections.

1. Conchal cartilage was harvested bilaterally during otoplasty, and an infundibulotomy was performed. A mucosal flap was taken from the lateral nasal wall. The septal cartilage was deepithelialized around the perforation on the left side, and the mucosa was glued to the left side and opposite side. The septal cartilage was exposed through an open approach, and a septal extension graft of conchal cartilage was placed to reconstruct the deficient anterior septal cartilage (**Fig. 19.6l**).

   The deviated rib graft was removed and "balanced." An onlay graft was fashioned from the conchal cartilage and portions of the rib graft. A columellar strut was fabricated from portions of the old rib graft, and an onlay graft from the old graft and conchal cartilage. A tip graft was placed, and the nasolabial angle was augmented with septal cartilage.

2. For refinement, retroauricular connective tissue was harvested and used to fill in the areas on both sides of the onlay graft.

Psychology, Motivation, Personal Background

The patient's strongest desire was to regain her original nose before the injury. In contrast to typical aesthetic motivations for a desired change, this patient wanted reconstructive surgery to restore the original status. In many cases, as in this one, rhinoplasty expectations include the desire for a rejuvenating effect.

Discussion

The goal of the revision was to restore symmetry by straightening and lengthening the nose. Many pathways lead to Rome, including the one taken in the present case.

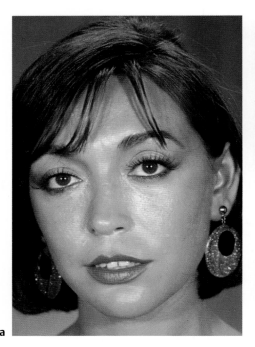
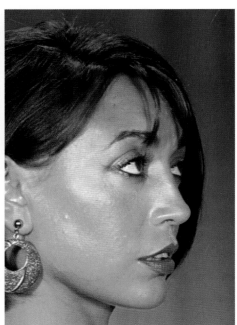

a   b

Fig. 19.6   (**a, b**) Frontal and profile views of the patient as a young woman.

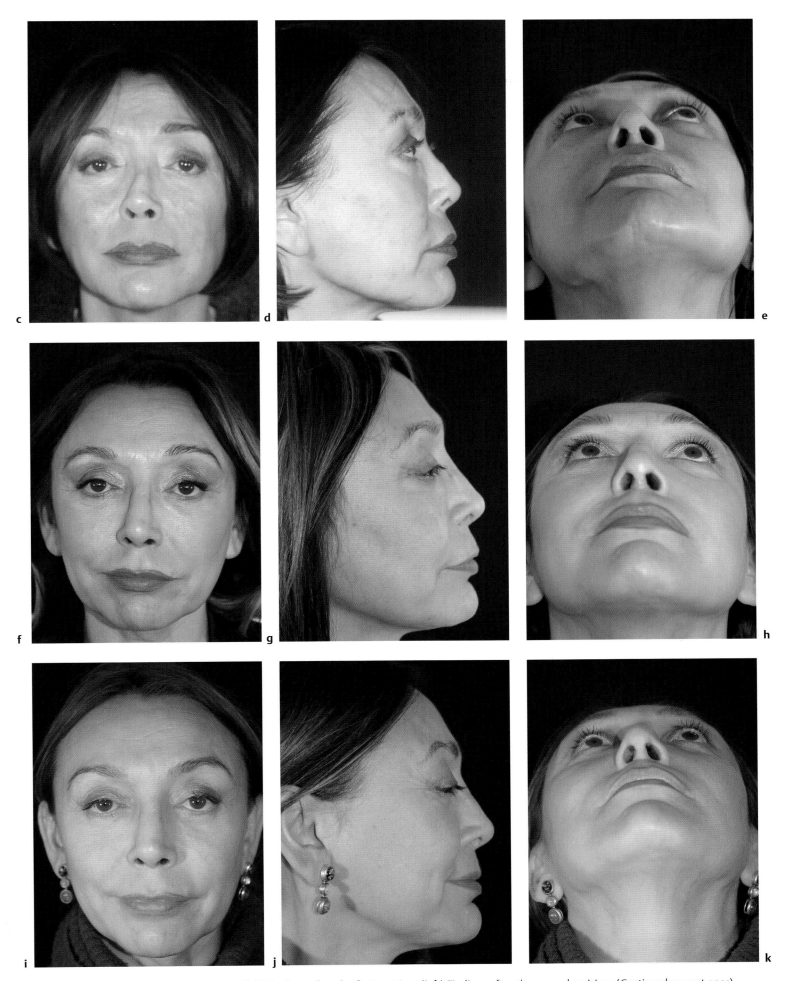

Fig. 19.6 (**c–e**) Findings before revision. (**f–h**) Findings after the first revision. (**i–k**) Findings after the second revision. (*Continued on next page*)

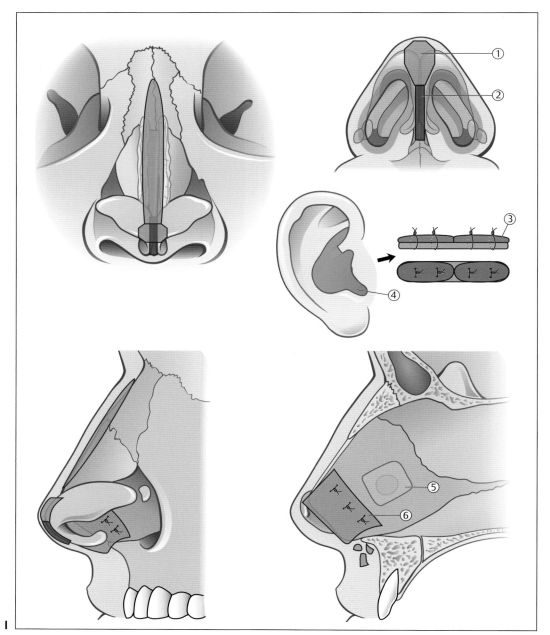

Fig. 19.6 (*Continued*)   (**I**) Surgical steps involved in the two revisions. 1, tip graft; 2, shield graft; 3, external making of long and thick dorsal onlay graft; 4, harvesting area of conchal cartilage; 5, closure of a septal perforation, mucosa patch on the left side; 6, septal extension graft.

References

1. Gunter JP, Rohrich RJ. Management of the deviated nose. The importance of septal reconstruction. Clin Plast Surg 1988;15(1):43–55

2. Johnson CM Jr, Anderson JR. The deviated nose—its correction. Laryngoscope 1977;87(10 Pt 1):1680–1684

3. Shipchandler TZ, Papel ID. The crooked nose. Facial Plast Surg 2011;27(2):203–212

4. Sykes JM, Kim J-E, Shaye D, Boccieri A. The importance of the nasal septum in the deviated nose. Facial Plast Surg 2011;27(5):413–421

5. Shah AR, Constantinides M. Aligning the bony nasal vault in rhinoplasty. Facial Plast Surg 2006;22(1):3–8

6. Zoumalan RA, Carron MA, Tajudeen BA, Miler PJ. Treatment of dorsal deviation. Otolaryngol Clin N Am 2009:579–586

7. Toriumi DM. Management of the middle nasal vault. Oper Tech Plast Reconst 1995;2:16–30

8. Wagner W, Schraven SP. Spreader grafts in septorhinoplasty [in German]. Laryngorhinootologie 2011;90(5):264–274

20 Multiple Nasal Injuries

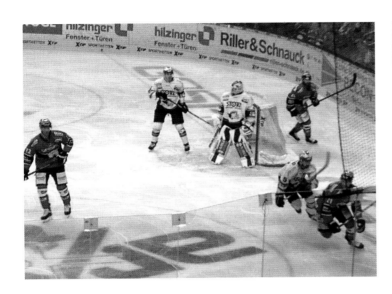

Multiple injuries to the nose create a special set of tissue circumstances involving the postoperative consolidation of fractures in a more or less optimal position, the presence of organized hematomas, and periosteum that is thickened and obliterated due to scarring.[1] These changes are typical of injuries sustained in contact sports such as boxing, ball sports, and ice hockey, which typically lead to repetitive trauma that includes fractures of the nasal bones and cartilage. The surgical correction of these noses follows special laws that relate to problems of tissue memory. Emphasis is placed upon wide undermining of the soft-tissue envelope with the division of adhesions and the resection of excess scar tissue. Posttraumatic humps should be removed in continuity with the periosteum, which is fixed by scar tissue and generally cannot be dissected. Low lateral osteotomies may provide definitive closure of an open roof. If this is unsuccessful, the use of extended spreader grafts or closure with fascia lata or a cartilaginous onlay graft is indicated. **Fig. 20.1** illustrates the pathogenic mechanism of a posttraumatic periosteal reaction with the formation of a typical hump.

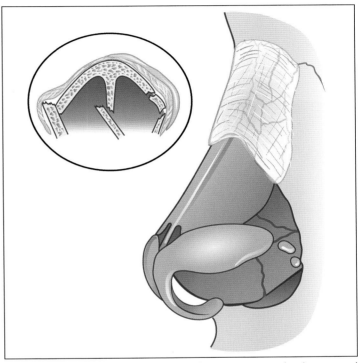

Fig. 20.1 Posttraumatic scar block formation over the bony nasal pyramid in patients with multiple nasal injuries.

Case 19

Introduction

A 22-year-old man sustained multiple nasal injuries resulting in a posttraumatic nasal hump and deviated septum.

Findings

Frontal view (**Fig. 20.2a**) shows a posttraumatic hump with asymmetric widening of the nasal pyramid. Profile view (**Fig. 20.2b**) and three-quarter view (**Fig. 20.2c**) show a bony dorsal hump.

Fig. 20.2d, **Fig. 20.2e**, and **Fig. 20.2f** show corresponding views taken 2 years after revision surgery.

Surgical Procedure

The deviated septum was removed through a hemitransfixion incision and straightened extracorporeally. The straight neoseptum was then reimplanted along with spreader grafts. The dorsal hump was removed en bloc, and medial and lateral curved osteotomies were performed (**Fig. 20.2g**).

Psychology, Motivation, Personal Background

Nasal airway obstruction can be a serious handicap, especially in competitive sports. Nasal bone fractures are a frequent occurrence in contact sports such as ice hockey, ball sports, boxing, and judo. The old maxim that a boxer's nose should be straightened only after retirement cannot be consistently followed. Repetitive trauma, dislocations, or posttraumatic epistaxis will often necessitate surgical intervention.

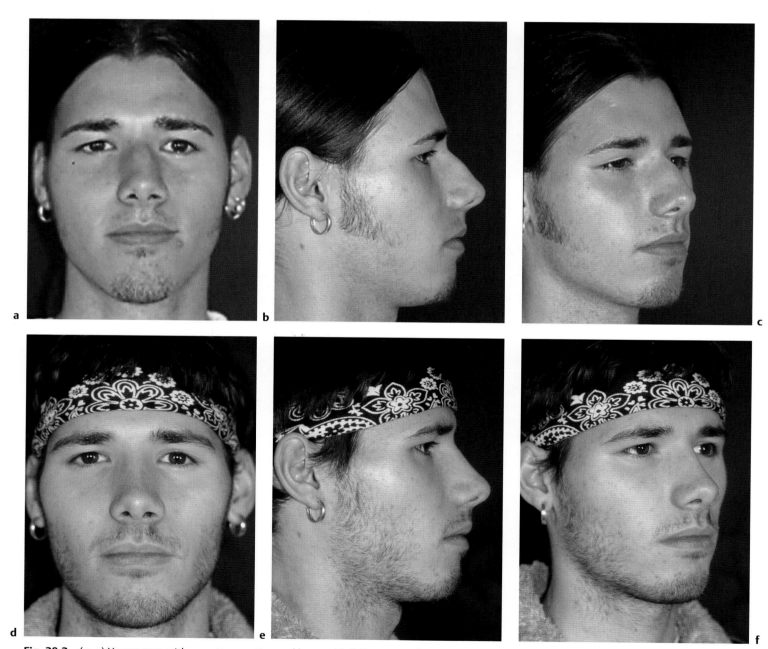

Fig. 20.2   (**a–c**) Young man with a posttraumatic nasal hump. (**d–f**) Two years after revision rhinoplasty.

Discussion

The greater the frequency of repetitive nasal injuries, the more likely it is that associated tissue changes will compromise wound healing and aesthetic outcome. Atraumatic elevators are available for fracture reduction and can often be used successfully for up to 10 days after the injury.[2] A definitive reduction may be done through an open or closed approach, depending on the fracture type and degree of displacement, and this should minimize subsequent nasal deformity.[3–5] Multiple nasal injuries lead to changes that may include dense scar tissue forming between all the layers of the soft-tissue envelope, bone thickening due to appositional bone growth, and greater tissue memory.

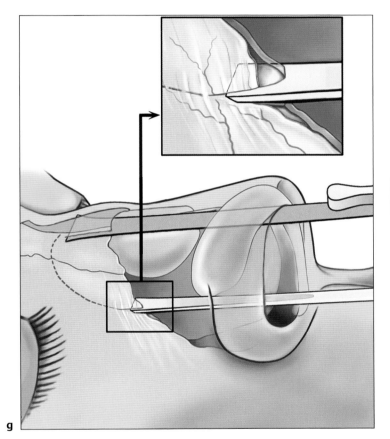

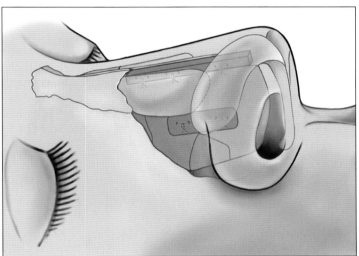

g   h

Fig. 20.2 (**g**) Removal of the posttraumatic hump and scar block formation. (**h**) Reconstruction of the nasal septum and dorsum with cartilaginous struts and spreader grafts.

Case 20

This case involves a severely twisted and short saddle nose with complete absence of the medial and intermediate crura (operation by Jacqueline Eichhorn-Sens).

Introduction

The patient sustained severe nasal trauma with a major loss of bony and cartilaginous framework. In recent years he had undergone 12 nasal operations elsewhere to improve the functional and aesthetic outcome. When seen at our department, he had a severe deformity of the nasal dorsum, painful columellar scars, and obstructed nasal breathing. He presented a severely twisted and short nose with complete loss of the nasal septum and a massive septal perforation.

Findings

Inspection revealed a conspicuous twisted and short nose with an S-shaped dorsum (**Fig. 20.3a**). A saddle nose deformity was visible in profile (**Fig. 20.3c**). The tip looked very wide and the tip defining points were asymmetric (**Fig. 20.3a**). Several deep scars were present in the dorsum. Also, two contracted scars were atypically located in the columella (**Fig. 20.3b**). That area was very tender to palpation, which disclosed a hard, extremely retracted columella. On palpation of the nasal dorsum, the old rib graft was found to be broken and deviated. Also, the nasal bones were absent and had been replaced by dense scar tissue. Endonasal inspection revealed a massive septal perforation. Except for the anterior septal support, no septal material could be found.

Surgical Procedure

An open approach was done through the cranially contracted scar. A scar revision was also done. Massive scars were found at the nasal tip and retracted columella. On dissecting the tip, we found a complete absence of both the medial and intermediate crura (**Fig. 20.3g**). Only a small remnant of the original anterior septal border was still in place. The "septum" consisted entirely of a rib graft splint, held in place by dense scar tissue.

The anterior nasal spine was missing. It was difficult to remove the broken and deviated dorsal rib graft (**Fig. 20.3h**). We found dense scar tissue in place of the lateral nasal bones. We attempted to release the scar tissue at the narrow right aperture. Costal cartilage was harvested and customized to reconstruct the nasal dorsum. The rib graft was sutured to the nasal root above and to a remaining straight piece of old costal cartilage below. The dorsum was additionally reconstructed with diced costal cartilage wrapped in a tube of autologous deep temporal fascia (DCF, diced cartilage in fascia). The alar cartilages were reconstructed with strips of costal cartilage using the bending technique[6,7] (**Fig. 20.3i**). Due to the brittle consistency of the costal cartilage and the thick skin over the nasal tip, a dome division technique had to be used to reconstitute the dome. Then the tip was configured with transdomal and interdomal sutures, a spanning suture, and finally a tip graft and two shield grafts made of costal cartilage, resulting in a longer columella (**Fig. 20.3j**). Silicone film was placed for two weeks to maintain patency of the corrected right vestibule.

Psychology, Motivation, Personal Background

The patient suffered from a poor functional and aesthetic outcome after 12 previous operations for severe nasal trauma. He was an avid diver and complained that he could not dive with a mask because of the extremely retracted, stiff, and painful columella. Thus, he was highly motivated to undergo another revision rhinoplasty. At 18 months postoperatively the patient is very pleased with the functional outcome and appearance of his nose (**Fig. 20.3d–f**) and has no problems with his mask while diving.

Discussion

The ideal solution would have been to correct the hidden columella with a double-layer conchal sandwich placed as a septal extension graft. Unfortunately, that option did not exist in this case due to heavy scarring of the columella, which made it impossible to move the columellar tissues to a more caudal position.

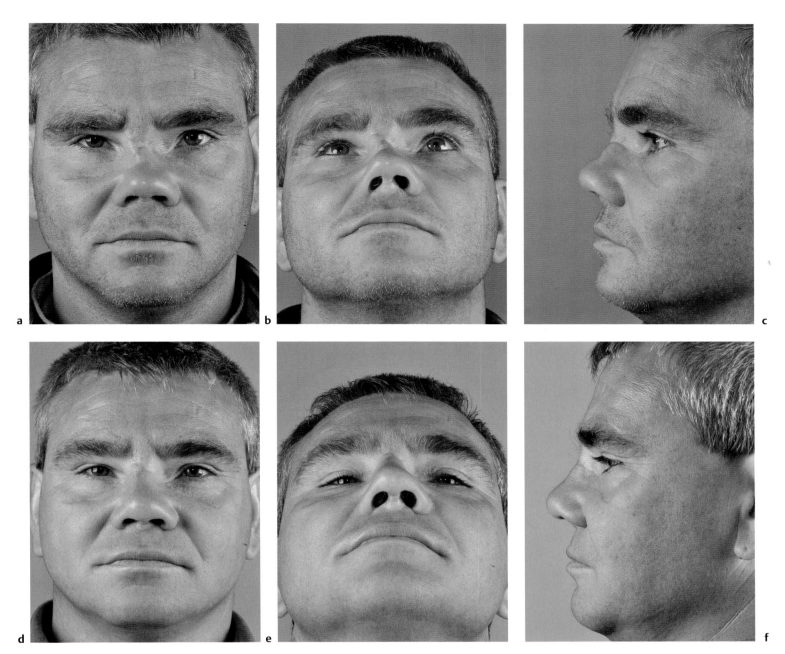

Fig. 20.3 Pre- and postoperative views. (**a**) The short, twisted nose is clearly evident in the frontal view. The nasal tip is undefined. The tip defining points are asymmetric and widely spaced. (**b**) Undefined tip in the basal view. The nostrils are asymmetric. The twisted dorsum and old scars over the nasal dorsum are visible. (**c**) The profile view shows a short saddle nose. The columella is not visible, and the tip is overrotated and over-projected. (**d**) Frontal view 18 months after revision rhinoplasty shows a straight nasal axis. The tip defining points are symmetric and the tip has a more harmonious look. (**e**) Basal view after revision rhinoplasty shows symmetrical nostrils. (**f**) Postoperative profile view at 18 months shows restoration of a normal nasal length. The saddle nose has been corrected and the tip is well projected and supported. (*Continued on next page*)

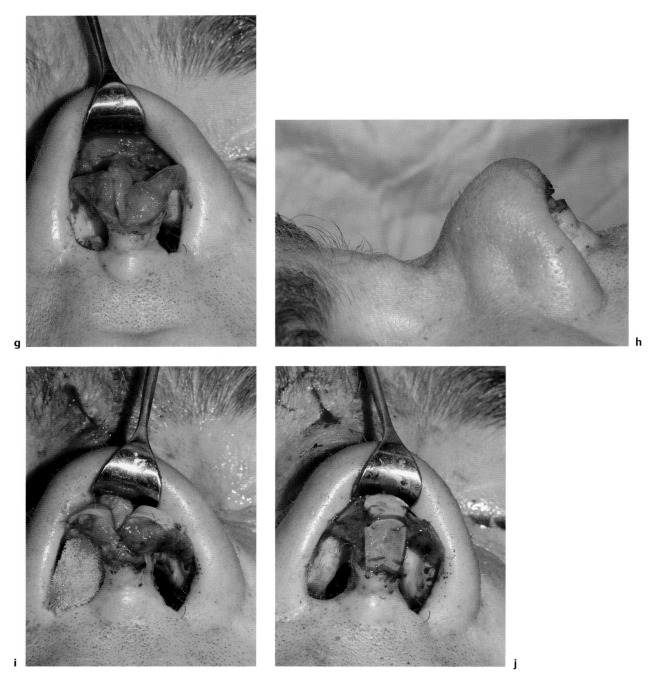

Fig. 20.3 (*Continued*)   (**g**) At operation the medial and intermediate crura were found to be absent on both sides. This view also shows that the right vestibule is obstructed by strictures and a narrow piriform aperture. (**h**) The fractured and deviated dorsal rib graft has been removed, leaving an extreme saddle nose deformity and severe irregularities in the nasal dorsum. (**i**) The missing portions of the lower cartilages are reconstructed with strips of costal cartilage using the bending technique. (**j**) The tip is reconfigured with transdomal and interdomal sutures and refined with a tip graft and shield graft fashioned from costal cartilage.

References

1. Kaschke O. Nasal trauma. In: Behrbohm H, Tardy ME, eds. Essentials of Septorhinoplasty. New York, NY: Thieme; 2003:220–231

2. Behrbohm H, Kaschke O. Elevatorium für Frakturen des Os nasale und des Arcus zygomaticus. Laryngorhinootologie 1998;77(1):52–53

3. Renner GJ. Management of nasal fractures. Otolaryngol Clin North Am 1991;24(1):195–213

4. Rohrich RJ, Adams WP Jr. Nasal fracture management: minimizing secondary nasal deformities. Plast Reconstr Surg 2000;106(2):266–273

5. Simmen D. [Nasal fractures—indications for open reposition]. Laryngorhinootologie 1998;77(7):388–393

6. Gubisch W, Eichhorn-Sens J. Overresection of the lower lateral cartilages: a common conceptual mistake with functional and aesthetic consequences. Aesthetic Plast Surg 2009;33(1):6–13

7. Eichhorn-Sens J, Gubisch W. Ausgedehnte Resektion der Flügelknorpel —ein falsches Konzept zur Verschmälerung der Nase. HNO 2009;57(11): 113–120

21 Nasal Refinement with Minimal Changes

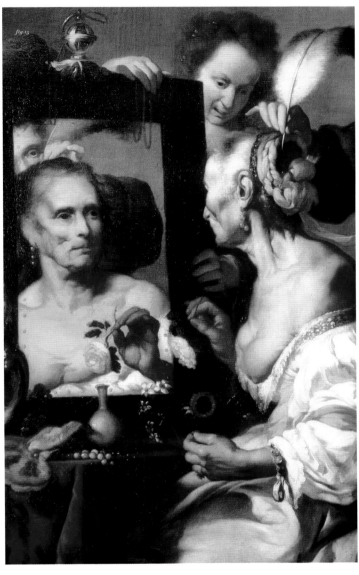

Fig. 21.1 *Vanity* by Bernardo Strozzi (1630).

Small morphologic changes can lead to major complaints and significant functional problems. They should not be taken lightly, because patients expect a perfect result and the devil is often in the details.[1] A good rule to remember: the smaller the anatomic problem, the greater the aesthetic expectations.

Case 21

Introduction
A 19-year-old woman presented 8 months after a functional and aesthetic rhinoplasty with hump removal, complaining of an unsightly step deformity in the left bony nasal pyramid. She also claimed that she had more difficulty breathing through the left side of her nose than through the right side.

Findings
Frontal view (**Fig. 21.2a**) shows a displaced osteotomy fragment on the left side. Profile view (**Fig. 21.2b**) shows a small residual hump. The step deformity is clearly visible in the overhead view (**Fig. 21.2c**).

Fig. 21.2d, **Fig. 21.2e**, and **Fig. 21.2f** show corresponding views taken 2 years after revision rhinoplasty.

Surgical Procedure
The soft-tissue envelope was sparingly undermined, and a reosteotomy was performed on the left side (see Case 20). A spreader graft was placed on the left side through an endonasal approach (**Fig. 21.2g, h**).

Psychology, Motivation, Personal Background
The patient's initial joy over her "new nose" was soon dampened by a deformity of the nasal pyramid. She welcomed the recommendation to proceed with immediate revision surgery.

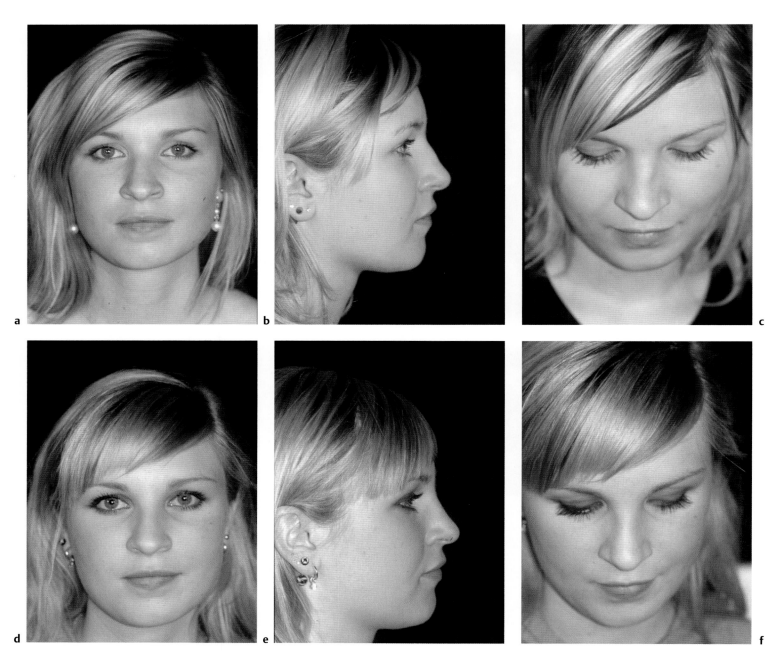

Fig. 21.2 (**a–c**) Findings 8 months after primary rhinoplasty. (**d–f**) Two years after revision rhinoplasty.

Discussion

The general recommendation is that osteotomies be used to completely mobilize and reposition the fragments. The medial and lateral osteotomy curves intersect at one point. In some cases the great mobility produced by osteotomies will allow the repositioned fragments to become displaced. It may be advantageous to leave a small, high bony bridge no more than 1 mm wide, which is audibly infractured at the end of the operation by pressing on it with the thumb. In this technique the surgeon leaves a fragment attached at least at one point so that it cannot "float." In the case described, a reosteotomy was performed to lateralize the medially displaced fragment. A spreader graft must be accurately placed in the extramucosal plane below the nasal dorsum and advanced to the piriform aperture.

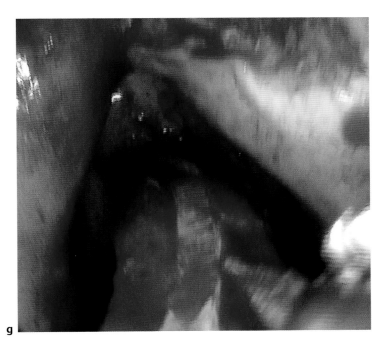

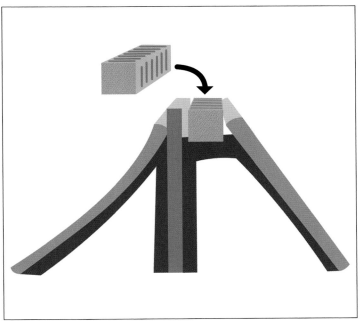

Fig. 21.2 (**g**) Endoscopic placement of a spreader graft. (**h**) Diagram showing the position and effect of a unilateral spreader graft.

Case 22

Introduction
A 42-year-old woman was concerned by a minor asymmetry in the right nasal pyramid left by a nasal injury that had occurred 20 years earlier. She had always been bothered by the slight deformity but never found the time to address it. Now she was finally resolved to take action.

Findings
Frontal view (**Fig. 21.3a**) shows an asymmetry on the right side of the nasal pyramid caused by a laterally displaced fragment. Profile view (**Fig. 21.3b**) shows a slightly overprojected nose. Basal view (**Fig. 21.3c**) shows asymmetry of the nasal base.

Surgical Procedure
A submucous septoplasty was performed with resection of a basal strip (see **Fig. 21.3g**). Medial and lateral curved osteotomies were performed on the right side (**Fig. 21.3g**).

Psychology, Motivation, Personal Background
Although the cosmetic flaw in this case was very minor, the patient had carried it with her for decades. Her desire for a "perfect nose" was very sincere and deeply held. In this respect a minor morphologic problem can sometimes assume major psychological importance. Here the patient and doctor embarked on a "quest" that would result in a happy or an unhappy patient.

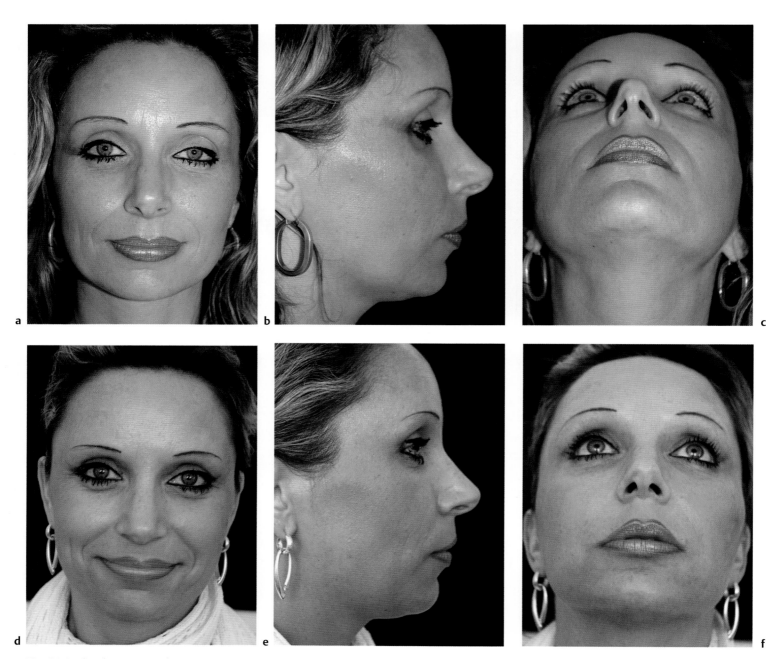

Fig. 21.3 (**a–c**) Woman with posttraumatic asymmetry of the nasal pyramid. (**d–f**) The patient 1 year after surgery.

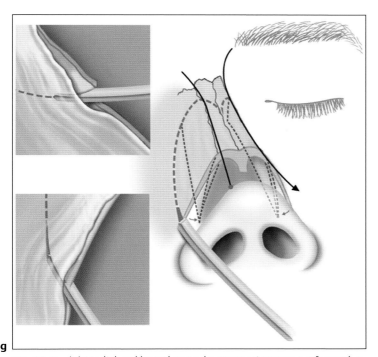

g

Fig. 21.3   (**g**) Medial and lateral curved osteotomies were performed on the right side using a mini-osteotome.

References

1. Tardy ME, Heinrich JA, Lindbeck EO. Refinement of the nasal tip. Rhinoplasty 2001. Chicago. Course Manual, 564–593

22 Functional Tension Nose and the Overprojected Nose

22.1 Functional Tension Nose

"Tension nose" is commonly associated with an overprojected nose or nasal tip. Due to the presence of excess cartilage, a functional tension nose is often disharmonious in relation to the face.

22.1.1 Measurement of Overprojection

Jacques Joseph used the profile angle as a measure of overprojection.[1] He defined it as the angle formed by the intersection of two straight lines: one drawn tangent to the glabella and chin, and one drawn tangent to the nasal dorsum. Joseph reported a normal range of 23 to 37 degrees. Richard Goode recommended the ratio of nasal length, measured as the distance between the nasion and pronasale, and projection, measured between the alar crease and the pronasale, for evaluating underprojection or overprojection of the nose and nasal tip. He defined the normal range as a ratio of 0.55–0.60.[2]

Charles Baud described a method of profile analysis in which he drew a circle around the face, using the distance from the external auditory canal to the pronasale (tip defining point) as the radius. He then assessed the relationship of three key profile points: the pronasale, the pogonium, and the frontal hairline (**Fig. 22.1**).[3] Ideally, these three key points are located on the path of the circle. In applying this method, we have developed our own modification of the "facial circle." In our experience the circle should be centered on the porion at the upper part of the tragus, or at the edge of the external auditory canal. We have had good results with this simplified and modified method in practice, as it permits a rapid assessment of nasal projection in relation to the chin and forehead. The following determinations can be made:

- Is the nose or tip overprojected?

- Does the patient have prognathism or a receding chin?
- How does the forehead affect the facial profile (high or sloped forehead)?

Aided by digital imaging and modern graphics software for aesthetic surgery, we can predict whether decreasing the projection of the nasal tip, and thus advancing the pogonion toward the reference circle, will provide adequate profile correction or whether it would also be advisable to perform a chin augmentation.

The revision of an overprojected functional tension nose always has both functional and aesthetic indications.[4,5]

22.1.2 Functional Indications

Typically the nostrils are narrow and elongated, presenting a slit-like rather than oval shape, and they open into a high "gothic arch" nasal vestibule. The crura of the upper and lower lateral cartilages are medialized, causing stenosis of the external and internal nasal valves. The internal nasal valve angle is less than 15 degrees. Alar collapse occurs on deep inspiration. Even a mild degree of high septal deviation in this situation will produce significant aerodynamic effects (**Fig. 22.2**).

22.1.3 Aesthetic Indications

Hyperplasia of the septal cartilage in its dorsobasal dimension tends to raise the cartilaginous nasal dorsum. As a result, the dorsum may appear convex or may form a cartilaginous hump that is continuous with a bony hump at the rhinion. The supratip point moves to the level of the tip defining points, and the tip loses definition. When the elastic fibers in the skin yield to the tension of the upper and lower lateral cartilages, the supratip point rises above the tip defining point. The nasal tip droops and becomes ptotic.

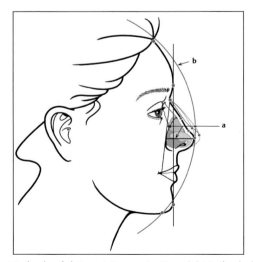

Fig. 22.1 Methods of determining projection. (**a**) Method of R. Goode. (**b**) Modified method of C. Baud. Within the facial circle = normal nose. Outside the facial circle = overprojected nose or tip. Black = normal nose; red = functional tension nose without overprojection; blue = overprojected tip; green = overprojected functional tension nose.

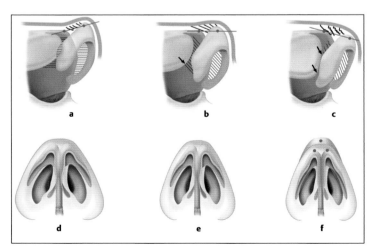

Fig. 22.2 Stages of tension nose. (**a**) Normal nose. (**b**) Compensated tension nose. (**c**) Decompensated tension nose with a ptotic tip. (**d**) Normal position of the alar cartilages. (**e**) Tension nose with elongated nares and incipient nasal valve obstruction. (**f**) Severe nasal valve obstruction with proneness to valve collapse and a ptotic tip.

Case 23

This case illustrates the management of a persistent overprojected tip (operation by Holger Gassner).

Introduction

A 23-year-old woman presented 4 years after undergoing an open-structure rhinoplasty. She sought correction of her persistent overprojected nasal tip and improvement of her predominantly right-sided nasal obstruction, which had been unresponsive to medical therapy.

Findings

Profile view (**Fig. 22.3b, c**) shows a step-off at the rhinion marking an incomplete reduction of the bony hump. The patient has an overprojected tip and slightly excessive columellar show. Frontal view (**Fig. 22.3a**) shows a C-shaped deviation of the rhinion to the left while the nasal tip is deviated to the right. The tip defining points are uneven, resulting in a complex asymmetry of

the nasal tip. Three-quarter profile (**Fig. 22.3d**) shows an overaccentuated alar crease, a rounded tip, and a scarred and retracted infratip lobule. Predominantly right-sided nasal valve collapse is noted on deep inspiration. Nasal endoscopy revealed an area 2 and 3 deviation to the right.

Surgical Procedure

The author reserves the open approach for complex revision procedures. The tipping point for electing an open approach in this case was the very firm and scarred infratip lobule. The old scar lines were followed in reopening the nose. After release of the upper lateral cartilages from the septum, the dorsal line was reduced and the middle vault was reconstructed with an autospreader graft on the right and a conventional spreader graft on the left (**Fig. 22.3e**). The deviated anterior septal angle was stented with a caudal septal extension graft (**Fig. 22.3g**). The nasal tip was reshaped with a combination of inter- and intradomal sutures. Due to the required strength of the repair, 5–0 Prolene was used in this case instead of the usual 6–0 Prolene. All suture ends were trimmed short before closure to minimize visibility through the skin.

Psychology, Motivation, Personal Background

This case illustrates the significant role that the nose plays in the self-image of young women (**Fig. 22.3h–k**). The patient had undergone otoplasty as child with an unfavorable outcome, as illustrated in **Fig. 22.3a** and **Fig. 22.3h**. While the auricular defect was perhaps even more pronounced than the nasal deformities, the patient was bothered only by the appearance of her nose and did not request revision of her otoplasty.

Discussion

The open approach has important indications in rhinoplasty, especially for complex revisions of the nasal tip. In these cases the open approach provides better visualization of the tip position, which may outweigh the drawbacks of the transcolumellar incision and the increased stiffness of the nasal tip.

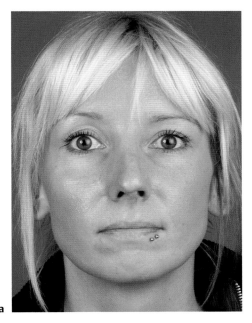
a

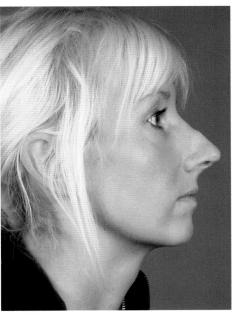
b

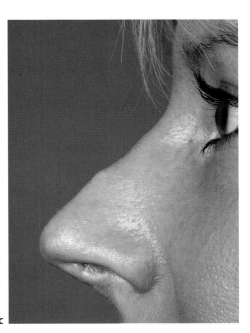
c

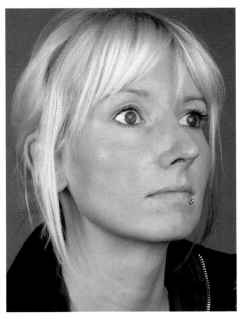
d

Fig. 22.3 (**a–d**) Preoperative views. (**a**) Frontal view shows tip asymmetry, a bossa on the right side, columellar shift, and a narrow, asymmetric middle vault. (**b**) Profile view shows residual overprojection of the nasal tip, incomplete reduction of the cartilaginous dorsum, and blunting of the nasolabial angle with prominence of the nasal spine. (**c**) Close-up profile view shows the gross overprojection of the anterior septal angle. (**d**) Three-quarter view shows an overaccentuated horizontal alar crease and a retracted infratip lobule.

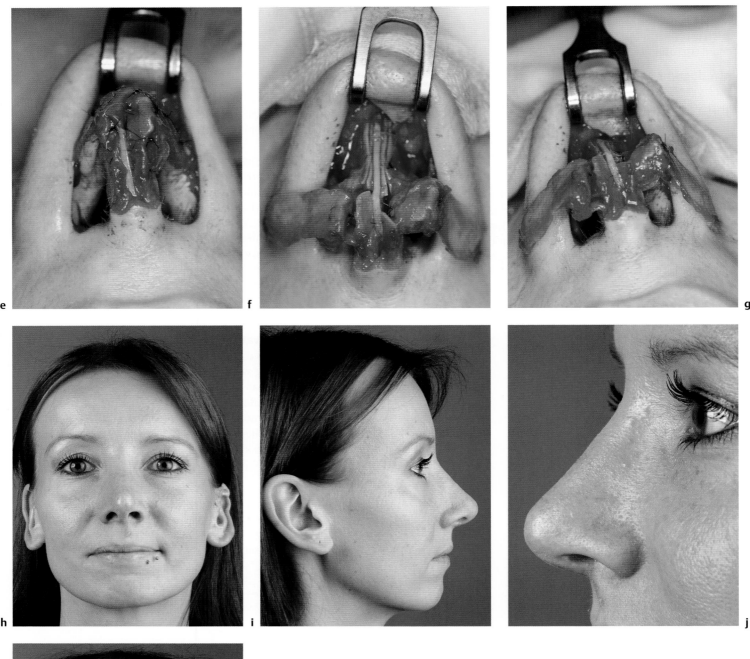

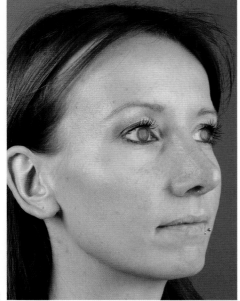

Fig. 22.3   (**e–g**) Intraoperative views. (**e**) Extensive grafting is performed through the open-structure approach. The columella is stented with a tongue-in-groove technique. There is only minimal preservation of the membranous septum. The middle vault is reconstructed with conventional spreader grafts. (**f**) Marked buckling of the medial crura, predominantly on the right side. (**g**) Multiple suture techniques are used to compensate for tip asymmetry. A caudal septal extension graft is fixed by suturing it to the medial crura. (**h–k**) Postoperative views. (**h**) Frontal view shows harmonious brow-tip aesthetic lines, symmetrical tip defining points, and a straight columella. (**i**) Profile view documents the correction of columellar show, a straight dorsal profile, and adequate rotation to avoid an operated, overrotated look. (**j**) Close-up profile view shows the gentle shadowing of the brow-tip aesthetic line curving smoothly down the dorsum to the tip-defining point. (**k**) Three-quarter view shows a straight dorsal line, a mild supratip break, and subtle filling of the horizontal alar fold.

Case 24

Introduction
A 39-year-old woman had undergone septoplasty 5 years earlier, at which time she had noticed a deformity above the nasal tip. She stated that she still had difficulty breathing through her nose. She now desired functional improvement, deprojection, and profile correction with removal of a nasal hump. She was also bothered by excessive nostril show when viewed from the side.

Findings
Frontal view (**Fig. 22.4a**) shows alar asymmetry and a long infratip triangle. Profile view (**Fig. 22.4c**) shows a bony and cartilaginous nasal hump, a hanging columella, overprojection, and vestibular skin show. Basal view (**Fig. 22.4b**) shows a taut vestibule with residual septal deviation, predominantly to the right, and stenosis of the nasal valve area.

Views in **Fig. 22.4d**, **Fig. 22.4e**, and **Fig. 22.4f** were taken 3 years after revision rhinoplasty. **Fig. 22.4g** and **Fig. 22.4h** are endoscopic views of the internal nasal valve before (**g**) and after (**h**) the operation.

Surgical Procedure
The main problem was that the septum was too long in its dorsobasal and craniocaudal dimensions. The key steps in the operation were shortening, relaxing, and medializing the nasal septum (**Fig. 22.4i–n**).

Psychology, Motivation, Personal Background
The patient came to surgery with well-defined aesthetic and functional concept and goals.

Discussion
See p. 148.

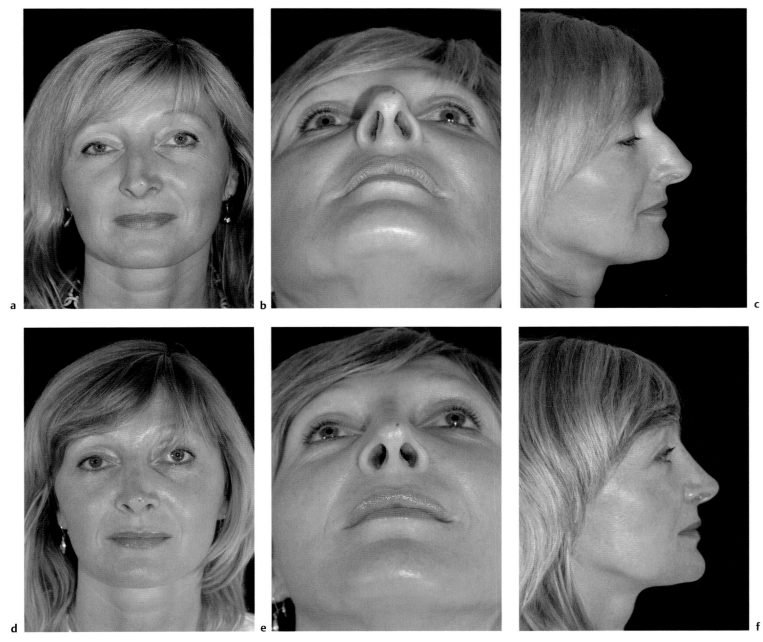

Fig. 22.4 (**a–c**) Findings before revision rhinoplasty. (**d–f**) Three years after revision rhinoplasty. (*Continued on next page*)

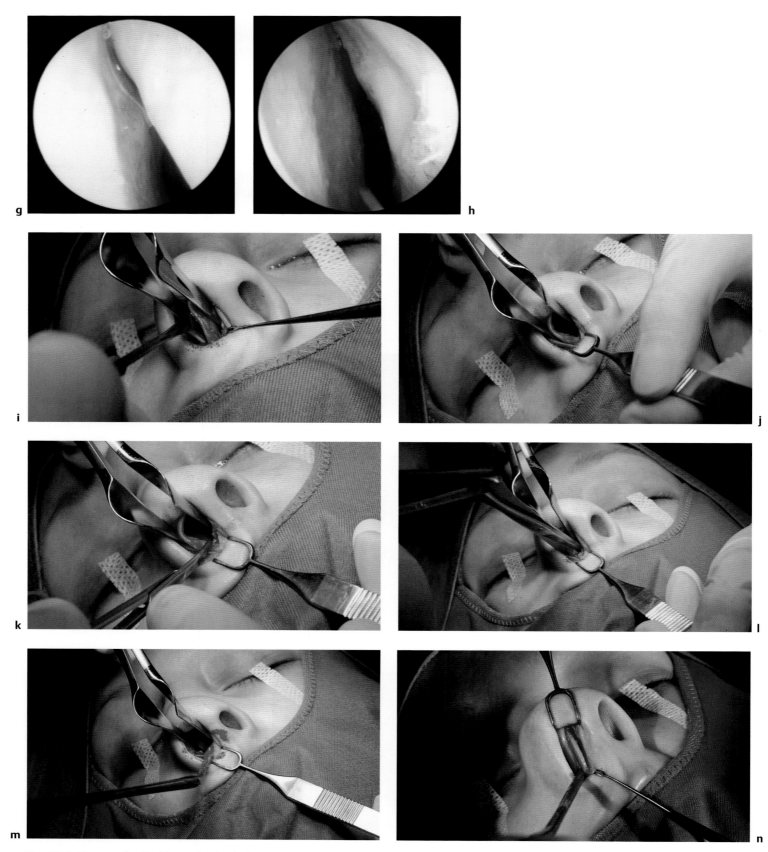

Fig. 22.4 (*Continued*)   (**g, h**) Nasal valve before and after revision rhinoplasty. (**i**) Exposure of the septal cartilage. (**j**) Visualization of the basal septum. (**k**) Detachment of the cartilage from the "septal table."

(**l**) Shortening of the septum. (**m**) Resection of a basal strip. (**n**) Shortening of the anterior septum, followed by tension-free fixation in the midline.

References

1. Joseph J. Nasenplastik und sonstige Gesichtsplastik nebst einem Anhang über Mammaplastik. Leipzig, Germany: C Kabitzsch; 1931

2. Presentation GR. "Nose and Face," Berlin 2005

3. Baud C. Harmonie der Gesichtszüge. La Chaux de Fonds, Switzerland: Clinique de la Tour; 1967

4. Parell GJ, Becker GD. The "tension nose," anatomy and surgical repair. Facial Plast Surg 1984;1(2):81–86

5. Tardy ME, Walter M, Patt B. Overprojection of the nose: an anatomic approach. Rhinoplasty 2001. Chicago, Course manual, 688–700

23 Problems Involving the Nasal Vestibule

Scar induration and distortion, stenosis, asymmetry, retraction, and recurrent or residual deviation of the anterior septum are not uncommon findings in previously operated noses. The nasal vestibule is the site for placing incisions for both endonasal and open approaches.[1] Unfavorably placed incisions or displaced alar cartilages may lead to contractures and troublesome step-offs or distortions in the "gull in flight" configuration of the alar cartilages. Individual findings will determine the specific corrective approach that should be used in any given case. It is usually sufficient to make minimally invasive corrections based on individual findings (**Fig. 23.1**).[2]

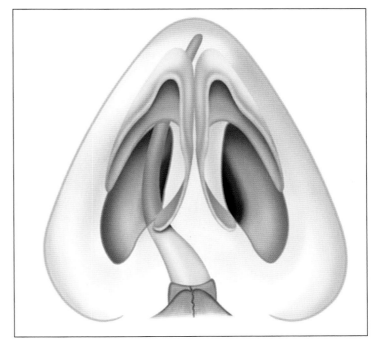

Fig. 23.1 The construction of the nasal vestibule. There are similarities to a turbine. The air will be accelerated, laminarized, and condensed by the nasal isthmus.

Case 25

This case involves an extracorporeal septoplasty with repositioning of the deviated nasal spine and a lateral sliding technique (operation by Wolfgang Gubisch).

Introduction

After six previous operations elsewhere, the patient was dissatisfied with the functional and aesthetic outcome of her procedures. She had a deviated nose with a displaced anterior nasal spine. The vestibule and nasal tip were asymmetric, and the patient had breathing problems due to a deviated septum and tight internal valves.

Findings

Inspection of the nose in the frontal view (**Fig. 23.2a**) showed disharmony of both brow-tip aesthetic lines. In the profile view (**Fig. 23.2c**), several conspicuous irregularities were apparent in the nasal dorsum. The nasal tip was asymmetric and undefined (**Fig. 23.2a, b**). The bony pyramid was deviated. In the basal view, the columella was deviated to the right and its base was to the left of the midline. The anterior nasal spine was also found to be off-midline when palpated. Endonasal inspection revealed a deviated septum. Manual expansion of the internal nasal valve with a glass rod immediately improved nasal airflow, confirming that the internal valves were stenotic and required reconstruction.

Surgical Procedure

An open approach was performed through the old scar using a standard inverted-V midcolumellar incision. Tip dissection was very difficult due to heavy scarring in that area (**Fig. 23.2g**). On dissecting the scars, we found an old cartilage graft on the right dome. When that graft was removed, it was apparent that the left

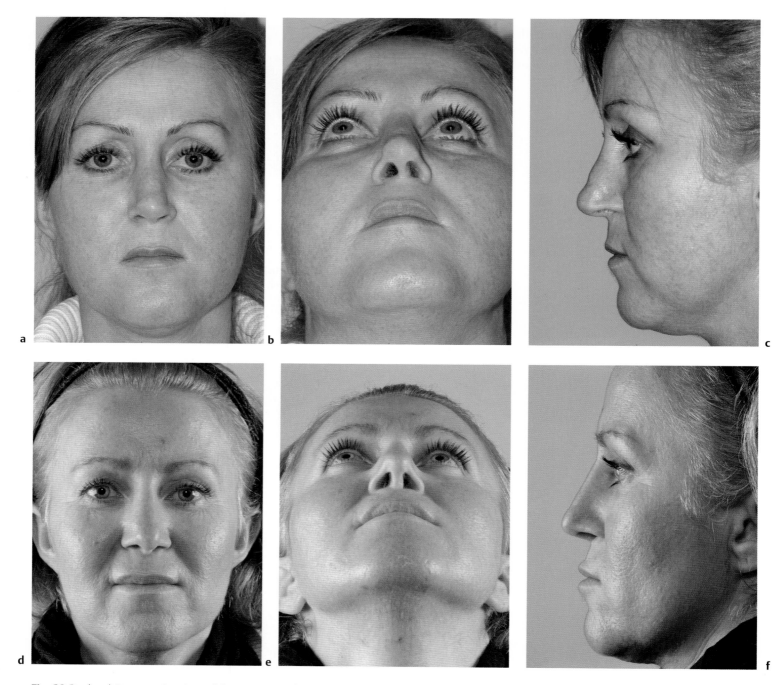

Fig. 23.2   (**a–c**) Preoperative views. (**a**) Preoperative frontal view shows a deviated nose and disharmonious brow-tip aesthetic lines. (**b**) Basal view shows the columella deviated to the right. Its base is to the right of the midline. The nostrils are asymmetric, and the tip has an undefined, asymmetric look. (**c**) Profile view shows irregularities of the dorsum and a small nasolabial angle. (**d, e**) At 3 years postoperatively the nose appears straight in the frontal and basal views. Nasal breathing is normal. (**f**) The nasal axis is straight and the tip is well defined.

dome occupied a higher position. For that reason a lateral sliding technique was performed on the left side (**Fig. 23.2j**). The nasal septum was deviated, especially in its anterior cartilaginous part. The septum was also highly unstable due to extensive cartilage resections in previous operations. Therefore we decided to remove the septum in one piece and perform an extracorporeal septal reconstruction (**Fig. 23.2h**). After smoothing all irregularities and thinning out the thickened portions of the perpendicular plate, we fixed the thin bony part of the septum to the cartilaginous part for straightening and stabilization (**Fig. 23.2i**). Because the anterior nasal spine was 8 mm to the left of the midline, we had to fracture the spine, return it to the midline, and secure it with a microplate. Conchal cartilage taken from the right ear was used to fashion a sandwich graft, which was placed as a columellar strut to stabilize the anterior septum. Conchal cartilage was also used to make spreader grafts, which were fixed to the dorsal border of the reconstructed septum to reconstitute the internal valves. Then the straight neoseptum was returned and fixed dorsally to the upper lateral cartilages with multiple back-and-forth sutures. It was also fixed to the repositioned anterior nasal spine with several sutures. We performed direct lateral, paramedian, and transverse osteotomies on both sides to correct the bony pyramid. The irregularities in the bony dorsum were smoothed out. The dorsum was additionally covered with three layers of homologous fascia lata. Finally we corrected the nasal tip with transdomal sutures, a spanning suture, and a tip suspension suture.

Psychology, Motivation, Personal Background

The patient worked in the fashion industry and was unhappy with the results of her six previous operations, especially in an aesthetic sense. Three years after the revision the patient is pleased with the functional outcome and with the aesthetic improvement in the appearance of her nose (**Fig. 23.2d–f**).

Discussion

A straight septal framework is the prerequisite for a straight nose. Therefore, every effort must be made to straighten the septum. In this case we found that an extracorporeal septoplasty was the best way to straighten the septum and the nose. We also corrected the position of the anterior spine, which we feel is also a prerequisite for keeping a reimplanted septum permanently in the midline. This in turn is key to achieving symmetry of the nostrils and nasolabial complex.

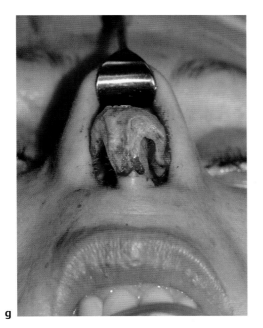

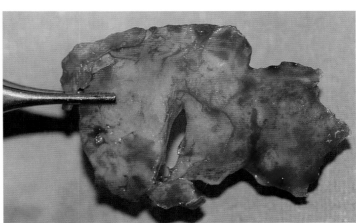

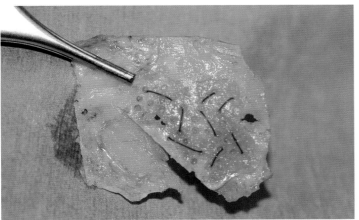

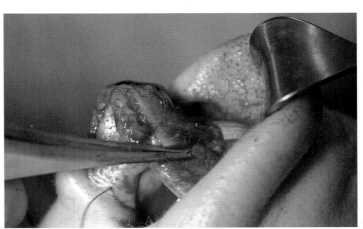

Fig. 23.2 (**g–j**) Intraoperative views. (**g**) Six previous operations had resulted in heavy scarring. (**h**) The rest of the deviated septum was removed in one piece. The deviation involved both the cartilaginous and bony portions of the septum. (**i**) A thin perpendicular plate was used to straighten the cartilaginous part of the reconstructed septum. (**j**) A lateral sliding technique was used on the left side to restore nasal tip symmetry.

Case 26

Introduction
A 51-year-old woman presented with residual septal deviation and nostril asymmetry 6 years after a previous septoplasty. The patient desired selective correction of the nostrils on functional and aesthetic grounds and did not specifically request any other corrections.

Findings
Frontal view (**Fig. 23.3a**) shows slight deviation of the cartilaginous septum to the right. Profile view (**Fig. 23.3b**) shows a bony and cartilaginous hump. Basal view (**Fig. 23.3c**) shows pronounced deviation of the anterior septum with distortion of the cartilaginous nose.

Fig. 23.3d, **Fig. 23.3e**, and **Fig. 23.3f** show corresponding views taken one year after revision surgery.

Surgical Procedure
A submucous septoplasty was performed in which the septum was returned to the midline and the nasal valve areas were opened on both sides (**Fig. 23.3g–o**).

Psychology, Motivation, Personal Background
The patient had a good awareness of the scope of the desired aesthetic changes. She wanted to reestablish nostril symmetry and aesthetics without altering her nasal profile.

Discussion
Positioning the septum on the midline can significantly improve the cartilaginous nose from both a functional and aesthetic standpoint.

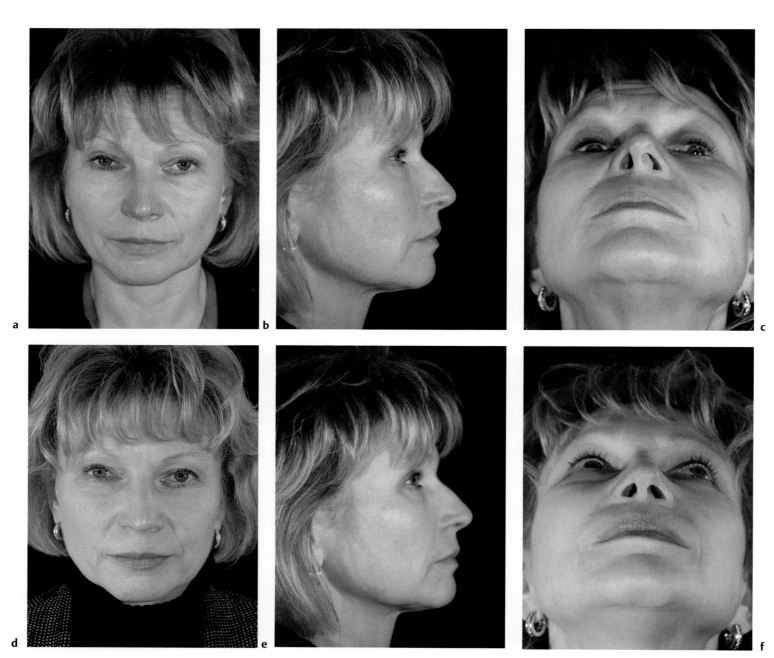

Fig. 23.3   (**a–c**) The patient 6 years after primary septorhinoplasty. (**d–f**) One year after revision rhinoplasty.

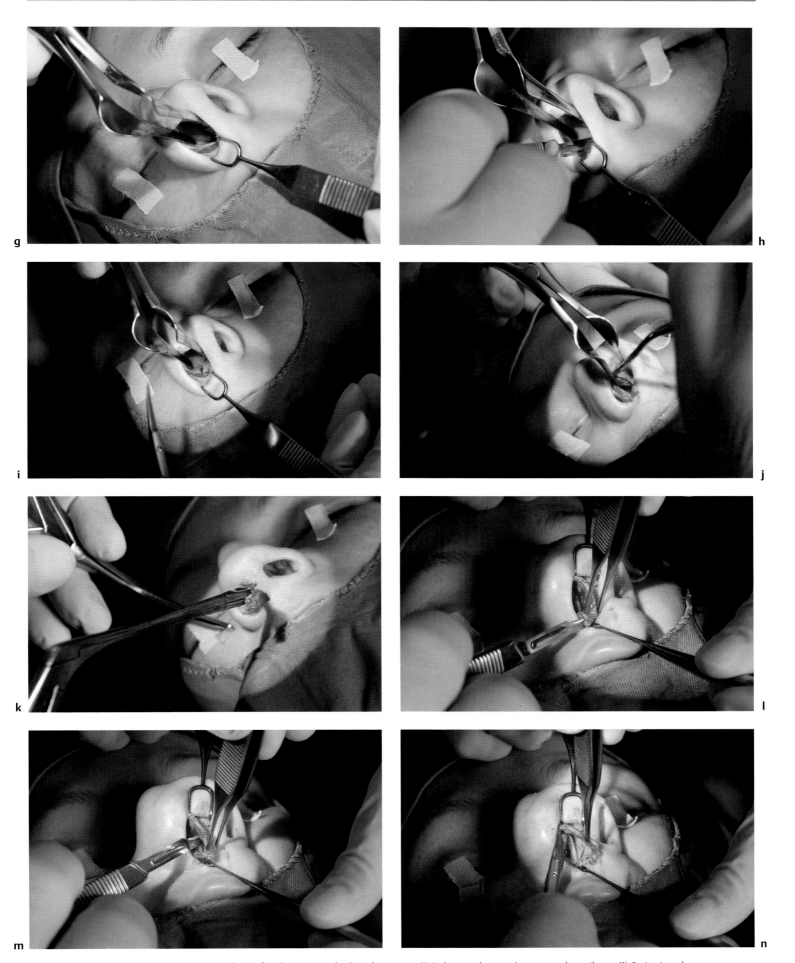

Fig. 23.3 (**g**) Exposure of the septal cartilage. (**h**) Shortening the basal septum. (**i**) Relaxing the too-long septal cartilage. (**j**) Swinging door maneuver. (**k**) Removal of resected cartilage. (**l–n**) Shortening the anterior septum. (*Continued on next page*)

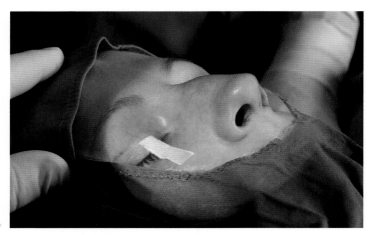

o

Fig. 23.3 (*Continued*)   (**o**) Findings at the end of the operation.

Case 27

Introduction
A 46-year-old woman presented 8 months after undergoing rhinosurgery in another country. While the initial aesthetic result was good, a noticeable deformity of the nasal dorsum developed over a period of several months. The patient continued to have nasal breathing problems.

Findings
Frontal view (**Fig. 23.4a**) shows asymmetry of the supratip area and nasal tip with excessive nostril show viewed from the front. Profile view (**Fig. 23.4b**) shows a hump over the rhinion, vestibular skin show, and an unfavorable columellar-lobular relationship. Basal view (**Fig. 23.4c**) shows stenosis of the internal nasal valve, septal deviation, and a slanted nasal base.

Photos in **Fig. 23.4d**, **Fig. 23.4e**, and **Fig. 23.4f** were taken 2 years after revision rhinoplasty.

Surgical Procedure
Two complete mucosal tunnels were developed through a hemitransfixion incision. A basal cartilage strip was resected, followed by a swinging door maneuver and vomer osteotomy. Deviated posterior portions of the septum were removed. The septum was straightened extracorporeally and reimplanted, and the anterior septal cartilage was relaxed by making scoring incisions on the concave side. A columellar pocket was developed, and the anterior septal cartilage was positioned on the midline.

Intercartilaginous incisions were made on both sides. The soft-tissue envelope was elevated from the dorsum, and irregularities were removed from the superior borders of the septum and upper lateral cartilages. The bony nasal dorsum was smoothed with a No. 2 scraper blade, and the superior cartilage borders were approximated with two all-layer 5–0 PDS sutures. The hemitransfixion incision was extended to a transfixion incision. The membranous septum was shortened by 1 to 2 mm, followed by wound closure (**Fig. 23.4g**).

Psychology, Motivation, Personal Background
Though initially pleased with what she considered a good result, the patient later felt a strong need to improve her nasal breathing and optimize the outcome of the previous surgery.

Discussion
The indication for revision rhinoplasty was based on both functional and aesthetic problems:

- Functional problems: septal deviation and bilateral nasal valve stenosis.
- Aesthetic problems: slight overprojection, vestibular skin show, recurrent hump in the nasal dorsum, and dorsal asymmetry.

Deprojection of the nose was achieved in this case by reducing the height of the anterior septum and releasing the medial crural footplates from the anterior septal border (weakening two tip-support mechanisms).

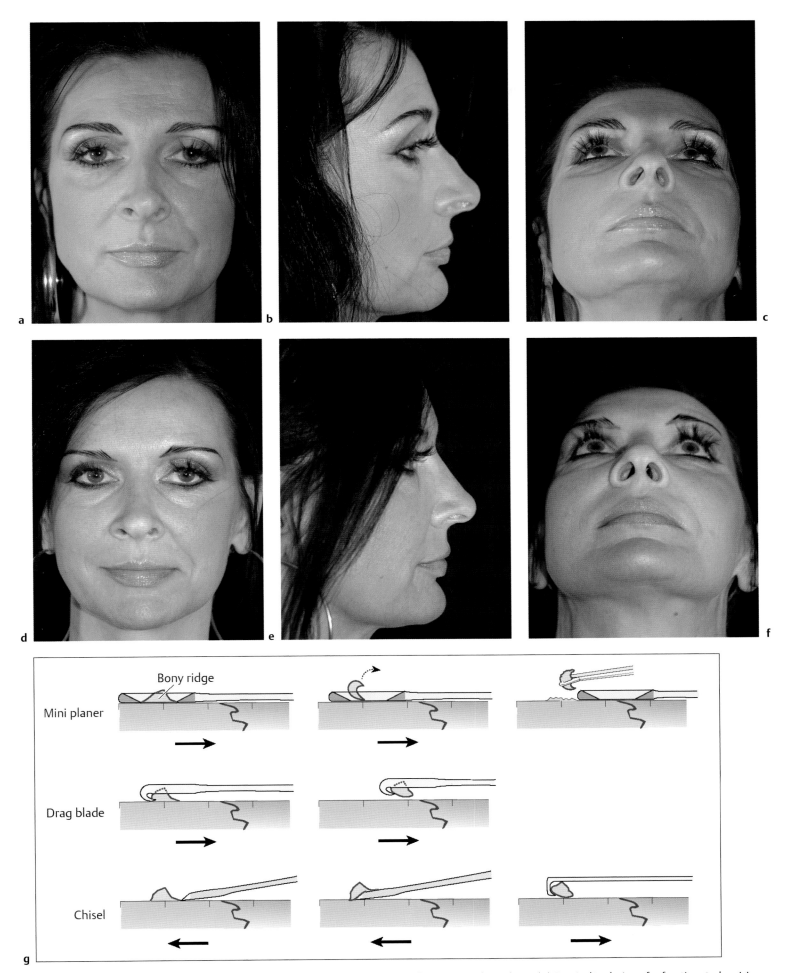

Fig. 23.4   (**a–c**) The patient before her secondary operation. (**d–f**) Two years after revision rhinoplasty. (**g**) Surgical technique for fractionated revision of the nasal dorsum, using special instruments after H. Behrbohm (Karl Storz, Tuttlingen).

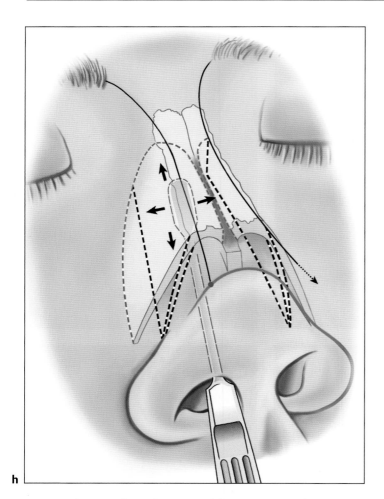

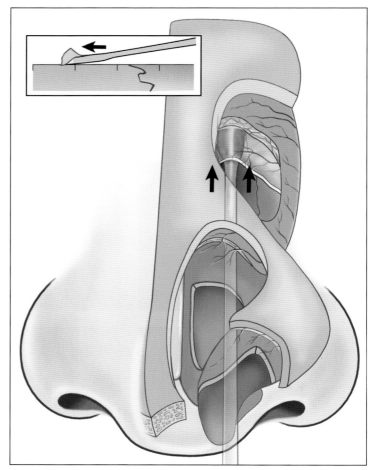

Fig. 23.4 (*Continued*)   Different possibilities to smooth the bony nasal dorsum. (**h**) With a mini-diamant rasp (after H. Behrbohm, Karl Storz, Tuttlingen). The advantage is the large and free working radius in all directions. (**i**) With a chisel.

References

1. Eichhorn-Sens J, Gubisch W. Sekundäre Rhinoplastik. In: von Heimburg D, Lemperle G, eds. Ästhetische Chirurgie, vol. 3. Heidelberg, Germany: ecomed Medizin; 2010:1–25

2. Fedok FG. Revision rhinoplasty using the endonasal approach. Facial Plast Surg 2008;24(3):293–309

24 Saddle Nose after Septoplasty or Trauma

Saddling of the nasal dorsum may result from a septal perforation or nasal trauma. Both etiologies involve mechanical weakening of the anterior septal cartilage. Besides functional problems, cartilaginous deviation, or a perforated septum, postoperative saddle nose is the most important complication of septal surgery. Destruction of the supportive function of the anterior septum for the nasal dorsum leads to collapse of the cartilaginous nasal dorsum. Bony saddle nose, a hallmark of tertiary syphilis decades ago, has become rare today (**Fig. 24.1**).

There may be lateralization, spreading, or separation of the upper lateral cartilages, depending on the depth of the saddling. With depression of the dorsal septal border, an important tip support mechanism is compromised. This leads to collapse of the supratip area and anterior septal angle. The nasal tip becomes amorphous. The loss of tip support leads to cephalic rotation of the tip. The tip may even rotate downward if the anterior septal margin is lost. Cephalic rotation also leads to loss of tip projection. The nasolabial angle is blunted (> 110 degrees). The loss of structural support allows the caudal portions of the upper lateral cartilages to sag, deforming and dilating the internal nasal valve. The alar cartilages spread laterally, resulting in a wide and bulbous nasal tip. The special aspects of septal surgery in children are reviewed on p. 21. **Fig. 24.2**, **Fig. 24.3**, and **Fig. 24.4** illustrate the three different pathogenic mechanisms of saddle nose deformity.

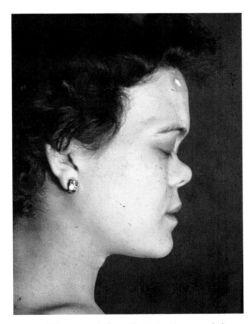

Fig. 24.1   Bony saddle nose deformity in tertiary syphilis.

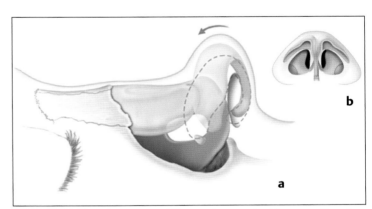

Fig. 24.2   (**a**) Cartilaginous saddle nose has resulted from cartilage loss (cartilage = blue) in the area indicated, with preservation of the anterior septal border. Note the collapse of the cartilaginous nasal dorsum and the cephalic tip rotation with loss of projection. (**b**) Typical changes in the nasal base with broadening of the nasal valve and compensatory hyperplasia of the inferior turbinate.

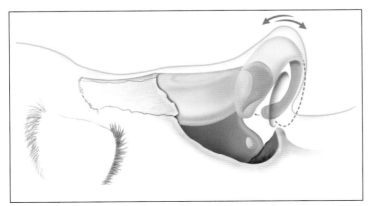

Fig. 24.3   Cartilaginous saddle nose with destruction of the causal septal border. The lower columella is retracted upward, creating a hidden columella, and the alar-columellar complex is deformed.

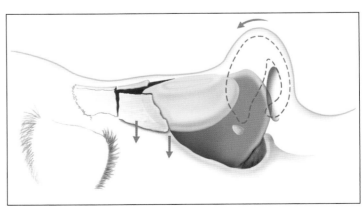

Fig. 24.4   Posttraumatic saddle nose with an open roof, displacement of nasal bone fragments, and disruption of the bony and cartilaginous junction at the rhinion (keystone area) with an inverted V.

Case 28

Introduction

A 21-year-old woman presented with the concern of a marked change in nasal shape one year after sustaining nasal trauma.

Findings

Frontal view (**Fig. 24.5a**) shows a broadened nasal tip with a wide dorsum. Profile view (**Fig. 24.5b**) shows a postoperative saddle nose deformity with saddling in the supratip area, a loss of tip projection with cephalic rotation, and loss of structural support due to overresection. Oblique view (**Fig. 24.5c**) shows a hidden columella due to loss of the anterior septal cartilage.

Fig. 24.5d, **Fig. 24.5e**, and **Fig. 24.5f** show corresponding views 2 years after revision rhinoplasty.

Surgical Procedure

Variant A: the destroyed or mechanically deficient septal cartilage is reconstructed like a mosaic, followed by the placement of a conchal cartilage onlay graft (**Fig. 24.5g**).

Variant B: interposition of a neoseptum (**Fig. 24.5h**).

Psychology, Motivation, Personal Background

Saddling of the nasal dorsum leads to a variety of changes that alter facial appearance in a way that is distressful for most patients. The facial appearance becomes coarser, the nose too short and too broad. The loss of projection causes a relative advancement of the chin. The wish to return the nose to its "old shape" usually reflects a desire to restore individual physiognomy and relieve the pain of its loss.

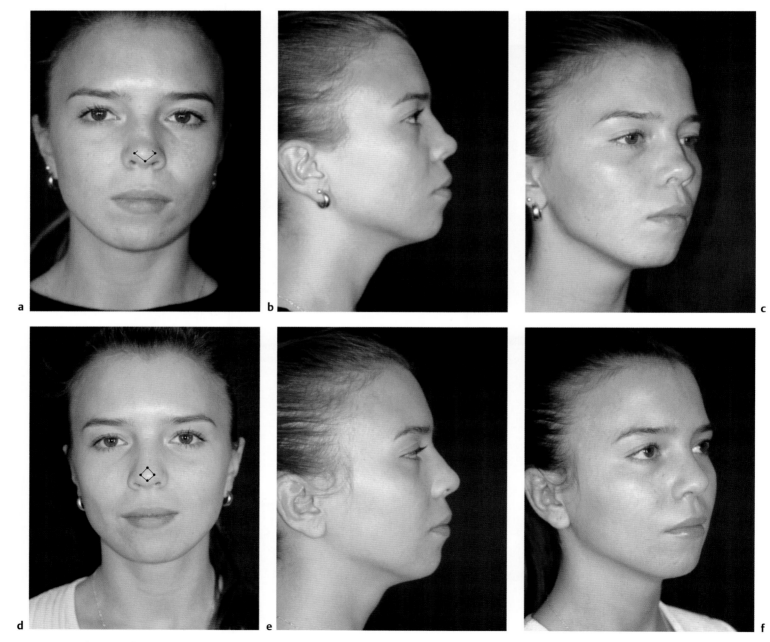

a   b   c

d   e   f

Fig. 24.5   (**a–c**) Findings before septorhinoplasty. (**d–f**) Two years after revision rhinoplasty. (*Continued on next page*)

Discussion

The main goal in the revision of postoperative or posttraumatic saddle nose is to reconstruct a stable septum. All additional steps such as fixing the upper lateral cartilages to the superior septal border and placing spreader grafts to reinforce the dorsal septal border are done in service to that goal.[1,2] Given the tendency of the nasal dorsum to contract after surgery, it is always recommended that an onlay graft be placed in the supratip area as an adjunct to the static reconstruction.[3]

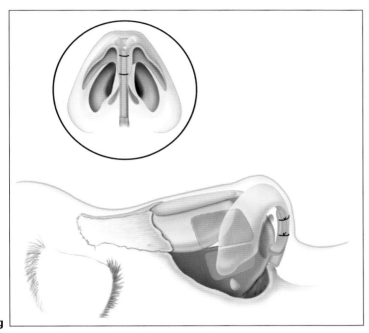

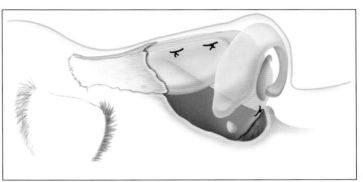

Fig. 24.5 (*Continued*)   (**g**) Surgical procedure, variant A: A columellar strut may be necessary in patients who lack tip projection. This was not necessary in the case shown. (**h**) Surgical procedure, variant B: Replacement of the anterior septum with conchal or rib cartilage. The upper lateral cartilages are fixed to the dorsal edge of the neoseptum, and the septal cartilage is fixed basally with a suture passed through the nasal spine.

Case 29

Case elements: nasal growth disturbance with a short nose, a hypoplastic nasal dorsum, facial asymmetry, overresection of the right alar cartilage, and severely impaired nasal breathing due to septal deviation following a septorhinoplasty in childhood (operation by Jacqueline Eichhorn-Sens).

Introduction

A 35-year-old man sustained nasal trauma at 12 years of age, followed by a septorhinoplasty performed elsewhere. He presented now with a short nose, a hypoplastic nasal dorsum, and severe breathing problems due to septal deviation and hypertrophy of the inferior turbinates.

Findings

Inspection showed impairment of nasal growth following trauma and septorhinoplasty in childhood, with conspicuous hypoplasia of the nasal dorsum and an extremely short nose with an overrotated tip (**Fig. 24.6a–c**). The length of the nose and size of the nasal tip appeared disharmonious. The bony pyramid was wide and deviated, and the brow-tip aesthetic lines were asymmetric. Palpation disclosed absence of the anterior septum. The septal border was palpable far behind the anterior nasal spine. The anterior nasal spine itself was palpable just behind the midline. Endonasal inspection revealed extreme septal deviation and hypertrophy of both inferior turbinates.

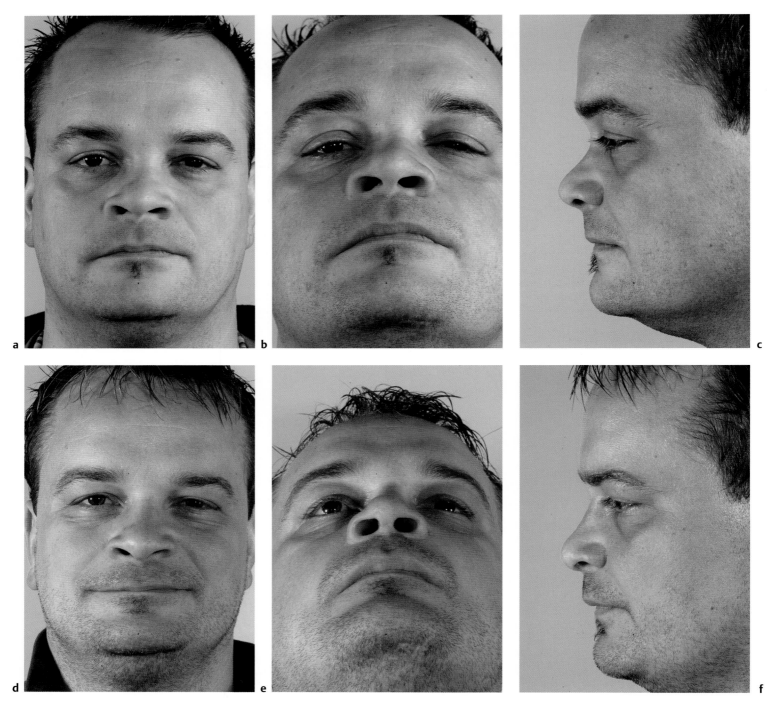

Fig. 24.6 (**a–f**) Pre- and postoperative views. (**a**) Preoperative frontal view shows a deviated nose and facial asymmetry. The nose is too short, resulting in disharmony between the dorsum and nasal tip size. (**b**) Basal view displays the dorsal deviation and a wide nasal base. (**c**) The severely hypoplastic nasal dorsum is conspicuous in the profile view. For a male, the nasolabial angle is too long and the tip is overrotated. (**d**) Result at 1 year. The nasal axis has a harmonious appearance. (**e**) Basal view shows nostril symmetry. (**f**) Viewed in profile, the dorsum and nasolabial angle show a stable, harmonious result. (*Continued on next page*)

Surgical Procedure

An open approach was done through a standard inverted-V mid-columellar incision. Dissection of the tip was very difficult due to massive scar formation, especially over the right alar cartilage. It was found that all of the right alar cartilage had been resected in the previous operation. Dissection of the septum was also very difficult due to heavy scarring. Analysis showed a major loss of septal material in the complete anterior portion and caudal portion of the dorsal septum. Fragments of septal cartilage were found just behind a displaced anterior nasal spine, causing obstruction of nasal airflow in that area. The anterior spine was very broad, and bone was burred from one side to recenter the remaining spine in the midline. When the septal cartilage was released from the dense scar tissue, the originally deviated septal cartilage became straight. We were able to harvest a piece of cartilage from the middle of the septum without compromising a stable cartilage framework. The harvested cartilage was used to fashion a septal extension graft and two extension spreader grafts. The L-shaped framework was fixed to the anterior spine with several sutures passed through a small drill hole. The septal extension graft was also fixed through the drill hole in the anterior spine and sutured to the anterior border of the remaining septum (**Fig. 24.6h**). The extension spreader grafts were fixed to the dorsal part of the reconstructed septum. The complete septum was suspended from the upper lateral cartilages with multiple forth-and-back sutures. Submucous turbinectomy was performed on both sides. The bony vault was straightened by lateral, transverse, and paramedian osteotomies. The resected intermediate part of the alar cartilage on the right side was reconstructed by the bending technique[4] with a strip of septal cartilage (**Fig. 24.6g, h**). A cephalic reduction of the alar cartilage was performed on the left side (**Fig. 24.6g**). Then transdomal sutures and a spanning suture were placed. A columellar strut made of septal cartilage was also inserted. Conchal cartilage was harvested from one site and used to make diced cartilage (**Fig. 24.6j**), which was wrapped in a tube of homologous fascia lata (**Fig. 24.6i**) and used to reconstruct the nasal dorsum. A conchal onlay graft was also placed on the caudal edge of the dorsum. Finally, a shield graft and tip graft made of conchal cartilage were used to reconfigure the tip.

Psychology, Motivation, Personal Background

With subsequent growth since undergoing a septorhinoplasty in early childhood, the patient developed typical functional and aesthetic problems that included a short nose, hypoplasia of the nasal dorsum, and increasing airway problems. One year after revision surgery the patient is very pleased with the functional and aesthetic outcome (**Fig. 24.6d–f**).

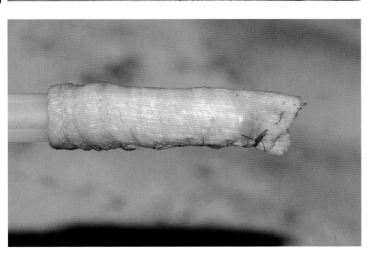

g

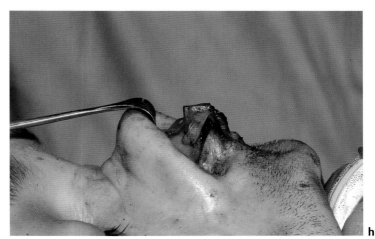

h

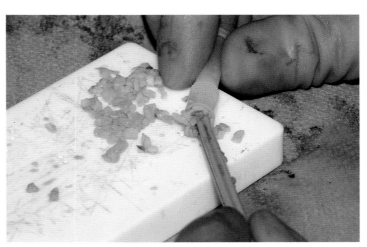

i

j

Fig. 24.6 (*Continued*) (**g–j**) Intraoperative views. (**g**) The intermediate part of the right alar cartilage is reconstructed with a strip of septal cartilage using the bending technique. Considerable cephalic reduction has already been done on the left alar cartilage. (**h**) The septal extension graft has been placed, as has the graft for reconstructing the resected intermediate crus of the right alar cartilage. (**i**) Homologous fascia lata is fashioned into a tube. (**j**) Cartilage is diced and packed into the fascia lata tube for reconstructing the nasal dorsum.

Discussion

The correction of wide nostrils is also a consideration in cases of this kind. That option was discussed but the patient declined it.

References

1. Riechelmann H, Rettinger G. Three-step reconstruction of complex saddle nose deformities. Arch Otolaryngol Head Neck Surg 2004;130(3):334–338

2. Rettinger G. Rekonstruktion ausgeprägter Sattelnasen. Laryngorhinootologie 1997;76(11):672–675

3. Wang TD. Augmentation des Nasenrückens. HNO 2010;58(9):907–911

4. Gubisch W, Eichhorn-Sens J. Overresection of the lower lateral cartilages: a common conceptual mistake with functional and aesthetic consequences. Aesthetic Plast Surg 2009;33(1):6–13

25 Augmentation of the Nasal Dorsum

The nasal dorsum runs from the root of the nose (radix) to the nasal tip. It extends over the bony and cartilaginous portions of the nasal pyramid. The area of the rhinion, or keystone area, has a major role in providing structural support. The internal nasal valve has special functional importance. Between the keystone area and nasal valve region is the middle vault, which is formed chiefly by the upper lateral cartilages. The upper lateral cartilages curve toward the nasal dorsum like the arches of a Gothic cathedral and are supported there by the septal cartilage. Together the upper lateral cartilages and septal cartilage comprise an anatomic unit.[1,2]

Saddling, irregularities, and deviations may be congenital, postinflammatory, posttraumatic, or iatrogenic due to previous surgery. Before reconstructing the nasal dorsum, the surgeon should first evaluate how the dorsum and tip are contributing to structural support.[3] This is done by inspection and especially by palpating the nasal tip and assessing supratip recoil. Augmentation is sufficient in noses with adequate protection and projection. If the nasal tip is not stable enough, it should be supported with a columellar strut to create an anterior pillar for the nasal dorsum.

Case 30

Introduction

The patient, now 38 years of age, underwent a septoplasty in 1990. Two years later she developed saddling of the nasal dorsum. She had surgery to correct the saddle nose in 1992, and another revision was done in 1999 for the same indication. Later the patient sustained facial trauma that included an open wound over the nasal dorsum. In 2004, an implant was placed to support the nasal dorsum and a scar revision was performed. She presented now with a persistent saddle nose deformity.

Findings

Posttraumatic saddle nose after four previous nasal operations, bilateral otoapostasis, and bilateral acute recurrent rhinosinusitis.

Frontal view (**Fig. 25.1a**) shows marked saddling of the middle vault and supratip area with a scar over the nasal dorsum.

Profile view (**Fig. 25.1b**) shows a pseudohump with cephalic tip rotation and an obtuse nasolabial angle. Basal view (**Fig. 25.1c**) shows a somewhat broadened nasal tip due to lateralization of the alar cartilages.

Fig. 25.1d, **Fig. 25.1e**, and **Fig. 25.1f** show the corresponding views 2 years after revision surgery. Tip recoil indicates satisfactory tip protection.

Surgical Procedure

A setback otoplasty was performed, and a revision rhinoplasty was performed through an intercartilaginous approach. Bilateral spreader grafts were placed to stabilize a weak "septal bridge." An onlay graft was placed in the supratip area, and the entire middle vault was augmented. Medial and lateral curved osteotomies were performed on both sides. Sinus problems were addressed by performing an infundibulotomy and supraturbinate antrostomy and establishing frontal sinus drainage with a Draf IIa procedure (**Fig. 25.1g**).

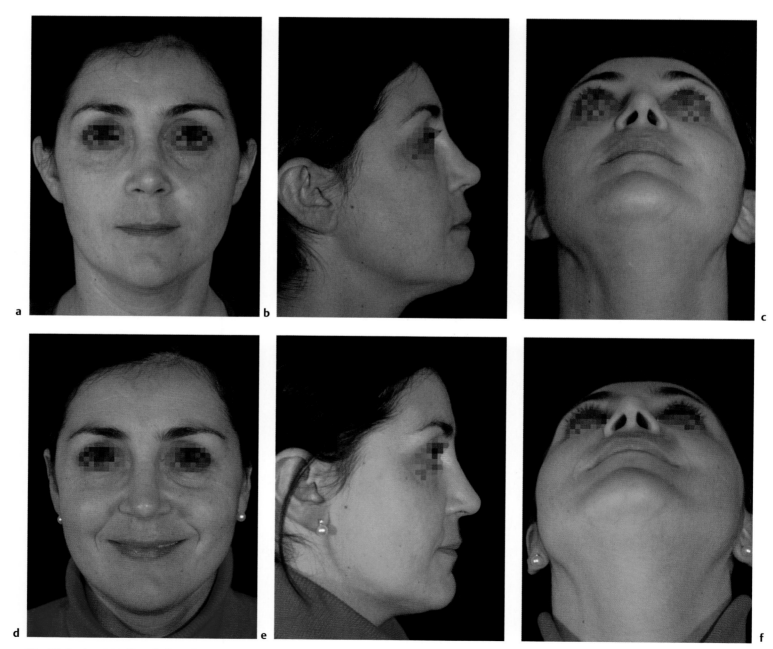

Fig. 25.1 (**a–c**) Findings before the third revision rhinoplasty. (**d–f**) Two years after the revision. (*Continued on next page*)

Psychology, Motivation, Personal Background

The odyssey of nasal operations, disappointments, and then a successful revision ruined by nasal trauma had left the patient with a "psychic wound." So while she wanted definitive closure on her nasal and sinus issues, she was reluctant to subject herself to another nasal operation and was pessimistic about the outcome.

Discussion

The decision to use autologous conchal cartilage was facilitated by the patient's desire for an otoplasty. Given her prior history, rib cartilage with its high mechanical stability would have been an option. The advantage of elastic conchal cartilage is its flexibility and its association with a thick layer of connective tissue, which can provide soft, harmonious support for the nasal dorsum. A stiff costal cartilage graft is bothersome for some patients, even with a good aesthetic outcome.

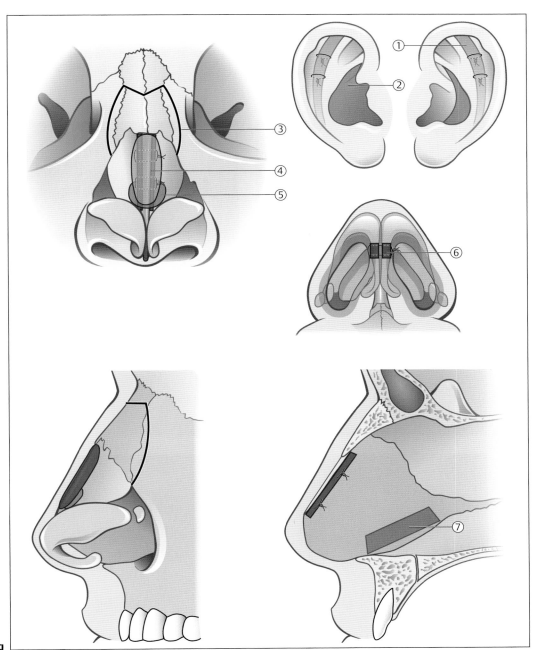

g

Fig. 25.1 (*Continued*) (**g**) Intraoperative details. Red = resections, black = osteotomies, blue = cartilage implants (spreader grafts, dorsal and supratip onlay grafts). 1, otoplasty, combined section suture technique; 2, harvesting area of conchal cartilage; 3, lateral curved osteotomies; 4, dorsal onlay graft; 5, onlay graft of the supratip area; 6, spreader grafts; 7, harvesting area of septal cartilage for the spreader grafts.

Case 31

Introduction
A 32-year-old man had sustained nasal trauma 6 years earlier. Although the injury had been reduced, he later noticed a significant change in the external shape of his nose. He also claimed difficulty breathing through the right side of the nose.

Findings
Frontal view (**Fig. 25.2a**) shows saddling of the bony nasal pyramid, an inverted-V and open-roof deformity, and posttraumatic dissection between the bony and cartilaginous nose. Profile view (**Fig. 25.2b**) shows a bony saddle nose and a polly beak deformity. Basal view (**Fig. 25.2c**) shows a wide nasal tip.

Fig. 25.2d, **Fig. 25.2e**, and **Fig. 25.2f** show the corresponding views 1 year after revision septoplasty. Tip recoil indicates satisfactory tip protection.

Surgical Procedure
Cartilage was harvested from the conchal bowl, and a submucous septoplasty was performed. A tailored onlay graft was fashioned from the conchal cartilage and connective tissue and sized with a Behrbohm caliper (**Fig. 25.2g**). A snug implant bed was developed. The implant was fitted into place and fixed with fibrin glue, followed by wound closure. The curved lateral osteotomies were marked and performed with a directional bevel osteotome (**Fig. 25.2h**).

Psychology, Motivation, Personal Background
The young man, who had a fine aesthetic sense owing to his work as a carpenter, desired a reconstruction that would restore an intact nasal contour.

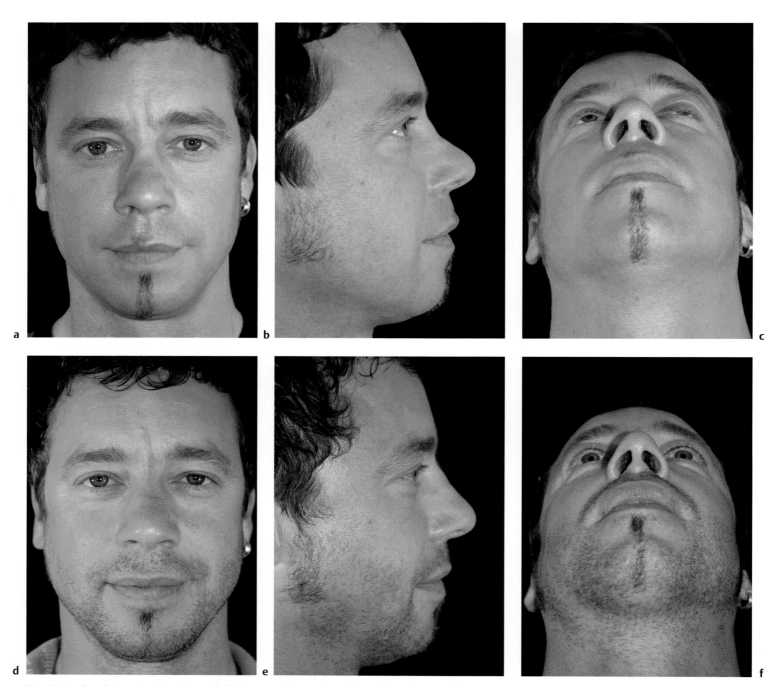

Fig. 25.2 (**a–c**) Preoperative views. (**d–f**) One year after revision rhinoplasty. (*Continued on next page*)

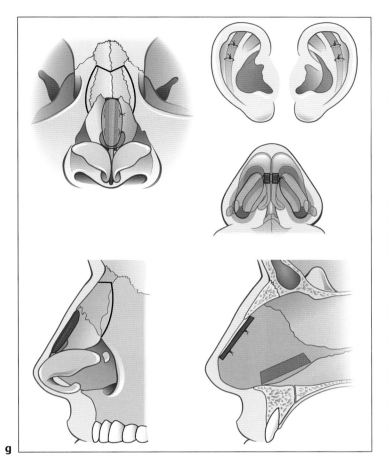

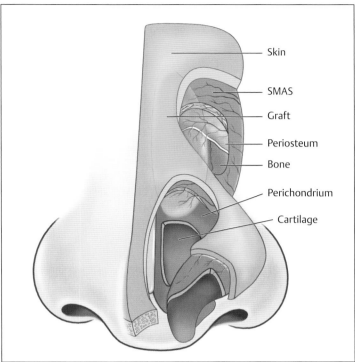

- Skin
- SMAS
- Graft
- Periosteum
- Bone
- Perichondrium
- Cartilage

Fig. 25.2 (*Continued*)   (**g**) Surgical procedure. (**h**) Implantation of a dorsal onlay graft in a tight implantation bed.

Case 32

Introduction

A 60-year-old woman had undergone a rhinoplasty many years ago. She had wanted just a slight reduction of her nasal dorsum, as she had "always had a pretty nose, as you can see in my wedding picture" (**Fig. 25.3**). She was unhappy with the result. "I'm not myself anymore. I want my nose high and straight like it used to be."

Findings

The nose appears normal in the frontal view (**Fig. 25.4a**). The profile view (**Fig. 25.4b**) shows an "anteface" profile with overresection of the nasal dorsum. Basal view (**Fig. 25.4c**) shows slight underprojection of the nasal tip.

At postoperative follow-up 3 years later, the frontal view (**Fig. 25.4d**) shows marked telangiectatic skin changes after the augmentation. The profile view (**Fig. 25.4e**) documents the restoration of a high, straight nasal dorsum.

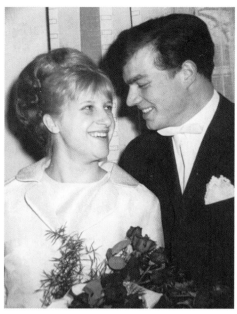

Fig. 25.3   "My nose" as it appeared in the patient's wedding picture.

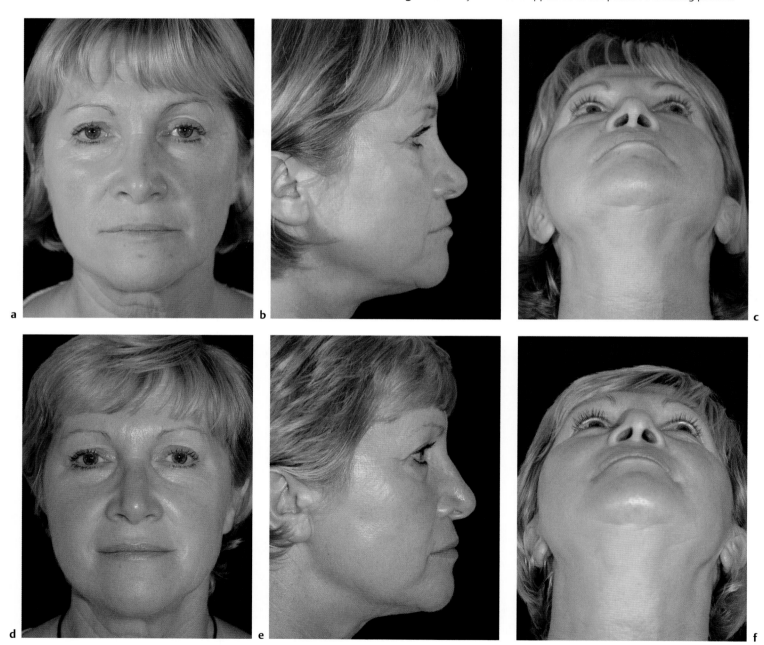

Fig. 25.4   (**a–c**) Preoperative views. (**d–f**) Views after revision rhinoplasty. (*Continued on next page*)

Surgical Procedure

The nasal dorsum was augmented with an implant fashioned from conchal cartilage and connective tissue. **Fig. 25.4g** shows the mechanism that may have been responsible for the telangiectatic skin changes over the nasal dorsum.

Psychology, Motivation, Personal Background

Although her first rhinoplasty had been performed decades ago, the patient was unable to identify with her "new nose." Faulty surgical goals are always the result of a communication problem between the doctor and rhinoplasty candidate. Especially in operations that will alter facial type, the intended result of the surgery should always be thoroughly discussed with the patient and visualized in advance to avoid misunderstandings.

Discussion

The more tissue is implanted, in this case for augmentation, the greater the risk of vascular congestion and ingrowth into the facial skin. This phenomenon is intensified by thin skin that has already sustained trophic damage due to subcutaneous scarring. Small areas can be cleared by obliterating the vessels with an argon or Nd-YAG laser, but it is difficult to treat larger areas by this method.

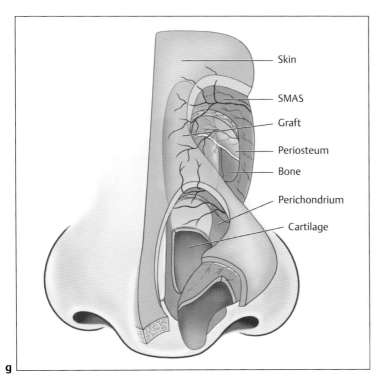

g

Fig. 25.4 (*Continued*) (**g**) Pathogenic mechanism of postoperative telangiectasia.

Case 33

Introduction

An 18-year-old male stated that he had suffered a nasal injury at 5 years of age. That had been followed by the formation of a septal abscess and by a gradual collapse of the nasal dorsum in subsequent years. Since then the patient has had great difficulty breathing through his nose. He also claimed to have been teased increasingly about his nasal deformity, giving rise to emotional problems.

Findings

An 18-year-old male with postinfectious saddle nose deformity. Frontal view (**Fig. 25.5a**) shows a general collapse of the cartilaginous nose. The nose is broad and has an amorphous, caudally rotated tip that overhangs the upper lip. Profile view (**Fig. 25.5b**) shows a cartilaginous saddle nose with a pseudohump

and ptotic tip. Basal view (**Fig. 25.5c**) shows deprojection due to a loss of tip protection and collapse of the cartilaginous nose. Tip recoil maneuver indicated a complete loss of tip protection.

Fig. 25.5d, **Fig. 25.5e**, and **Fig. 25.5f** show the patient 2 years after reconstruction of the cartilaginous nasal framework.

Surgical Procedure

Rib cartilage was harvested and used to fashion a balanced graft. A stable columellar strut was made from the rib cartilage and inserted, and a dorsal graft was rounded at the sides and placed abutting the nasal pyramid. Both grafts were joined together in a groove-and-tongue fashion (**Fig. 25.5g**).

Psychology, Motivation, Personal Background

The young man had been the brunt of relentless teasing about his nose while at school. This had already given rise to emotional problems requiring therapy. Correction of his nasal deformity has given the patient hope for a happier life.

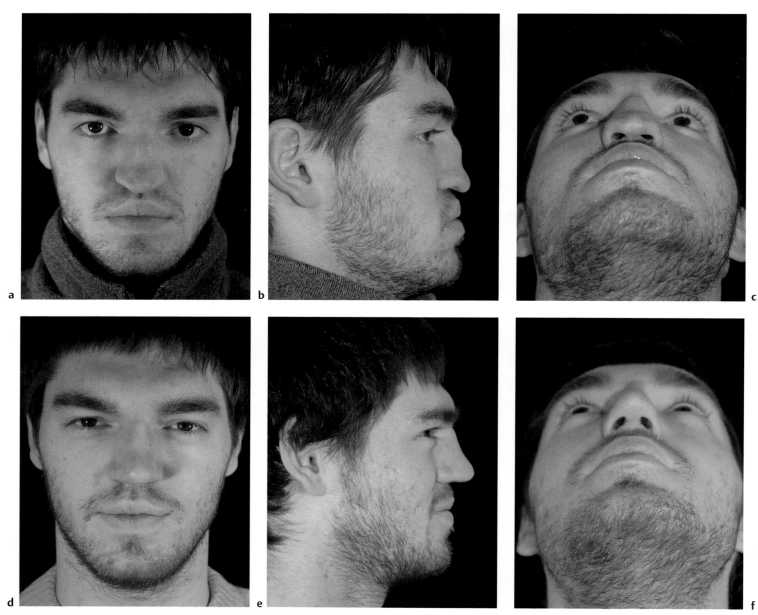

Fig. 25.5 (**a–c**) Preoperative views. (**d–f**) Two years after revision rhinoplasty. (*Continued on next page*)

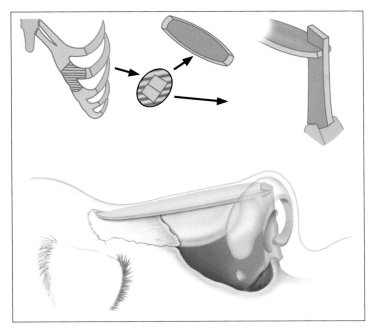

Fig. 25.5 (*Continued*) (**g**) Complete static reconstruction of the supportive framework of the nose. Rib cartilage was harvested, followed by carving and balancing of the graft. A dorsal graft and columellar strut were placed and joined together in a tongue-and-groove fashion.

Discussion

Reconstruction with autologous rib cartilage is the method of first choice in patients who have a complete loss of projection and protection.

References

1. Rettinger G. Rekonstruktion ausgeprägter Sattelnasen. Laryngorhinootologie 1997;76(11):672–675

2. Riechelmann H, Rettinger G. Three-step reconstruction of complex saddle nose deformities. Arch Otolaryngol Head Neck Surg 2004;130(3): 334–338

3. Bateman N, Jones NS. Retrospective review of augmentation rhinoplasties using autologous cartilage grafts. J Laryngol Otol 2000;114(7): 514–518

26 Over- and Underresection of the Alar Cartilages

26.1 Alar Retraction

"Always leave behind more than you remove." Despite this sound recommendation on how much tissue to resect during a rhinoplasty,[1] overresections of the alar cartilages are still common. They are done in the belief that reducing the cartilages will narrow the nasal tip. Unfortunately, the result is a cascade of problems that are difficult to correct.[2] Weakening the cartilage destabilizes the external nasal valve, resulting in inspiratory collapse. It also deforms the vestibule as an aerodynamic body, hampering or preventing lamination and acceleration of the inspired air toward the nasal isthmus.[3] Deformation of the alae may also cause too much nostril show in the profile view, while the symmetry and configuration of the nasal tip are lost. The condition that we call "vestibular skin show" is present if more than 1.5 to 3 mm of vestibular skin can be seen when the nostril is viewed from the side.

Alar retraction may also result from overtightening the sutures during the closure of intranasal incisions.

Reconstructive options range from replacement of the missing alar cartilage with alar rim grafts or composite grafts placed through an endonasal approach to a complete reconstruction of the alar cartilages with the bending technique.[4–7]

The scope of the necessary and desired reconstructions will depend on the aesthetic and functional findings and on the desires of the patient.

The replacement of alar cartilage with rim grafts presumes that the alar cartilage still has a caudal margin to which a graft can be applied. Alar retraction almost always results from the overresection of cephalic alar cartilage. Scar contractions then deform the ala and deflect the remaining cartilage cephalad. The cartilage bed necessary for the placement of alar rim grafts is not always still present. The implants, fabricated from septal or conchal cartilage, are inserted lateromedially through a lateral stab incision into a pocket that should fit the graft snugly. Ideally, the implant should not create a visible step in the alar contour. Its effect is immediately apparent.[4,7]

A composite graft made from auricular cartilage is a sound conceptual solution that carries other risks. The graft must be fitted precisely and sutured so firmly in place that it will not be displaced medially by scar traction. Fixation with all-layer mattress suture placed under tension and tied over a soft, malleable piece of metal foil (from the suture package) for six days will improve the chances for rapid vascularization.

Complete reconstruction of the alar cartilage by the bending technique, for example, is available as a last resort and is the logical solution if it appears that plan A or B would be unsuccessful.

Case 34

This case involves overresection of the alar cartilages, septal perforation, an open roof, saddle nose deformity, and an empty columella (operation by Jacqueline Eichhorn-Sens).

Introduction

After two previous operations performed elsewhere 37 years ago and 8 years ago, the patient had breathing problems due to a large anterior septal perforation and dysfunction of both internal nasal valves. She also suffered from aesthetic issues consisting of an open roof, a deviated and undefined round nasal tip, a hidden columella, and saddle nose deformity.

Findings

The brow-tip aesthetic lines appear disharmonious in the frontal view (**Fig. 26.1a**). The profile view (**Fig. 26.1c**) shows a saddle nose and hidden columella. The undefined nasal tip is deviated to the left and appears off-center relative to the axis of the nose and face (**Fig. 26.1a**). The nasal tip has an unnatural appearance at the level of the alar cartilages. It was suspected that the alar cartilages had been overresected in the previous operations, and palpation confirmed it. An open roof was palpable on the nasal dorsum, and the anterior septum felt empty. The frontal view shows deviation of the nasal pyramid (**Fig. 26.1a**). The columella is deviated to the left in the basal view (**Fig. 26.1b**). Endonasal inspection revealed a large anterior septal perforation measuring 12 × 12 mm. The septal mucosa was dry and fragile. The internal nasal valves were stenotic.

Surgical Procedure

An open approach was done through a standard inverted-V mid-columellar incision. On dissecting the tip, we found that both alar

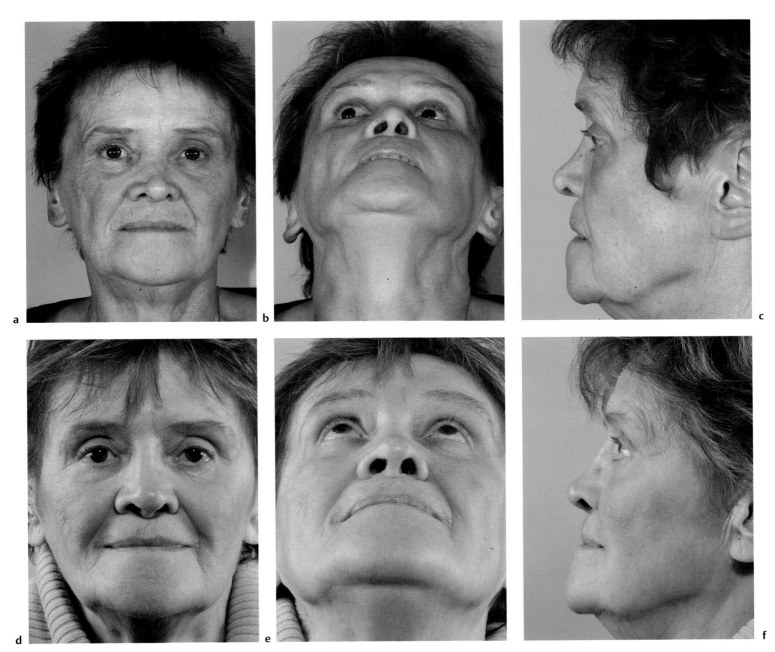

a b c
d e f

Fig. 26.1 (**a–f**) Pre- and postoperative views. (**a**) Preoperative frontal view shows a deviated nose. The cartilaginous dorsum is depressed, and the nasal tip is undefined and deviated to the left. (**b**) Basal view shows deviation of the columella to the left. (**c**) Profile view shows a saddle nose deformity and hidden columella. (**d–f**) At one year the nose is straight and nasal breathing is normal. (**d**) The nasal axis is straightened and the tip is well defined. (**e**) Basal view shows symmetric nostrils and nasal tip and a straight columella. (**f**) In the profile view, the dorsum and nasolabial angle show a stable result.

cartilages had been overresected and that the dome area was asymmetrical on both sides (**Fig. 26.1g**). Dissecting the dorsum in a submuscular plane was difficult due to the irregularities in the dorsum and the open roof. Analysis showed that the anterior septal border was missing. The remaining cartilaginous framework was only 6.0 mm wide and was absolutely unstable. After mobilizing the septal mucosa and the mucosa at the nasal base, we used a four-flap technique to close the septal perforation on both sides. A small residual defect on the right side was additionally closed with a piece of mucosa from the turbinate. Conchal and tragal cartilage were harvested from both ears. Flat tragal cartilage was used to fill the cartilaginous defect between the reconstructed mucosal layers over the previous septal perforation.

A double-layer sandwich graft was used to construct a straight anterior septal border (**Fig. 26.1h**). It was sutured through a drill hole in the anterior spine and to the rest of the original septal framework. Additionally, extended spreader grafts were fashioned from conchal cartilage. They were sutured together at the upper anterior angle of the sandwich graft and between the nasal bones using nonabsorbable sutures passed through small drill holes. The alar cartilages were reconstructed with batten grafts made from conchal cartilage, which were fixed in overlapping fashion in the dome area (**Fig. 26.1i**). The tip was corrected by scarring the dome on the right side and placing a transdomal suture, spanning suture, and finally a shield graft

and tip graft (**Fig. 26.1i**). The nasal dorsum was reconstructed with diced cartilage wrapped in autologous deep fascia from the temporalis muscle (**Fig. 26.1j**).

Psychology, Motivation, Personal Background

After two previous operations elsewhere, the patient had increasing breathing problems due mainly to a large anterior septal perforation. She suffered from dry vestibular skin and recurrent bleeding from the fragile septal mucosa. She was also distressed by the appearance of her nose. She was a heavy smoker, and we told her that a revision rhinoplasty had a chance of success only if she stopped smoking. She was so determined to have the revision rhinoplasty that she finally quit smoking.

The patient was very pleased with the outcome at 1 year (**Fig. 26.1d–f**). She had no breathing problems, and the anterior septal perforation was still closed. The patient has remained a nonsmoker.

Discussion

It is possible to use rib cartilage instead of harvesting conchal cartilage from both ears. But the risk of infection may be higher when costal cartilage is used. Especially in this case, which featured a large septal perforation and fragile mucosa, we preferred to use conchal cartilage. It is important to preserve the inner perichondrium of the conchal cartilage as a barrier against infection.

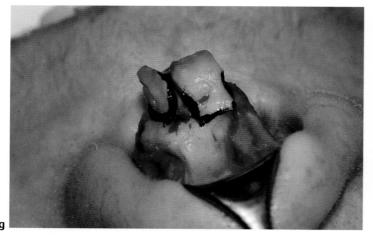

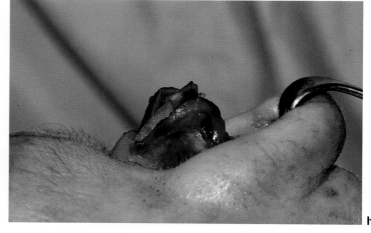

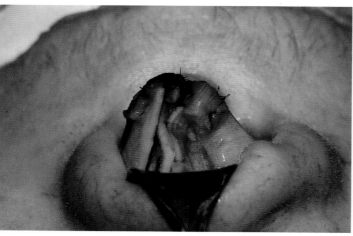

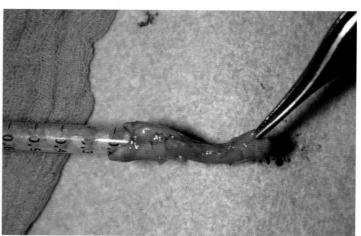

Fig. 26.1 (**g–j**) Intraoperative views. (**g**) Intraoperative view of asymmetrically overresected alar cartilages and bilateral asymmetry of the domes. (**h**) A double-layer conchal graft (sandwich graft) is used to reconstruct a straight anterior septal border and provide columellar support. (**i**) Conchal cartilage batten grafts are placed for nasal tip correction, with bilateral reconstruction of the alar cartilages. (**j**) Nasal dorsum is reconstructed with diced conchal cartilage wrapped in a tube of deep temporalis fascia.

Case 35

Introduction

A young woman underwent a rhinoplasty with profile correction two years ago. Marked retraction of the nasal alae developed after the surgery. The patient was bothered by the length of her nose, which she considered too short, and by excessive vestibular skin show when her nose was viewed from the front and side.

Findings

Frontal view (**Fig. 26.2a**) shows a short nose with excessive nostril show. Profile view (**Fig. 26.2b**) shows a polly beak deformity and alar retraction with considerable vestibular skin show. Alar retraction in the three-quarter profile view (**Fig. 26.2c**) imparts a beak-like shape to the nose.

Fig. 26.2f, **Fig. 26.2g**, and **Fig. 26.2h** show the patient 2 years after revision surgery.

Surgical Procedure

Alar retraction was corrected by the insertion of auricular composite grafts (**Fig. 26.2j**). Alternatively, alar rim grafts are a suitable technique (**Fig. 26.2e**).

Psychology, Motivation, Personal Background

The primary rhinoplasty did not give the patient the desired result and caused her many months of severe emotional distress. Since the deformity appeared to be correctible, the patient was advised to have revision surgery. It is still unclear at present whether the positive outcome of the revision surgery will improve the patient's psychological state. This is common when a failed primary rhinoplasty affects a mentally unstable personality.

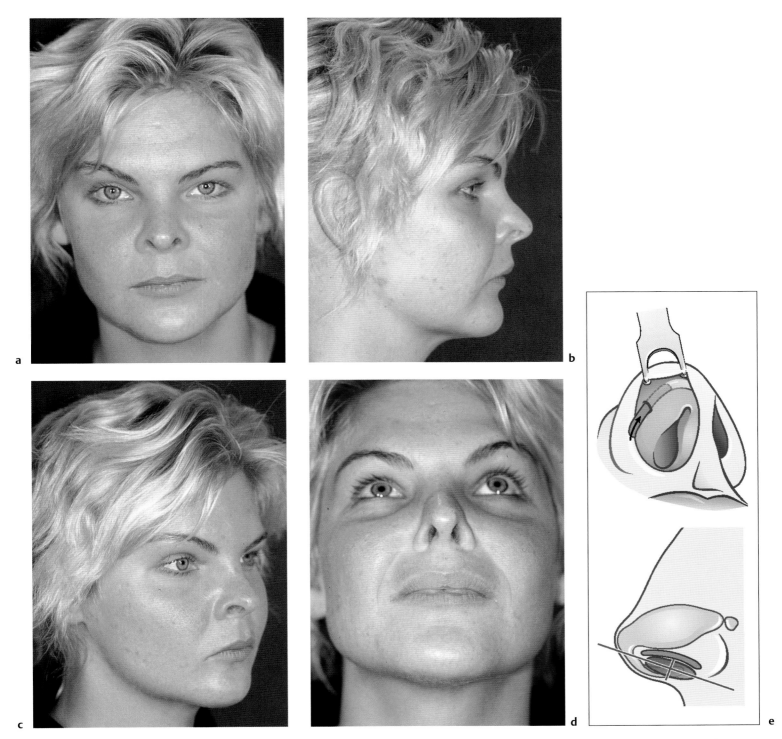

Fig. 26.2 (**a–d**) Findings before revision rhinoplasty. (**e**) Alternative technique in this situation: rim grafts. Positioning of alar rim grafts; rim grafts in situ.

26.2 Underresection of the Alar Cartilages

In some cases the desire of a rhinoplasty candidate for "hump removal" is met too literally, resulting in a nose that is structurally unbalanced. The aesthetic results are particularly unfavorable in cases where markedly hyperplastic structural components remain untouched. The solution in these cases is to "complete" the previous operation. The case below illustrates the complex deformities that may result from a simple hump removal.

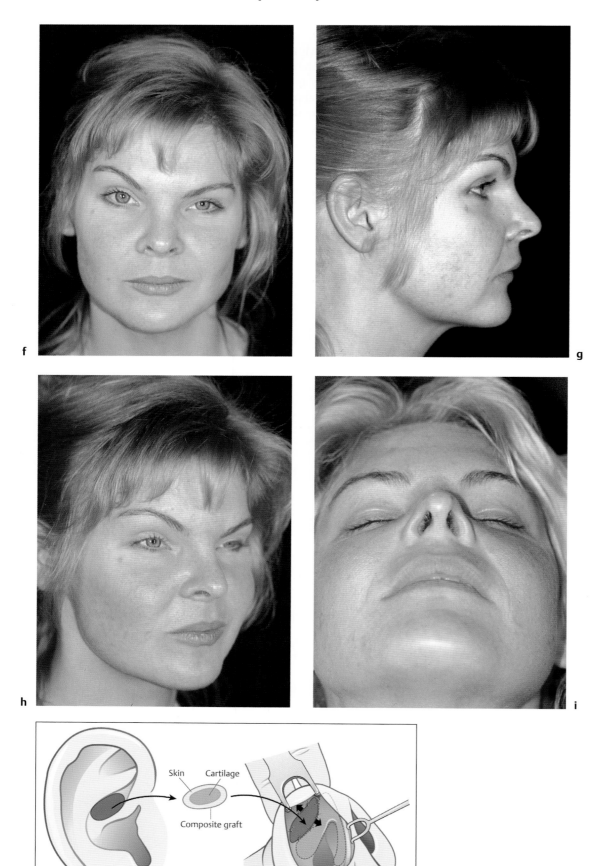

Fig. 26.2 (**f–i**) Two years after revision rhinoplasty. (**j**) The donor site is marked, and the composite graft is inserted. The implant should "abut" the anterior edge of the alar cartilage and should not slip over it or dislodge. That is the main problem.

Case 36

Introduction

A 26-year-old woman presented 7 years after undergoing a rhinoplasty with hump removal at a university hospital in 2001 at 18 years of age. She now sought aesthetic improvement of her nasal tip. She also wanted her nose shortened and her profile improved.

Findings

Frontal view (**Fig. 26.3a**) shows asymmetric brow-tip aesthetic lines and disproportion between the nasal dorsum and tip and between the bony and cartilaginous portions of the nasal vault. Profile view (**Fig. 26.3b**) shows a long nose with polly beak deformity, lack of projection and protection, a residual hump, and a poorly defined, droopy tip. Basal view (**Fig. 26.3c**) shows subluxation with nostril asymmetry.

Fig. 26.3d, **Fig. 26.3e**, and **Fig. 26.3f** show the corresponding views 2 years after revision rhinoplasty.

Surgical Procedure

Intraoperative details: high transfixion incision, posterior septoplasty with local grafts, shortening the anterior septal border, cephalic trimming of the alar cartilages, elevation of the soft-tissue envelope, removal of scars and residual hump, and the placement of flaring sutures to control the shape and position of the lateral alar cartilages on both sides (**Fig. 26.3g–n**).

Psychology, Motivation, Personal Background

The decision to undergo a second rhinoplasty was a long and difficult one for the patient. This process included seeking expert advice and receiving various opinions. But the patient had a deep-seated desire to improve the outcome of the primary rhinoplasty and its effect on her face. After several consultation visits, the patient had realistic expectations and a good understanding of the surgical procedure.

Discussion

The goal of the revision was to address structural components of the nose that had been given little or no attention in the primary rhinoplasty and thus, in a sense, to "complete" the previous operation.

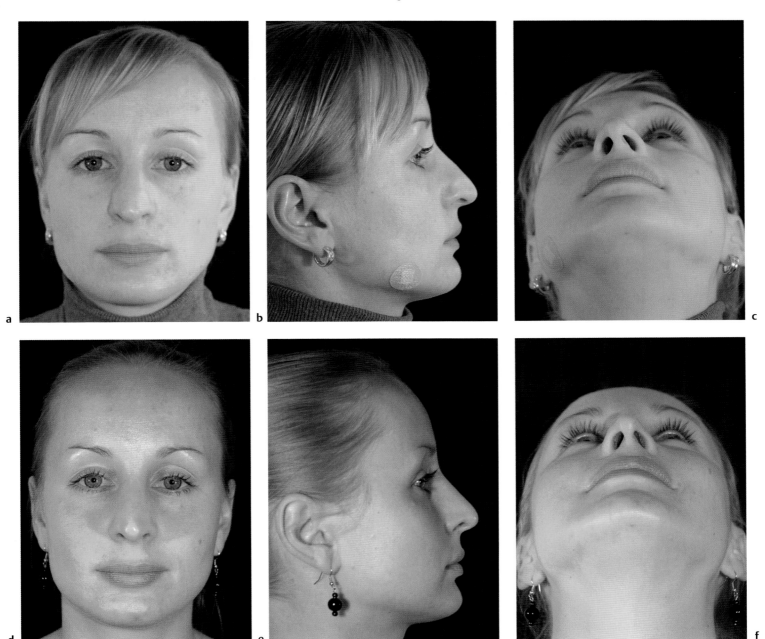

Fig. 26.3   (**a–c**) Findings 7 years after primary rhinoplasty. (**d–f**) Findings 2 years after revision rhinoplasty.

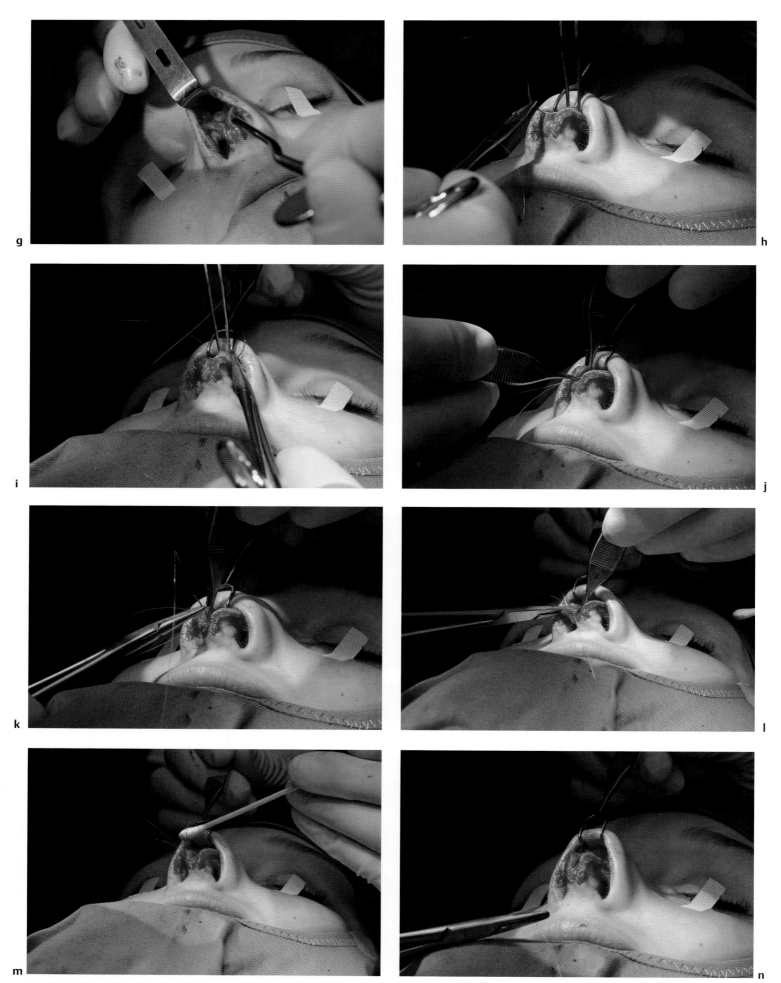

Fig. 26.3 (**g–n**) Steps for the placement of flaring sutures to exert controlled tension on the lateral alar cartilages.

Case 37

Introduction

The patient, a 50-year-old woman, was a popular ballet dancer in her home town. After undergoing two previous functional-aesthetic rhinoplasties at a university hospital at 20 and 32 years of age, she presented now with a desire to deproject her nasal tip. She approached this goal with mixed feelings because she had previously doubted that the shape of her nose could be further improved and, as a stage performer, had perceived this as a handicap. An old photograph shows the young, attractive woman before her first operation (**Fig. 26.4a**). The patient brought along plaster models of her face that had been used in planning the previous surgery (**Fig. 26.4b, c**).

Findings

Frontal view of the patient (**Fig. 26.4d**) shows a narrow, tense nasal tip with excessive nostril show. Profile view (**Fig. 26.4e**) shows an overprojected nasal tip and large nasolabial angle.

The postoperative views (**Fig. 26.4f, g**) show the patient 3 years after revision rhinoplasty.

Surgical Procedure

The revision was performed through an open approach and included basal shortening of the septum at a basal ridge, cephalic volume reduction, and medial and lateral sliding techniques (**Fig. 26.4h–j**).

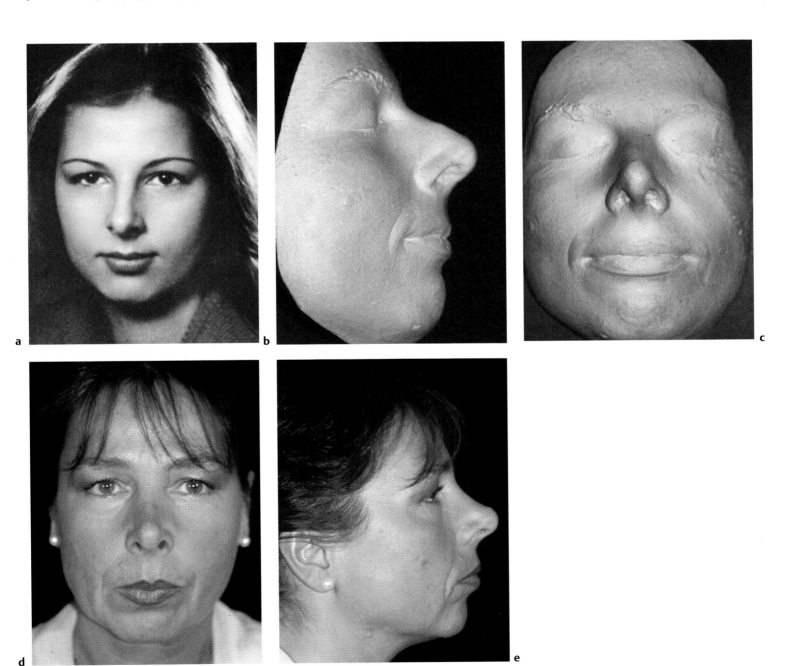

Fig. 26.4 (**a**) Photograph of the patient as a young woman before her first rhinoplasty. (**b, c**) Plaster molds taken before the initial rhinoplasty. (**d, e**) Appearance before the third rhinoplasty.

Psychology, Motivation, Personal Background

The patient had been unhappy with the results of two previous rhinoplasties. She had been told in further visits that her nose could not be improved and she would have to live with it. The patient was reconciled to her "fate." In one last attempt, we advised her to have a revision rhinoplasty.

Discussion

The decision for an open approach was based on the degree of overprojection and the steps that would be needed to reduce the various structural elements of the nose. In our experience, more than 6 mm of deprojection requires an open approach so that the structural elements can be reduced with maximum visibility.

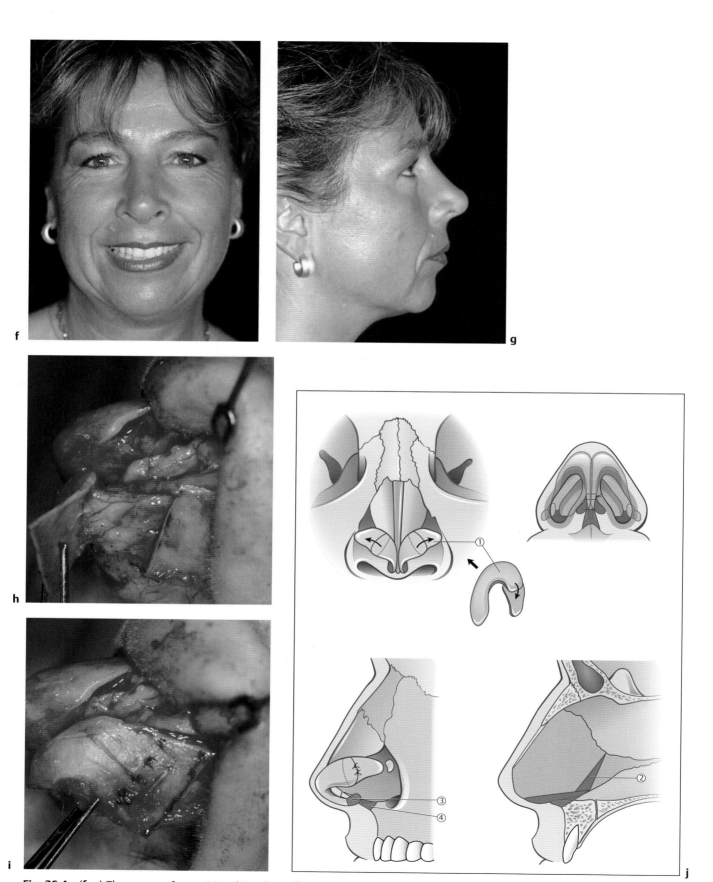

Fig. 26.4 **(f, g)** Three years after revision rhinoplasty. **(h, i)** Lateral sliding technique. **(j)** Individual steps in the operation. 1, lateral conchal overlapping, sliding technique; 2, shortening of the basal septal cartilage; 3, footplate resection; 4, shortening of the anterior nasal spine.

References

1. Pastorek NJ. Surgery of the nasal tip. Rhinoplasty 2001, Chicago

2. Eichhorn-Sens J, Gubisch W. Ausgedehnte Resektion der Flügelknorpel. Häufige Ursache für Revisionen nach Rhinoplastiken. HNO 2009;57(11): 1113–1120

3. Bull TR, Mackay IS. Alar collapse. Facial Plast Surg 1986;3(4):267–276

4. Boahene KD, Hilger PA. Alar rim grafting in rhinoplasty: indications, technique, and outcomes. Arch Facial Plast Surg 2009;11(5):285–289

5. Eichhorn-Sens J, Gubisch W. Die Sliding-Technik. HNO 2009;57: 1262–1272

6. Tardy ME, Toriumi D. Alar retraction: composite graft correction. Rhinoplasty 2001. Chicago, Course manual, 579–585

7. Toriumi DM, Josen J, Weinberger M, Tardy ME Jr. Use of alar batten grafts for correction of nasal valve collapse. Arch Otolaryngol Head Neck Surg 1997;123(8):802–808

27 The Nasal Tip

27.1 Boxy Tip

An aesthetic disproportion between a thin nasal pyramid, a narrow middle vault, and a wide, boxy nasal tip following primary rhinoplasty may have two different causes. Either the nasal tip was ignored in the previous operation—a common oversight in isolated hump removals—or the surgical measures failed to produce the intended result.[1,2] Helpful aids in making this determination are the initial photographs taken before the primary rhinoplasty and the surgical report. It is important to analyze the morphologic problem. Were the resections inadequate? Were sutures loosened by the tension from thick alar cartilages? Is there an open dome angle? Is the tip shape compromised by flaring lateral crura?[2,3]

Based on the broad spectrum of potential causes, a large palette of corrective options are available that depend in part on the patient's skin and connective-tissue type. In patients with thick or moderately thick skin, tip refinement can be achieved with tip and shield grafts. Corrections in patients with thin skin should be limited to suture techniques.[4,5]

If no previous surgery has been done on the nasal tip, the surgeon has the advantage of being able to perform a "primary" rhinoplasty in that area, free from scar contractions and deformities. But if, say, multiple previous operations have been done that involved the tip area, the surgeon will face the challenging problem of altered tip anatomy due to scarring. This may be so pronounced in extreme cases that it is impossible to dissect in normal tissue planes. Revision surgery then requires a dissection technique that I call "carving." Using a sharp No. 11 or No. 15 blade, the surgeon carves the shape of anatomic structures out of blocks of scar tissue. In most cases the carved structure should be camouflaged with a suitable material such as perichondrium.

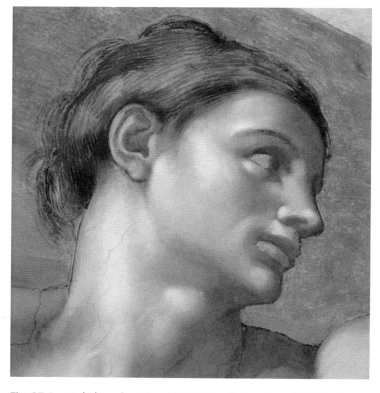

Fig. 27.1 Michelangelo, Adam (detail), The Sistine Chapel, Edizioni Musei Vaticani.

Illustrative Case 38

Introduction

A 34-year-old woman had undergone rhinoplasty for hump removal 9 years ago. As a fashion model, she felt that her wide nasal tip was unphotogenic and that her nose had an unsightly appearance in photographs of her face (**Fig. 27.2a, b**).

Findings

Frontal view (**Fig. 27.3a**) shows a wide nasal tip, a wide nasal pyramid with an open-roof deformity, a mild inverted-V deformity, and a washed-out transition from supratip area to tip. Profile view (**Fig. 27.3b**) shows a small residual hump with a polly beak deformity and a poorly defined tip. Basal view (**Fig. 27.3c**) shows a wide, boxy tip.

Surgical Procedure

A delivery approach was used, and the residual hump was removed with a Rubin osteotome. Medial and lateral curved osteotomies were performed. Transdomal sutures were placed to shorten the inter- and intradomal distance (**Fig. 27.3g–n**).

Psychology, Motivation, Personal Background

The patient had a clear and reasonable motive for seeking aesthetic revision. The individual critical points were clearly addressed, and an overall surgical goal was defined jointly by the patient and surgeon. All these elements provided a solid foundation for undertaking a revision rhinoplasty.

Discussion

In this case the nasal tip had been untouched in the previous operation, so all revision options were available to the surgeon. The suture technique was an obvious choice for narrowing the tip and moving the tip-defining points closer together. The nasal bones were of moderate length, suggesting that reosteotomies could be successfully used to narrow the bony pyramid and the brow-tip aesthetic lines. If the nasal bones had been short, the use of spreader grafts would have been considered.

27.2 Nasal Tip Asymmetry

Asymmetries and irregularities of the nasal tip may arise in various ways during and after previous surgery. A frequent cause is inadequate mobilization and asymmetric resections through a "minimal approach" that does not afford adequate exposure. In many cases, minor variants in the shape of the medial and intermediate crura of the alar cartilages will not affect the nasal tip shape. But if a deviated S-shaped intermediate crus has been mobilized in a previous operation and freed from its attachment by intercrural fibers, a previously nonexistent problem may become apparent after the surgery (see the case report below).

Uni- or bilateral asymmetric divisions of the alar cartilages are another potential cause of tip asymmetry. Reconstructive corrections with cartilage grafts or approximating suture techniques are appropriate in these cases (domal equalization sutures, interdomal sutures). The vault of the dome can be reconstituted with, say, domal creation sutures or lateral crural mattress sutures if the alar cartilages are sufficiently pliable. Asymmetric dome heights can be equalized by uni- or bilateral sliding maneuvers, the Lipsett maneuver (**Fig. 27.4a, b**), or by vertical lobule division. A columellar strut provides the main structural support for the creation of symmetrical domes (**Fig. 27.4c**).

A common problem is an amorphous nasal tip after primary rhinoplasty in a patient with thick skin and fragile cartilage. Cap and shield grafts may be useful for improving tip definition in these cases. The complete excision of subcutaneous scars may be advisable, but the skin should not be thinned too much, as this may cause trophic disturbances and acrocyanotic redness. Small injections of triamcinolone may be appropriate in patients with repeated strong connective tissue reactions or thick subcutaneous scarring. If tip support has been permanently destroyed by overresections, the only remaining option is to reconstruct the missing cartilage with implants (see Case 53).

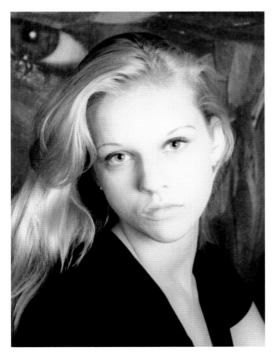
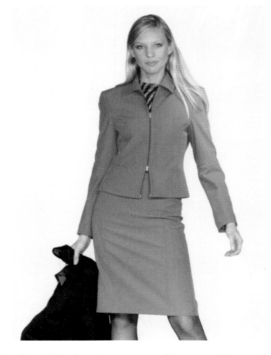

a   b

Fig. 27.2 (**a, b**) Images of the patient from earlier photo shoots. The face is overexposed to conceal the nasal tip.

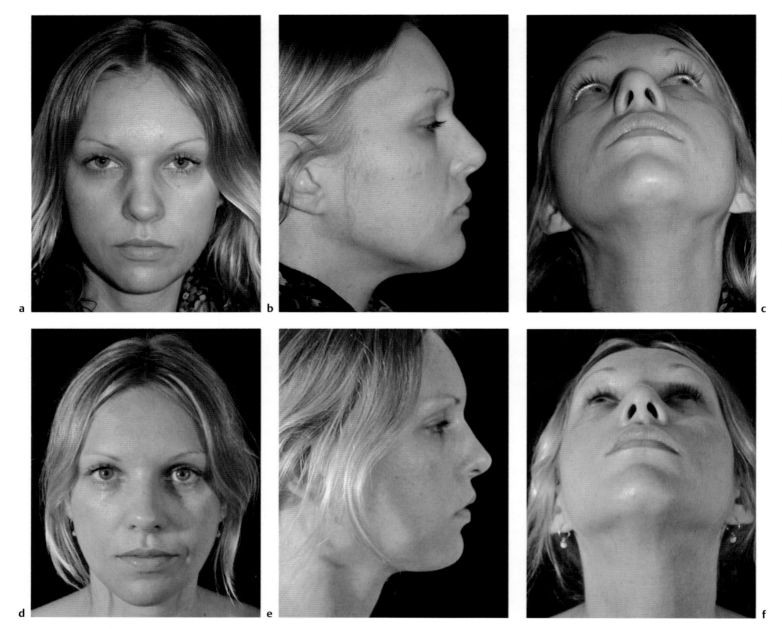

Fig. 27.3 (**a–c**) Before revision rhinoplasty. (**d–f**) Two years after revision rhinoplasty. (*Continued on next page*)

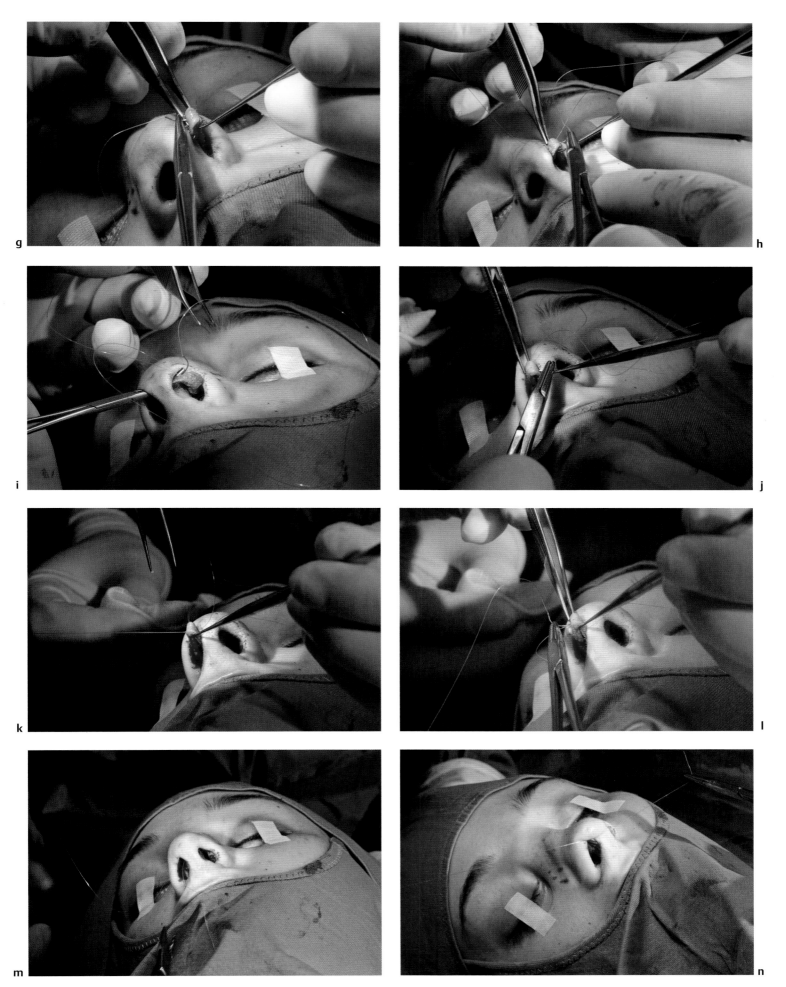

Fig. 27.3 (*Continued*)   (**g–n**) Sequence of transdomal suture placement for narrowing the nasal tip through a delivery approach.

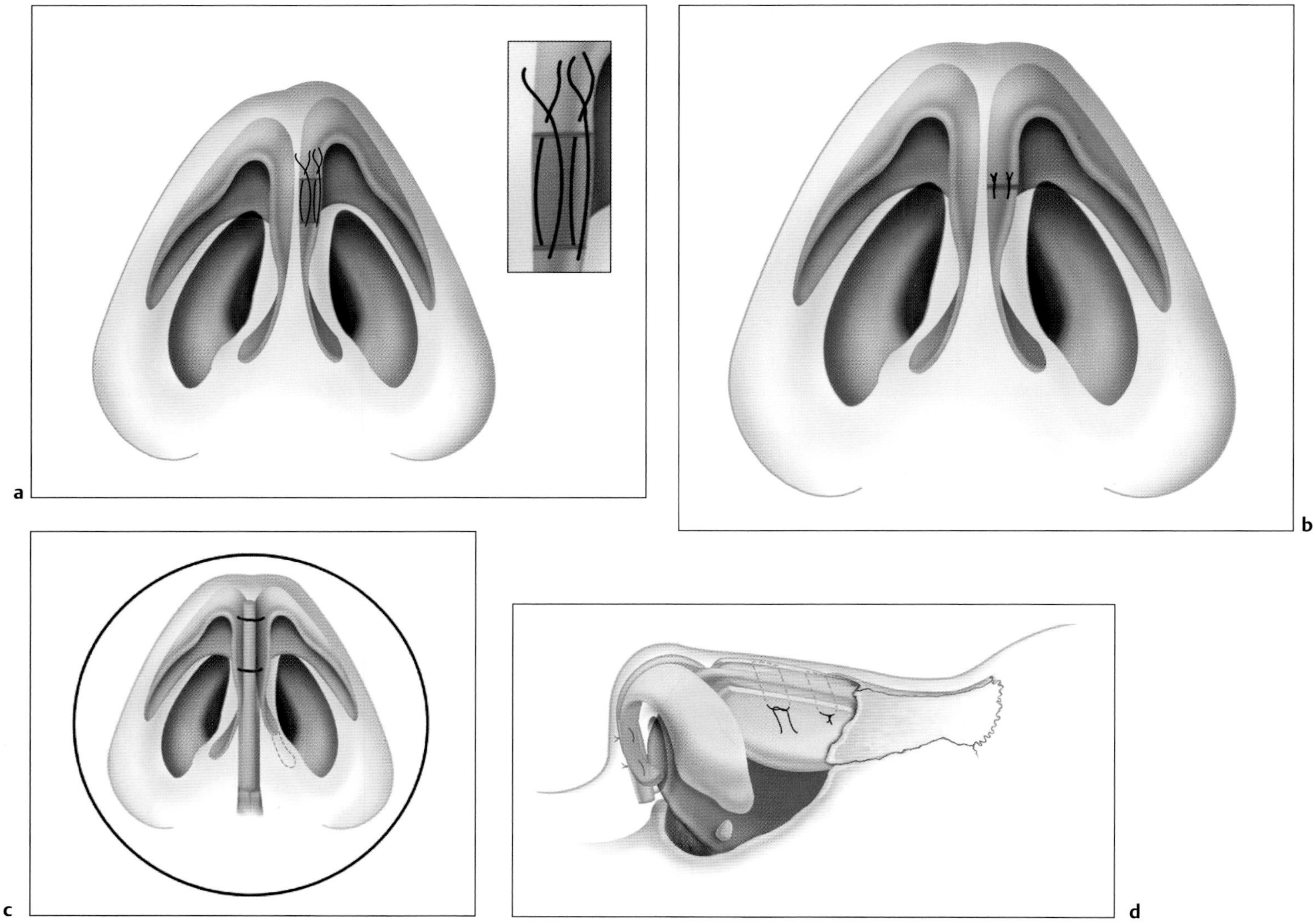

Fig. 27.4   (a, b) The Lipsett maneuver. **(c, d)** Restoring the symmetry of the nasal vestibule with a columellar strut.

Case 39

Introduction

A 35-year-old man stated that he had undergone a septorhinoplasty 3 years ago and that a nasal tip deformity had developed afterward. He now sought deprojection of the nasal tip, the creation of a round, harmonious shape, and elimination of the tip deformity.

Findings

Frontal view (**Fig. 27.5a**) shows asymmetry of the nasal tip, a bifid tip, and thin skin. Profile view (**Fig. 27.5b**) shows an overprojected nasal tip with an unnaturally pointed shape.

Fig. 27.5c and **Fig. 27.5d** show the patient 2 years after revision surgery.

Surgical Procedure

1. An open approach was used, exposing the anatomy of the nasal tip. The right alar cartilage has a pronounced, unilateral S-shaped curve in its intermediate portion. This explains the visible asymmetry.

2. The S-shaped deformity was resected and the crura approximated with 6–0 Prolene. A columellar strut from the nasal septum was inserted. A symmetrical nasal dome was constructed "from bottom to top" along the columellar strut with tragal cartilage. Thin needles can be used to fix the medial crus to the columellar strut and adjust its position. The tip was camouflaged with tragal perichondrium (**Fig. 27.5e, f**).

Psychology, Motivation, Personal Background

The motivation for revision rhinoplasty was based on objective local findings.

Discussion

In patients with a thin skin type, the only effective way to correct the nasal tip is by using suture techniques to reorient the alar cartilages. Grafts would be contraindicated in thin-skinned patients. The tip shape can be softened by camouflage with thin perichondrium.

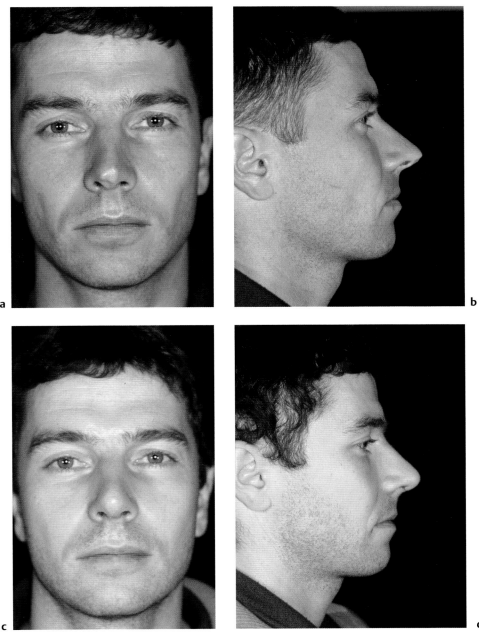

Fig. 27.5   (**a, b**) Before revision rhinoplasty. (**c, d**) Two years after revision rhinoplasty.

27.3 Bossae

The development of asymmetric prominences over the alar cartilages after rhinoplasty is a widely discussed and controversial phenomenon. The occurrence of these "bossae" depends mainly on the technique that was used for shaping the nasal tip in the previous operation. Various predisposing factors have been discussed: interrupted strip techniques, thin skin over the nasal tip, vertical dome division techniques, and the triad of thin skin, thick cartilage, and a bifid tip.[2] Other factors are postoperative scarring and long-term shrinkage of the connective tissue and soft-tissue envelope over the nasal tip. Sharp cut edges in thick cartilage after a cephalic volume reduction also lead to visible and palpable bossae. They may also reflect a lack of tissue tension between the medial and lateral crura.

Given the varied potential causes, only a correction based on etiology and individual findings can be successful. The range of options includes a delivery approach with the resection of asymmetries, weakening the dome area by gentle morselization, alar cartilage suture techniques (e.g., lateral crural mattress sutures), and tip stabilization with a columellar strut and domal fixation sutures. In most cases minor corrections will yield good results. If reorientation is unsuccessful, the only remaining option is a nasal tip reconstruction.

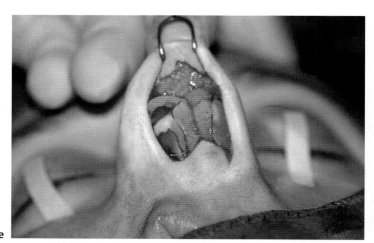
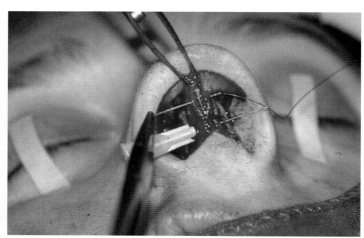

e   f

Fig. 27.5 (**e**) Visualization of the anatomy of the nasal tip. Large asymmetry of the lower cartilages in the tip area with a a cartilaginous hunchback. (**f**) Building up of symmetry from below to above, with a columella strut as a guideline and pillar.

Case 40

Introduction

A woman, then 34 years of age, presented with chronic recurrent sinusitis 7 years after undergoing a septoplasty. She sought a rhinoplasty for profile correction during the course of an ethmoid operation. Two years later she presented again with the concern of an asymmetric nasal tip with a bossa on the left side.

Findings

Frontal view before the primary operation (**Fig. 27.6a–c**). Frontal view before revision rhinoplasty (**Fig. 27.6d**) shows slight nasal tip asymmetry due to prominence of the left ala. Profile view (**Fig. 27.6e**) shows an undercorrected nasal hump. Basal view (**Fig. 27.6f**) shows a bossa on the left side.

Fig. 27.6g, Fig. 27.6h, and **Fig. 27.6i** show the corresponding views 6 years after revision rhinoplasty.

Surgical Procedure

An open approach was performed through a medial intercartilaginous incision on both sides. Scars were removed with the new microinstruments. A delivery approach was used on the left side to perform a cephalic volume reduction on that side. The dome area was weakened by gentle compression with a broad, blunt Adson forceps, followed by the placement of a 5–0 PDS interdomal suture (**Fig. 27.6j, k**).

Psychology, Motivation, Personal Background

Although the patient viewed the bossa as a "minor cosmetic flaw," she was still motivated to have it corrected.

Discussion

The different etiologies of the postoperative tip deformities called for different approaches and surgical techniques. The optimum approaches and techniques are determined by individual findings and often require improvisation (see above).

27.4 Dysmorphic Nasal Tip

Dysmorphia of the alar cartilages may cause the nasal tip to become a conspicuous facial feature that the patient may even perceive as disfiguring. Typical examples are a marked asymmetry or paradoxical shape of the alar cartilages.

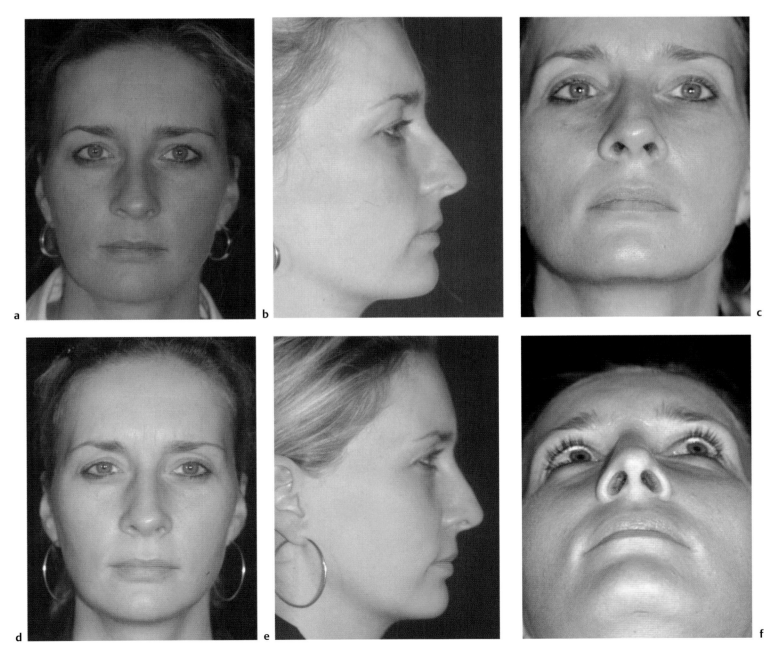

Fig. 27.6 (**a–c**) Findings before primary rhinoplasty. (**d–f**) Findings before revision rhinoplasty.

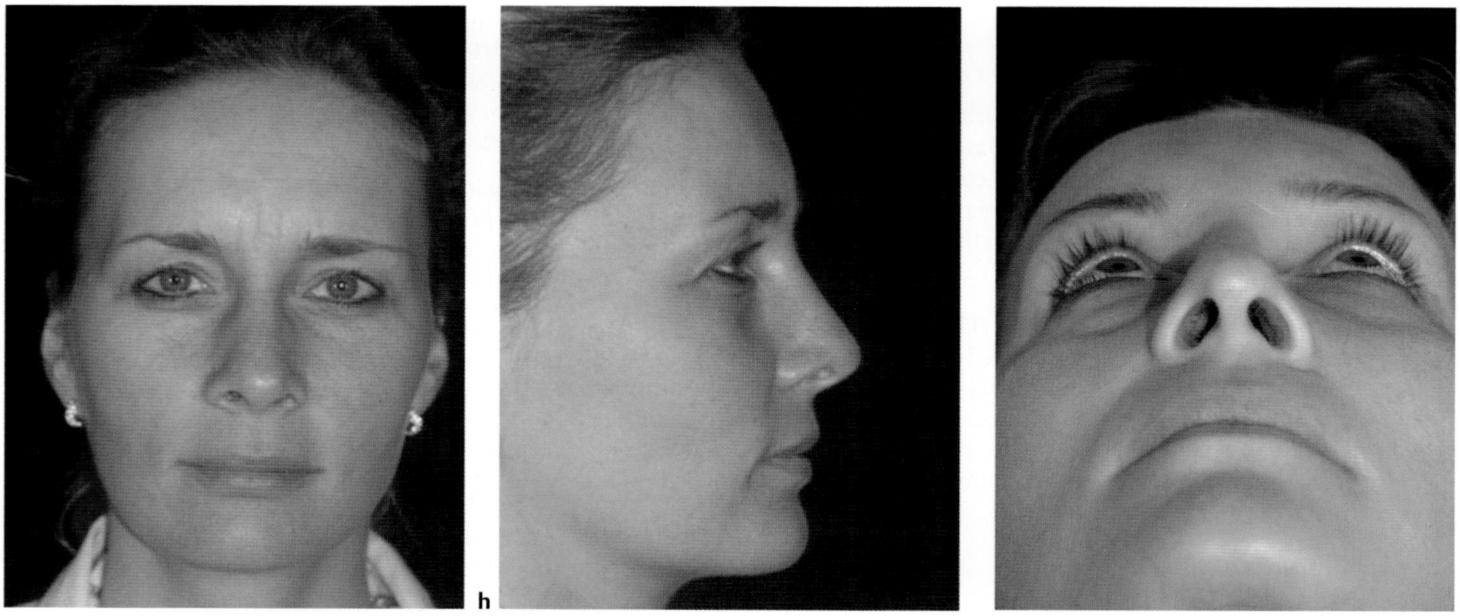

Fig. 27.6   (**g–i**) Findings after revision rhinoplasty. (**j, k**) After cephalic volume reduction, the dome is inspected by pulling up the mobilized alar cartilage with a single-prong hook, and the cartilage on both sides of the dome is gently morselize. Dome position and height are fixed with an interdomal suture.

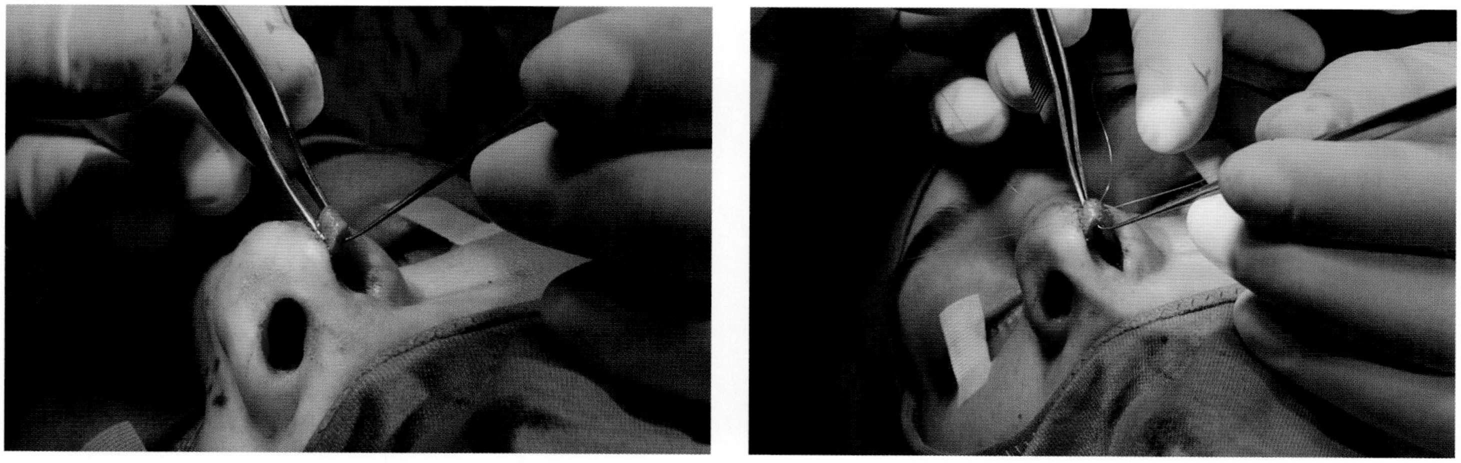

Case 41

This case involves persistent overprojection of the nasal tip (operation by Holger Gassner).

Introduction

A 40-year-old woman presented 6 years after open-structure rhinoplasty. She sought improvement of predominantly right-sided nasal obstruction that was unresponsive to medical therapy. She also desired revision to reduce her nasal hump and improve the appearance of her nasal tip. She was anxious to avoid an "artificial" look after surgery and did not want excessive reduction of her nasal dorsum.

Findings

The frontal and basal views (**Fig. 27.7a, d**) show a ptotic, asymmetric nasal tip with noticeable broadening and bifidity. **Fig. 27.7b** and **Fig. 27.7c** show a persistent bony and cartilaginous nasal hump and a ptotic tip.

Surgical Procedure

The open approach was re-accessed due to the preexisting transcolumellar scar and marked nasal tip asymmetry (**Fig. 27.7e**).

Inspection of the alar cartilages revealed a previous right dome division with the right dome overlapping the midline (**Fig. 27.7f**). The preexisting changes were reversed, all divisions were repaired, and then the tip was reshaped with a columellar strut plus bilateral alar strut grafts, lateral advancement of the lateral crura, and intra- and interdomal sutures.

Tip symmetry was enhanced by the revision. The appearance of the middle vault was improved, and normal nasal function was restored (**Fig. 27.7g–j**).

Psychology, Motivation, Personal Background

This patient was anxious about a possible overreduction of her nasal hump and having a "surgically altered" look. During computer simulation she opted for a slight residual dorsal convexity. This is not too unusual in the middle-aged female population. On the other hand, a young woman seeking rhinoplasty will typically request a perfectly straight or slightly scooped dorsum. It is important to inform these patients that even a slight concavity of the dorsum may give the face an unbalanced look as the patient ages. The scooped dorsum may look excellent in a 25-year-old but out of place in a 65-year-old face. Thus, the author tends to recommend a linear dorsal profile in younger women, which should give the nose more of a timeless elegance than a markedly concave dorsum.

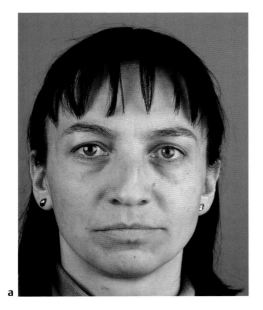

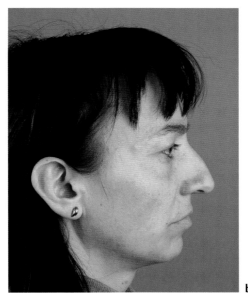

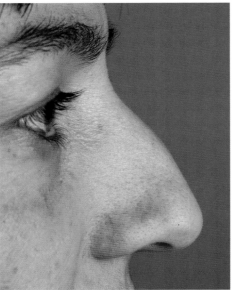

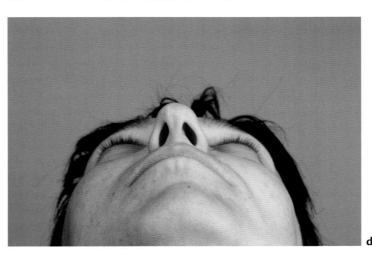

Fig. 27.7 (**a–d**) Preoperative photographs show marked asymmetry of the nasal tip, an overaccentuated intercrural groove, a right-sided bossa, moderate underrotation of the nasal tip, and a combined bony and cartilaginous hump.

Discussion

Revision surgery is often associated with dome division or other maneuvers that disrupt the anatomic continuity of the alar cartilages. In the vast majority of cases, the author preserves the anatomic continuity of the alar cartilages to minimize the risk of asymmetries, distortions, and irregularities of the nasal tip. In revision cases where these changes are identified, normal anatomy is restored first and then the nasal tip is shaped with more conservative techniques such as nasal tip recontouring.[6]

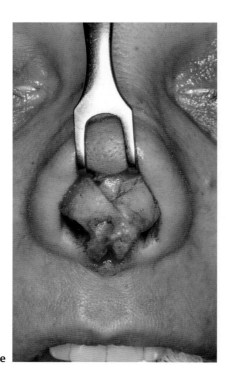
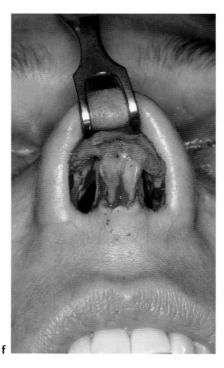
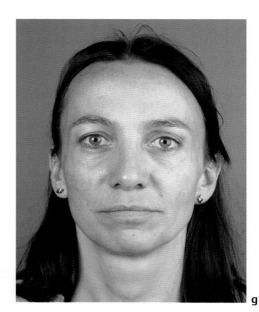
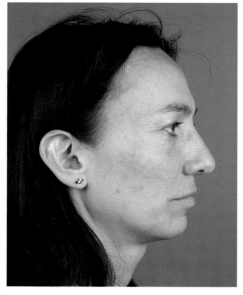
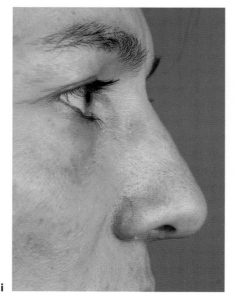
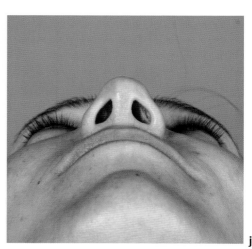

Fig. 27.7 (**e, f**) An unusual intraoperative finding: right-sided dome division with a suture in the right dome overlapping onto the left dome. Previously placed nonabsorbable suture material is still visible. (**g–j**) This middle-aged patient requested a revision to produce inconspicuous, natural-looking changes. Tip symmetry has been restored, tip rotation slightly increased, and the dorsal hump gently reduced.

Case 42

Introduction

A 30-year-old woman wanted to have her nasal tip corrected and her nose shortened. Nasal tip prominence had become an issue only after a septoplasty performed 4 years earlier.

Findings

Frontal view (**Fig. 27.8a**) shows thin skin, concave lateral crura, an asymmetric bifid tip, and disharmony between the nasal tip and pyramid. Profile view (**Fig. 27.8b**) shows an overprojected nasal tip with a definite anteface profile and mandibular prognathism. Basal view (**Fig. 27.8c**) shows an asymmetric bifid tip.

    Fig. 27.8d, **Fig. 27.8e**, and **Fig. 27.8f** show the patient 2 years after revision rhinoplasty.

Surgical Procedure

An open approach and "flip-flop" technique were used. The alar cartilages were divided at the level of the domes, mobilized, and flipped over. At that point they can be sutured back into place on the same side or, as in this case, sutured on the contralateral side as a crossover graft (**Fig. 27.8g, h**).

Psychology, Motivation, Personal Background

The revision was motivated for aesthetic reasons and also to relieve a sensitive, often painful nasal tip.

Discussion

This technique can be used on strongly concave alar cartilages with a paradoxical curve. The devil is in the details. Secure fixation is essential to counteract the tendency of the caudal cartilage edges to dislocate. An alternative in milder cases is to correct the convexity with alar button grafts. Another option would be lateral crural mattress sutures, or strut grafts could be used to secure the reoriented cartilages.

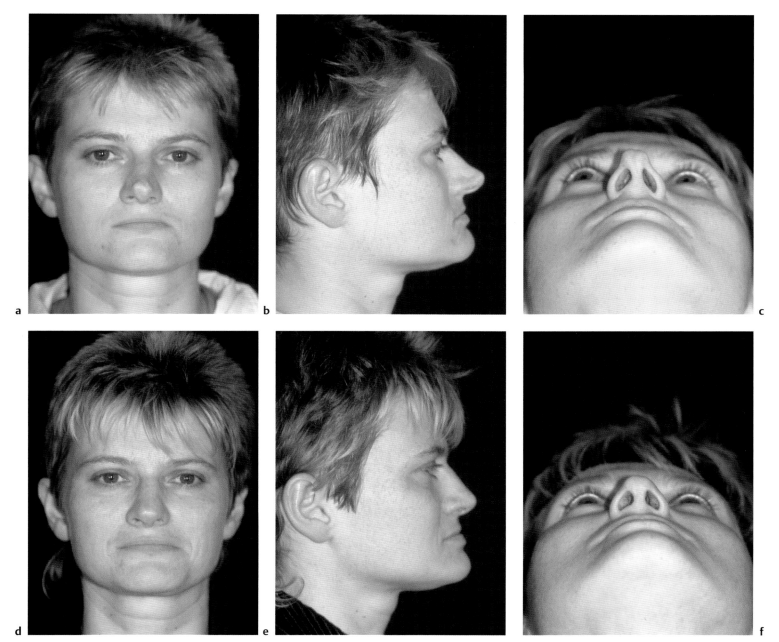

Fig. 27.8   (**a–c**) Before revision rhinoplasty. (**d–f**) Two years after revision rhinoplasty.

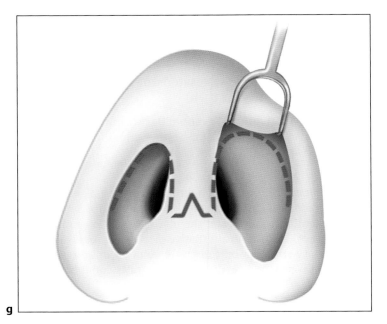

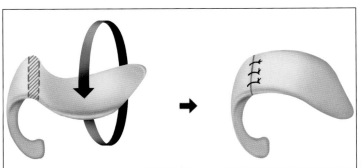

Fig. 27.8   (**g**) The flip-flop technique requires an open approach. (**h**) Principle of the flip-flop technique with the alar cartilages transposed to the contralateral side.

References

1. Eichhorn-Sens J, Gubisch W. Ästhetische Chirurgie der Nasenspitze. In: Von Heimburg D, Lemperle G, eds. Ästhetische Chirurgie, vol 2a. Heidelberg, Germany: ecomed Medizin; 2010:1–28

2. Kridel RWH, Yoon PJ, Koch RJ. Prevention and correction of nasal tip bossae in rhinoplasty. Arch Facial Plast Surg 2003;5(5):416–422

3. Gillman GS, Simons RL, Lee DJ. Nasal tip bossae in rhinoplasty. Etiology, predisposing factors, and management techniques. Rhinoplasty 2001, Chicago, Course Manual, 525–531

4. Tardy ME. Transdomal suture refinement of the nasal tip. Facial Plast Surg 1987;4:317

5. Tardy ME. Rhinoplasty, the Art and the Science, Vol. II. Philadelphia, PA: WB Saunders; 1997

6. Gassner HG, Mueller-Vogt U, Strutz J, Kuehnel T. Nasal tip recontouring in primary rhinoplasty: the endonasal complete release approach. JAMA Facial Plast Surg 2013;15(1):11–16

28 Reconstruction of Tissue Loss: Columella and Nasal Tip

Nasal cannulas are often used for oxygen administration in premature infants. Prolonged cannula pressure on the delicate nasal tissues of a newborn baby may cause injuries ranging from pressure sores to necrosis and superinfection. The following case involves a young woman who had two previous reconstructive operations for columellar necrosis.[1]

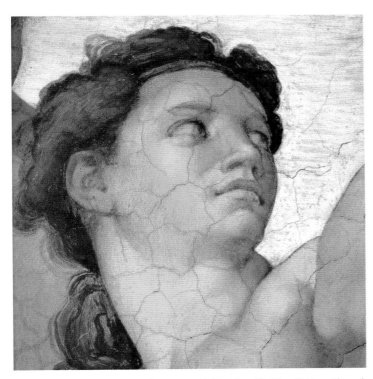

Fig. 28.1 Michelangelo, The Original Sin (detail), The Sistine Chapel, Edizioni Musei Vaticani.

Case 43

Introduction

This 20-year-old woman had undergone two previous operations. As a premature baby, this patient had a nasal tube for several weeks. During nasal intubation, necrosis of the columella occurred. During the first operation, simple stitches were placed to adapt the wound margins without reconstruction of the columella tissue defect. The second procedure was a VY plasty of the columella.

Findings

Frontal view (**Fig. 28.2a**) shows an amorphous nasal tip with poorly defined alar contours. Basal view (**Fig. 28.2b**) shows a scarred columella with a wide base. Profile view (**Fig. 28.2c**) shows unnatural cephalic rotation and shortening of the nose.

Fig. 28.2d, **Fig. 28.2e**, and **Fig. 28.2f** show corresponding views 4 years after revision rhinoplasty.

Surgical Procedure

The old scar was opened and scar tissue was resected by sharp dissection. Reconstruction of the columella was achieved with long shield grafts. To heighten the tip, a tip graft was used. The nostrils were opened by placing two alar rim grafts (**Fig. 28.2g**).

Psychology, Motivation, Personal Background

The young, attractive, and self-confident woman worked in the hotel industry and was comfortable in her interactions with the public. Despite the poor outcome of the previous operations, she had a self-confident personality. Nevertheless, she still wanted to have an improvement of the aesthetic appearance of the nasal tip–columella complex.

Discussion

The findings in this case suggested that, while the nose could be significantly improved, an ideal result probably could not be achieved. The revision plan consisted of resecting hyperplastic scars and contractures, thinning indurated areas, and reconstructing the structural components of the nasal tip.

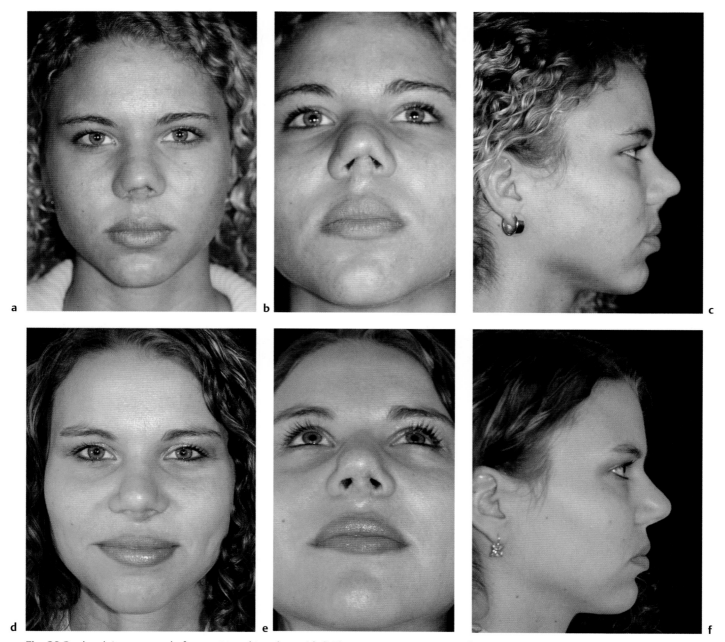

Fig. 28.2 (**a–c**) Appearance before revision rhinoplasty. (**d–f**) The young woman 4 years after surgery. (*Continued on next page*)

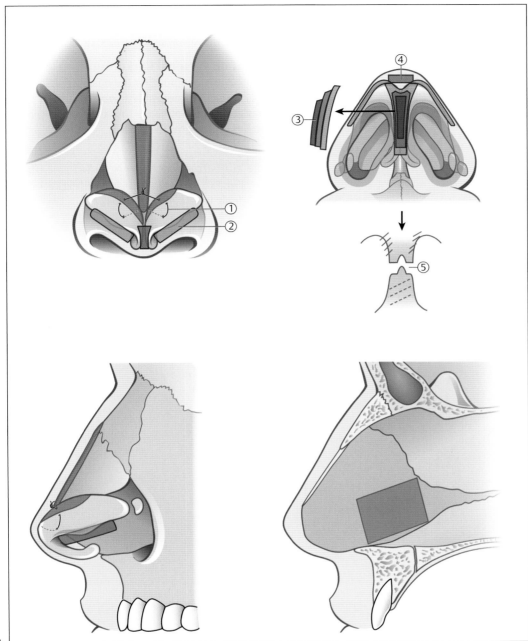

g

Fig. 28.2 (*Continued*)   (**g**) Alar rim grafts are placed in tight pockets along the anterior border of the alar cartilages. They form the contour line of the ala and open the external nasal valve. They can be used to correct alar collapse and retractions. They also form a smooth, elegant transition from nasal tip to nasal base. 1, intra-oral transdorsal sutures with spanning sling; 2, alar rim grafts; 3, shield grafts; 4, tip graft; 5, red, resections.

Case 44

Introduction

Resection of a basal cell carcinoma had resulted in loss of the nasal tip. The patient presented with the goal of restoring a normal-appearing tip. **Fig. 28.3a, d** shows the patient before (**a**) and immediately after (**d**) her cancer surgery.

Findings

In the frontal view (**Fig. 28.3b**) the nasal tip has a flat contour line following partial resection of the alar cartilages. Profile view (**Fig. 28.3c**) shows absence of the nasal tip.

Fig. 28.3e and **Fig. 28.3f** were taken 1 year after reconstruction.

Surgical Procedure

The nasal tip contour was reconstructed with a thick shield tip graft placed through an open approach (**Fig. 28.3g, h**).

Psychology, Motivation, Personal Background

The patient felt seriously handicapped by the nasal tip defect and suffered considerably from the deformity, which she felt to be disfiguring. She was strongly motivated to have the procedure, and she had realistic expectations.

Discussion

Autologous cartilage grafts from the septum, auricle, or rib are well suited for reconstructing tissue defects in the alar cartilages. A multilayer implant made from conchal cartilage was used in this case. To obtain a soft nasal tip, we recommend camouflaging the attached cartilage graft with a layer of perichondrium or fascia.

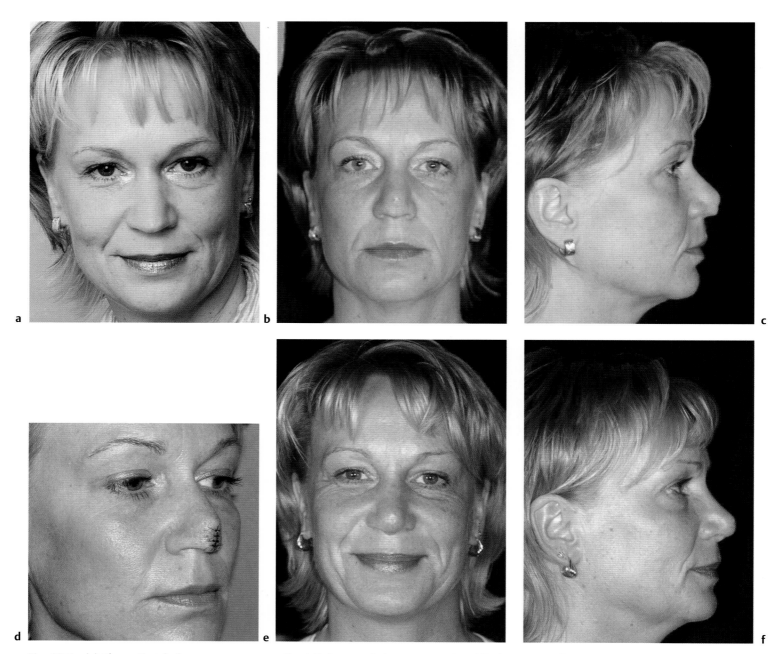

Fig. 28.3 (**a**) The patient before cancer surgery. (**b, c**) Before nasal tip reconstruction. (**d**) The patient after resection of basal cell carcinoma. (**e, f**) One year after nasal tip reconstruction. (*Continued on next page*)

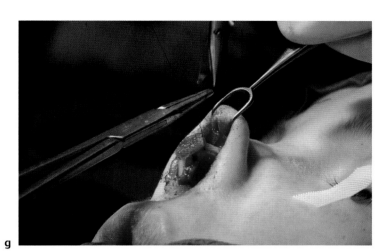

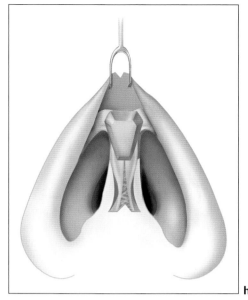

Fig. 28.3 (*Continued*)   (**g**) The nasal tip is reconstructed with a shield tip graft. (**h**) Position of the shield graft.

Reference

1. Menick F. Nasal Reconstruction: Art and Practice. Philadelphia, PA: WB Saunders; 2008

29 Rhinoplasty after Tumor Surgery

In cooperation with Johanna Brehm

The most common malignant tumors that occur in the nose and paranasal sinuses are epithelial tumors such as squamous cell carcinoma, adenoid cystic carcinoma, and adenocarcinoma. A rare malignant tumor arising from the olfactory epithelium is esthesioneuroblastoma. Mesenchymal tumors such as sarcomas are also rare. The closer the tumor is located to the skull base, the less favorable its prognosis. The nasal cavity is a relatively common site for squamous cell carcinoma arising from inverted papilloma, as in the case described below. The cardinal symptoms are nasal obstruction, epistaxis, hyposmia, headache, and possible earache due to impaired middle ear ventilation. Many patients seek medical attention too late, when the tumor has already reached an advanced size (T2 or larger). All possible oncologic treatment options such as adjuvant chemoradiation, conventional or fractionated radiation, and CyberKnife therapy should be discussed and coordinated in an interdisciplinary case conference before treatment is initiated. (Please find more information on this topic in chapter 34.)

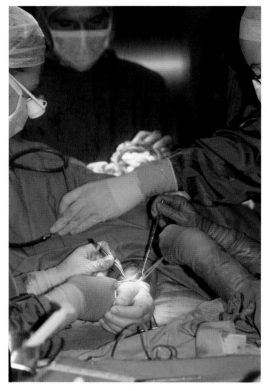

Fig. 29.1 Oncologic procedure with two surgical teams. The first team during tumor resection. The second team (in the foreground) is harvesting a free tissue radial flap for the microvascular anastomosis.

Case 45

Introduction
A 48-year-old woman presented in 2005 with a nasal septal mass encroaching on the undersurface of the middle vault. In 1999, she had undergone the resection of an intranasal inverted papilloma. The latest tumor resection was a histographically controlled excision that identified the lesion as adenoid cystic carcinoma. An R0 resection was achieved and was confirmed in histologic follow-ups. Postoperative care was followed by adjuvant radiation. Subsequent staging tests consistently confirmed an R0 M0 N0 status. The patient, a heavy smoker, died from an acute pulmonary embolism in 2011.

Findings
Frontal view (**Fig. 29.2a**) shows a deformed nasal dorsum following resection of the bony and cartilaginous nasal skeleton. Profile view (**Fig. 29.2b**) shows dorsal saddling of the nose with a pseudohump and alar retraction.

The patient 5 years after the revisions (**Fig. 29.2f**).

Surgical Procedure
1. Tumor resection: transfixion incision with complete removal of the anterior and posterior nasal septum. The alar cartilages and nasal vestibule were free of tumor. The upper lateral cartilages and caudal nasal bone were resected through an intercartilaginous approach along with portions of the maxillary frontal process on both sides, with negative margins. The right conchal cartilage was harvested, and a customized cartilage graft was sutured into place to replace the bony pyramid (**Fig. 29.2h**).

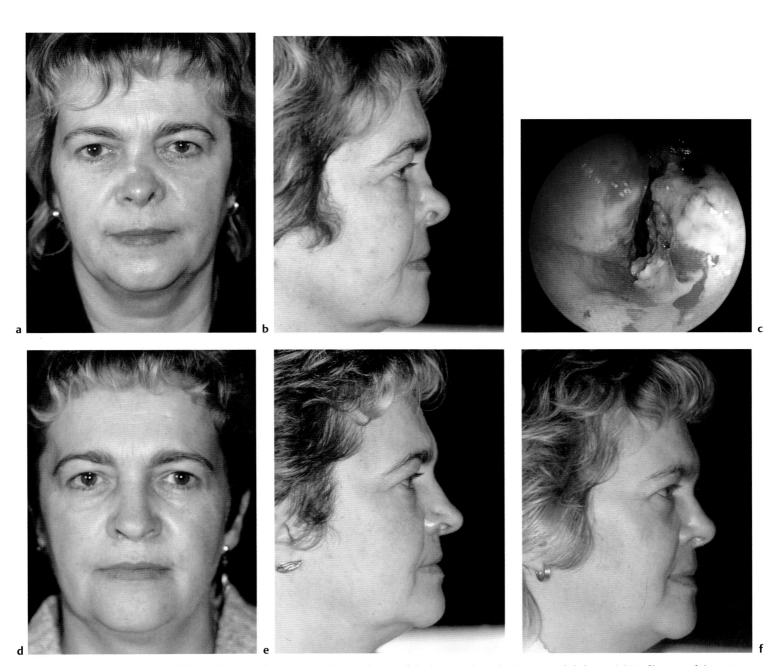

Fig. 29.2 (**a**) Frontal view and (**b**) profile view of the patient after endonasal tumor resection and radiotherapy. (**c**) Adenoid cystic carcinoma of the nasal cavity. (**d**) Frontal view of the patient 4 years after reconstruction of the bony and cartilaginous nasal skeleton. (**e**) Profile view of the patient 4 years after reconstruction; alar retraction. (**f**) Profile view of the patient 5 years after a second revision of the alar retraction with rim grafts.

2. Reconstructive surgery: The postoperative saddle nose was reconstructed in a total of three operations. First, one year was allowed for epithelialization of the nasal surface of the soft-tissue tube that formed the nasal dorsum.

- In an initial operation, cartilage from the conchal bowl was implanted into a prepared intradermal pocket. A columellar strut was also placed to increase the protection of the alar cartilages.

- The nasal pyramid was further stabilized by augmentation on the right side, and alar retraction was corrected with a composite graft inserted into the vestibule on each side.

Psychology, Motivation, Personal Background

The patient returned to her job as a nurse following surgery and radiation therapy. She was psychologically stable, and that status was supported by her disease-free survival and the gratifying results of reconstructive surgery.

Discussion

In patients with malignant tumors of the nasal cavity or septum, the decision whether to preserve the external soft-tissue envelope of the nose will depend on the intraoperative findings and frozen section histology.[1] It is important to respect the oncologic principles of *radicality, functionality,* and *aesthetics,* in that order. Of course, it is a great advantage both surgically and psychologically if the nose does not have to be completely reconstructed. Intranasal tumor clearance is regularly assessed by endoscopic follow-ups with tissue sampling and will direct the selection of adjuvant treatment options.[2] Aesthetic rehabilitation of the face is of fundamental importance because a patient who is oncologically cured but disfigured will be prone to psychosocial isolation.

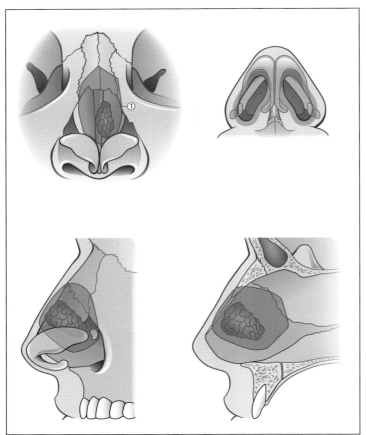

g

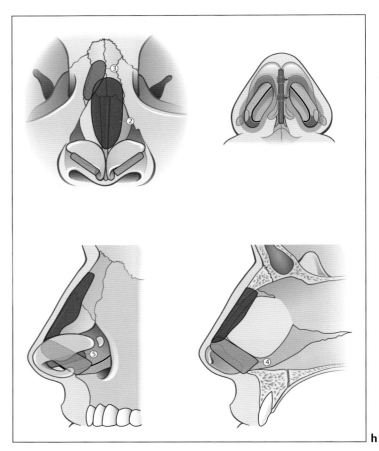

h

Fig. 29.2 (**g, h**) Steps involved in reconstructing the bony and cartilaginous framework of the nose. 1, histographic tumor resections; 2, intracutaneous conchal cartilage implant; 3, osseous replacement implant of conchal cartilage to reconstruct the lateral nasal pyramid; 4, structural collumellar strut; 5, alar rim grafts.

Case 46

This woman underwent the endonasal resection of a squamous cell carcinoma of the nasal septum that had destroyed significant portions of the septum. Endonasal resection of the bony nasal pyramid along with the upper lateral cartilages and septal cartilage had completely destabilized the nasal tip, which retracted far cephalad after radiotherapy. The actual defect involved the middle vault region. Reconstruction was withheld due to problems of radiogenic tissue changes, and the patient was fitted with an external nasal prosthesis (**Fig. 29.3a, b**).

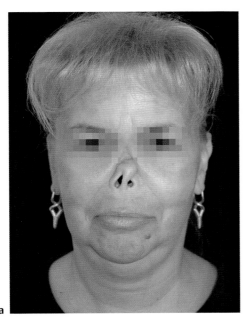
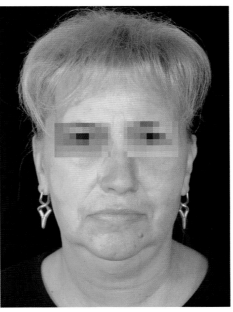

a   b

Fig. 29.3   (**a**) The patient after tumor resection and the conclusion of radiotherapy. (**b**) The patient fitted with a nasal prosthesis.

Case 47

Posttraumatic necrosis developed in the columellar region of a man well over 90 years of age (**Fig. 29.4a, b**). Plastic surgical repair in the first sitting did not provide definitive closure of the defect. The defect was therefore treated with a partial prosthesis (**Fig. 29.4c, d**), which was custom fitted to the patient (**Fig. 29.4e**).

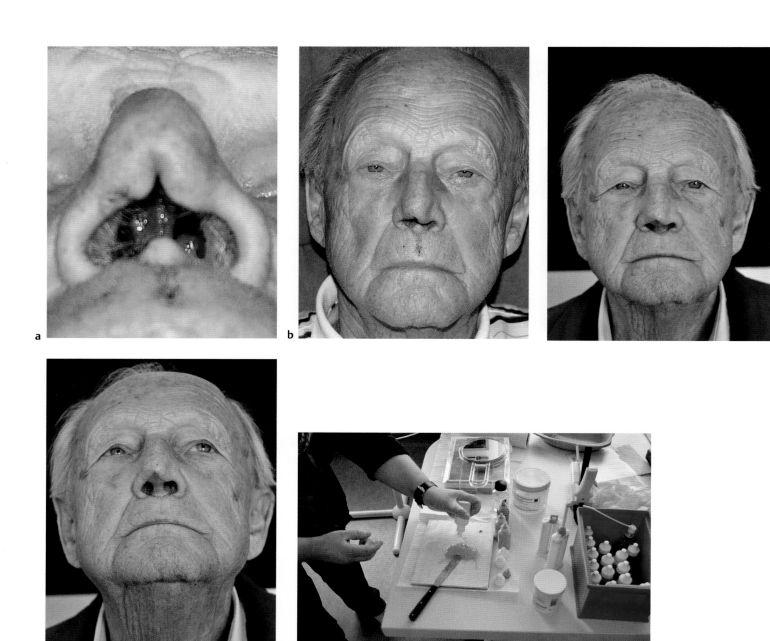

Fig. 29.4   (**a, b**) Defect in the columella. (**c, d**) The defect is closed with a prosthesis. (**e**) Fitting of the prosthesis.

References

1. Lund V, Howard DJ, Wei WI. Endoscopic resection of malignant tumors of the nose and sinuses. Am J Rhinol 2007;21(1):89–94

2. Lund VJ. Malignant sinonasal tumors. In: Kennedy DW, Hwang PH, eds. Rhinology. Diseases of the Nose, Sinuses, and Skull Base. New York, NY: Thieme; 2012:409–424

30 Rhinoplasty in Patients with Systemic Diseases

In cooperation with Johanna Brehm

There are various systemic diseases that have nasal and mucosal manifestations and may lead to a change in the external shape of the nose. Thus, the preoperative endonasal examination should include attention to possible septal perforations and particularly mucosal lesions, as they may be an initial manifestation of a previously undiagnosed systemic disease.[1] Especially in patients with a saddle nose deformity, it is important to look for a possible underlying disease and treat it before proceeding with reconstructive surgery. Some conditions would contraindicate operative treatment. Examples are malignant diseases such as primary nasal NK/T cell lymphoma (due to the severity of the underlying disease) and relapsing perichondritis (due to the recurring nature of the disease).

Systemic diseases that may cause nasal changes include infectious diseases such as tuberculosis or leprosy as well as immune deficiency syndromes (HIV), malignancies, and chronic inflammatory bowel diseases (Crohn disease, ulcerative colitis).[2,3] Other important diseases that may have nasal manifestations are granulomatous diseases (sarcoidosis), various forms of vasculitis (Wegener disease, Churg-Straus syndrome),[4] and relapsing polychondritis.[5,6] The possibility of cocaine abuse should be considered when the history is taken, as it may lead to mucosal granulomas.

In many of these systemic diseases, a cursory preoperative examination may reveal only mild mucosal lesions whose significance is not fully appreciated. But these lesions may lead to postoperative wound healing problems and even external deformities of the nose. If a systemic disease is suspected preoperatively, further tests should be done to avoid a failed operation and especially to direct the prompt treatment of a potentially severe systemic illness.[7-9] The workup should normally consist of serologic blood tests (pANCA, cANCA, ANA, IgG, IgE, etc.), biopsies with histologic evaluation, and imaging studies (chest radiograph, joint imaging, etc.). Ideally, the candidate for a reconstructive rhinoplasty should be in a state of full remission that is supported by long-term compliance with prescribed medications.

Case 48

Introduction

Ten years ago the patient, now 50 years of age, suffered an episode of suppurative rhinitis marked by the rapid development of a saddle nose deformity and perforated septum. Initially she was suspected of having Wegener vasculitis, but nasal mucosal biopsies did not confirm this. There was evidence of nonspecific rhinitis and perichondritis. With a presumptive diagnosis of p-ANCA-associated vasculitis, the patient was treated medically with prednisolone, acathioprin Endoxan, and MTX. She expressed a desire to have both the function and appearance of her nose improved.

Findings

Frontal view (**Fig. 30.1a**) shows an inverted-V deformity of the nasal dorsum. Profile view (**Fig. 30.1b**) shows a severe saddle nose deformity with ballooning, a perforated septum, and a pseudohump. The patient also suffered recurrent inflammatory swelling between revision procedures, at times with severe suppurative postsurgical complications. Photos were taken at the end of a 9-year reconstructive "odyssey" following the initial surgery.

Surgical Procedures

The nasal skeleton was reconstructed in four operations over the past 8 years:

1. In 2003: pseudohump removal plus bilateral medial and lateral curved osteotomies. The saddle-nose depression was augmented with conchal cartilage. The keystone area and piriform aperture were camouflaged with tragal perichondrium (**Fig. 30.1c, d**).

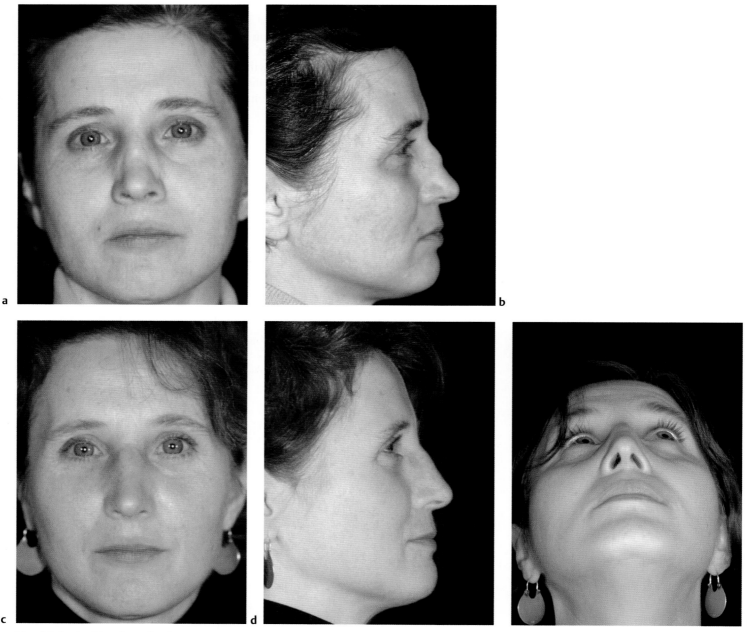

Fig. 30.1 (**a, b**) Before the first operation. (**c–e**) After the first revision. Marked, undulating inflammatory redness and swelling are visible over the nasal dorsum.

2. In 2004: The middle vault and bone-cartilage junction were augmented with conchal cartilage and connective tissue.

3. In 2005: Granulation tissue was removed from the nasal dorsum following a postoperative infection and granulating inflammation (*Staphylococcus aureus*) (**Fig. 30.1f**). **Fig. 30.1h**, **Fig. 30.1i**, and **Fig. 30.1j** were taken after the infection had resolved.

4. In 2006: Lysis of adhesions over the left nasal flank (**Fig. 30.1k–m**).

Discussion

This case illustrates the specific problems that may arise when reconstructive rhinoplasties are performed in patients with systemic diseases such as vasculitis, perichondritis, or Wegener granulomatosis. Although the serologic and histologic studies had a low yield, the clinical course illustrates the problems that can result from exuberant tissue reactions, marked by years of alternating inflammatory and edematous swelling, postoperative infections, and granulating inflammation.

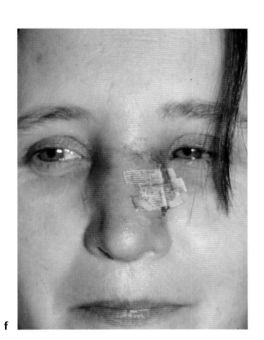

f

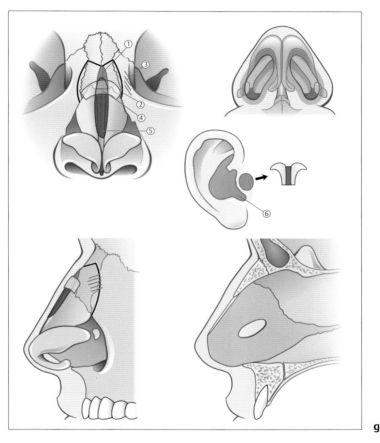

g

Fig. 30.1   (**f**) A postoperative wound infection developed, and a drain was placed. (**g**) Intraoperative details. Red = resected area, blue = areas augmented with cartilage, black = osteotomy, purple = camouflage with connective tissue, perichondrium, or fascia. 1, resection of the pseudohump; 2, lateral osteotomies; 3, green, loosen of adhesions and scars; 4, camouflage of the rhinion area; 5, dorsal onlay graft; 6, harvesting areas of conchal and tragus cartilage. (*Continued on next page*)

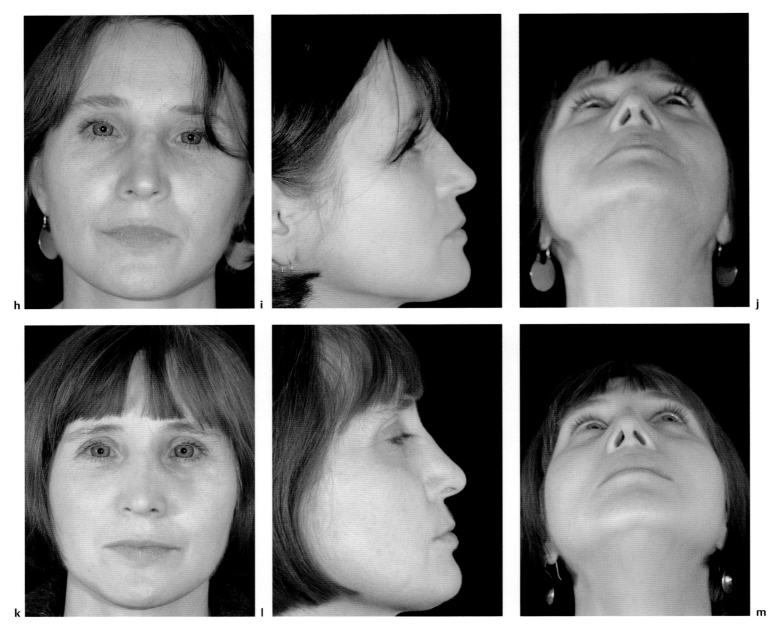

Fig. 30.1 (*Continued*)   (**h–j**) The patient after the third revision. (**k–m**) Final result after four revisions.

References

1. Døsen LK, Haye R. Nasal septal perforation 1981–2005: changes in etiology, gender and size. BMC Ear Nose Throat Disord 2007;7:1

2. Alic B, Askar I. Cutaneous tuberculosis on the nasal dorsum. Ann Plast Surg 2001;47(3):348–349

3. Merkonidis C, Verma S, Salam MA. Saddle nose deformity in a patient with Crohn's disease. J Laryngol Otol 2005;119(7):573–576

4. Paulsen JI, Rudert H. [Manifestations of primary vasculitis in the ENT region]. Z Rheumatol 2001;60(4):219–225

5. Buttgereit F, Kaschke O, Krause A, Burmester G-R. Protrahiert verlaufende Polychondritis als Ursache für progrediente Nasendeformität, subglottische Trachealstenose und Innenohrschwerhörigkeit. Laryngorhinootologie 1997;76(1):46–49

6. Lowry TR. Sarcoidosis of nasal ala and lower lip. Otolaryngol Head Neck Surg 2004;131(1):142

7. Sachse F, Stoll W. Rhinochirurgie bei Systemerkrankungen. Laryngorhinootologie 1999;78:307–312

8. Sachse F, Stoll W. Nasal surgery in patients with systemic disorders. Rhinologic functions—functional rhinosurgery. Current Topics in Otorhinolaryngology Head and Neck Surgery 2010;4:217–241

9. Pirsig W, Pentz S, Lenders H. Repair of saddle nose deformity in Wegener's granulomatosis and ectodermal dysplasia. Rhinology 1993;31(2):69–72

31 Paraffinomas (Lipogranulomas)

In cooperation with Johanna Brehm

Various materials can induce the formation of granulomas. It is known, for example, that exposure to talcum or aluminum can induce granuloma formation at various sites in the body. Mineral fats such as paraffin and petroleum jelly are of special significance in the nose. Paraffinomas have repeatedly been described after rhinoplasties and sinus operations.[1,2] Mineral fats are contained in ointments that are placed on postoperative intranasal packing. Paraffin, for example, may enter the subcutaneous tissue or muscle through dehiscent sites or osteotomies, inciting a granulomatous reaction with the formation of paraffinomas.[3] The latent period to paraffinoma formation is variable. The typical clinical presentation is that of a firm, slowly progressive swelling. Histology shows a foreign-body granuloma with abundant giant cells, and numerous cavities typically remain in the specimen after deparaffination.[4] Various ointments applied to wounds and muscles may incite a spherocytosis or myospherulosis.[5] Histology reveals cystic cavities of varying size surrounded by histiocytes and multinucleated giant cells. The pathogenic mechanism is similar to that of paraffinomas.

Case 49

Introduction

The patient, then 32 years of age, had undergone several nasal operations in her native country of Hungary: a septoplasty in 2003, hump removal in 2004, and another revision in 2008. The patient desired aesthetic improvement of her nasal shape and also sought treatment for multiple facial tumors that had formed since her second operation.

Findings

The frontal view (**Fig. 31.1a**) and view from above (**Fig. 31.1b**) show three smooth, firm, indolent tumors in the medial nasal flank, at the medial canthus, and in the left periorbital area. Associated findings include a wide nose with inverted-V deformity; asymmetry of the pyramid, middle vault, tip, and supratip area;

and postoperative telangiectasias. Profile view (**Fig. 31.3c**) shows a polly beak with a ptotic tip, a small nasolabial angle, and an impaired alar-columellar relationship.

Fig. 31.3d, **Fig. 31.3e**, and **Fig. 31.3f** show the patient 2 years after revision surgery.

Surgical Procedures

Two more revision operations were performed:

First operation:

1. Harvesting of conchal cartilage with connective tissue.

2. Midfacial degloving approach to expose and elevate the soft tissues of the face and both antral walls. The infraorbital nerve was exposed on both sides, and the tumors were excised under microscopic vision. Histology identified the lesions as paraffinomas. Intercartilaginous approach (**Fig. 31.1g**).

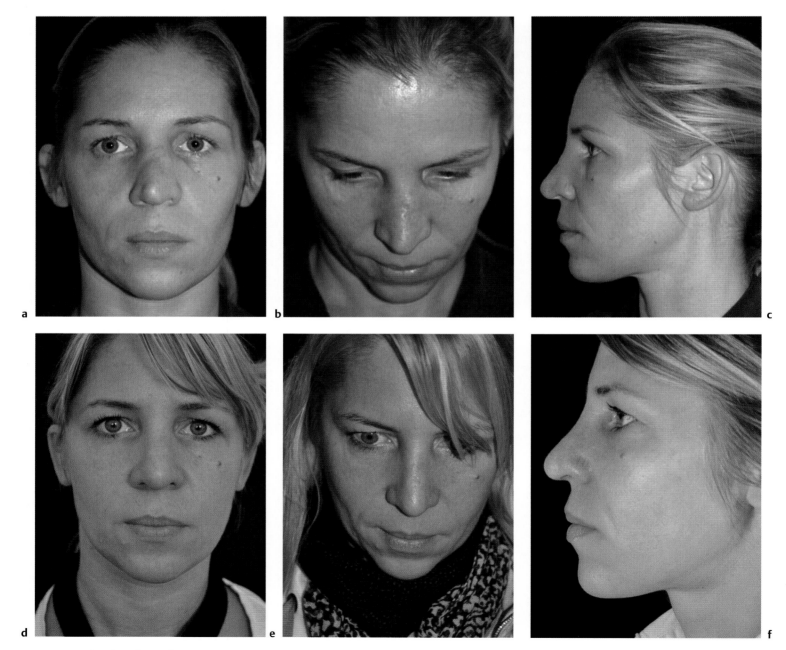

Fig. 31.1   (**a–c**) Findings after two rhinoplasties. (**d–f**) After two revision operations.

3. Intercartilaginous approach with elevation of the soft-tissue envelope. Asymmetric scar tissue was removed, and the keystone area was camouflaged with connective tissue from the concha. The lateral ala was augmented with conchal cartilage. Medial and lateral curved osteotomies were performed.

The second operation was for refinement. Tragal cartilage was harvested, and the anterior septum was reconstructed through a hemitransfixion incision. Scars were excised, and reosteotomies were done on both sides.

Discussion

The treatment of this patient had two goals. The first priority was definitive removal of the paraffinomas, and surgery was the only effective option. A midfacial degloving approach was used to provide adequate exposure. Then another operation was done to improve the aesthetic outcome. A good general rule is to avoid the use of intranasal ointments. Use gels only!

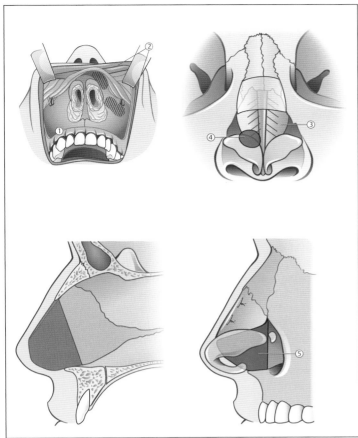

g

Fig. 31.1 (**g**) Midfacial degloving approach for removing the paraffinomas. 1, midfacial degloving; 2, resection of paraffinomas; 3, loosen and resection of scars and adhesions; 4, conchal cartilage augmentation; 5, extracorporeal septoplasty and fixation on the nasal pyramid, upper cartilages, and nasal spine.

References

1. Bachor E, Dost P, Unger A, Ruwe M. Paraffinoma—a rare complication following endonasal surgery [in German]. Laryngorhinootologie 1999; 78(6):307–312

2. Hintschich CR, Stefani FH, Beyer-Machule CK. Paraffinome als Spätkomplikation nach Nasennebenhöhlenoperationen. ORL Nova 1996;6:205–210

3. Becker H. Paraffinoma as a complication of nasal packing. Plast Reconstr Surg 1983;72(5):735–736

4. Rettinger G, Steininger H. Lipogranulomas as complications of septorhinoplasty. Arch Otolaryngol Head Neck Surg 1997;123(8):809–814

5. Weber R. Nasentamponaden und Stents. http://www.rainerweber.de/Nasentamponaden-und-Stents-Seite14.html. 1996; accessed 3 June 2013

32 Rhinoplasty after Cleft Lip Repair

Wolfgang Gubisch

In all cleft lip and palate (CLP) patients, a nasal deformity is part of the malformation and affects patients functionally as well as aesthetically. This complex deformity is due to a congenital anomaly and may partly be the result of previous surgical procedures. The nasal deformity in a unilateral cleft lip patient is totally different from that in a bilateral cleft lip patient.

32.1 Correction of Unilateral Cleft Lip Nasal Deformity

The nasal floor and the nostril sill are usually reconstructed during primary lip repair, which should be focused specifically on the repair of the divided oral ring muscle. The ala on the cleft side is repositioned symmetrically with the healthy side and sometimes also the lower lateral cartilages are fixed in a more symmetric way. Only a few surgeons try to position the dislocated anterior septum in the midline, which always follows the dislocated anterior nasal spine to the noncleft side. New concepts attempt to reach early symmetry of the nostrils and the tip through subtle techniques without interfering with cartilage growth and avoiding the typical severe nose deformities that stigmatize these patients.[1,2,3]

32.2 Surgical Anatomy

According to Huffmann and Lierle,[4] the classic cleft nose is characterized by 22 features, although not all of them are typically present in every patient.

The external examination reveals a deviated nose to the healthy side due to the characteristic septal deformity. The anterior septum follows the dislocated anterior nasal spine (ANS) to the noncleft side. Therefore, the caudal border is always subluxated to the noncleft side. Very often there is also an asymmetry of the nasal bones, so that not only the cartilaginous nose is deviated.

Because of the malposition of the ANS, and thereby induced deformity of the caudal septum, there is always an oblique columella with asymmetric nostrils. In addition, the columella on the cleft side is shortened and the lower lateral cartilage (LLC; alar cartilage) on the cleft side presents an S-shaped distortion and is flattened and displaced laterally and/or cranially. Therefore, the nostril on the cleft side is horizontally orientated and presents as an oval shape in contrast to the physiological oblique orientation of the nostril on the noncleft side.

The endonasal examination reveals a bowed septal deformity toward the cleft side, and the septum is deviated in all three planes—a so-called *difficult septum* being the result. Compensating for this typical deformity, the inferior turbinate of the noncleft side quite often shows a hypertrophy. The most lateral part of the lateral crus on the cleft side slants into the vestibule and forms the vestibular plica. The sill is often missing, depending on the effect of the alveolar bone grafting that is mostly performed at the age of 10 years. There might be a bony deficiency with a depression.

32.3 Indication

In many patients with a unilateral CLP deformity, the correction of the nasal deformity has a high priority because it produces characteristic stigmata in the middle of the face. Upon meeting another person, usually you look into their eyes, but with a conspicuous nose like a cleft nose, your gaze will be drawn to it. This is realized and noticed by these patients, and it affects them. But it is not only the typical distortion of the nose that worries them, it is also the functional impairment. Typically, there is a blockage in the cleft side and quite often breathing is blocked on both sides.

The nose correction is, therefore, an essential part in the rehabilitation of CLP patients.

32.4 Surgical Principles

The goal of surgery is straightening the deviated internal and external nose, creating symmetry of the nostrils, and giving a good contour to the tip. By correcting the anatomical deformities, good function can be achieved.

In our concept, most of these severely deformed septums need an extracorporeal septal reconstruction, which means a temporary explantation of the whole septum.[5] Because this drastically affects the growing zones, we only perform this kind of surgery one year after menarche in girls and one year after a change of voice in boys.

32.5 Operative Technique

Because of the complexity of surgery, we perform all cleft nose corrections under general anesthesia.

There are five complex problems that need to be addressed:

1. *The deformed septum.* To straighten the nose we need a straight septum. Because the septum presents mostly a three-dimensional deformity, in most cases we perform an extracorporeal septal reconstruction.

2. *The displaced ANS.* Not only must the septum stay in the midline, but the malpositioned ANS has to be fixed in its normal anatomical position. Therefore, in all major ANS displacements, we osteotomize the ANS, transfer it into the midline, and fix it there by microscrews and microplates.

3. *The deviated nose.* Because in most cases an asymmetric nasal pyramid is seen, we straighten the bony pyramid via parasagittal medial osteotomies as well as percutaneous lateral and transverse osteotomies.[6]

4. *The distorted ala and deformed nasal tip.* To reach symmetry of the nostrils we generally perform a lateral crural steal technique on the cleft side and then replace the missing lateral crus with a cartilage graft.

5. *The malposition of the alar base.* Correction of the ala base is optional because this deformity depends a great deal on the

previous surgery. There is a wide variety of typical ala base asymmetries, but in most cases the ala on the cleft side is too far lateral and too caudal.

32.6 Septal Correction, Part 1

Using an open approach we dissect the anterior septal angle, expose the caudal border, perform an extramucous dissection, and cut the upper lateral cartilage (ULC) from the septum. Then the upper and the lower tunnel of both sides are dissected. To remove the whole septum—if possible, take it out in one piece—a parasagittal medial osteotomy is performed. The author prefers a Lindemann fraise for that maneuver because an exact, straight bone cut can be achieved with this tool, while simultaneously removing some bone that otherwise might block the bone fragments during repositioning.[6] To avoid any bad fractures, which might extend into the cribriform area, we make a bone cut downward from the bony dorsum with an angle of about 60 degrees. After dissecting out the base of the septum from the maxillary crest, we fracture the bony septum by pressing with a 5 mm chisel. It is important that the whole mucosal wall be freed from the septum before this step so that the mucosa will not tear during its removal.

To achieve a straight neoseptum, or at least a straight L-shaped frame with the adequate dimensions, the length of the original dorsum and of the original caudal border have to be measured. Very often the explanted septum can be rotated 90 degrees so that the bony–cartilaginous junction becomes the new dorsum and the original dorsum gets the caudal septal border. Bent or weak parts are best splinted with thinned ethmoid bone. For reconstruction of the internal nasal valves and for keeping the neoseptum straight we always apply spreader grafts. The use of spreader flaps is possible, but in these cases it is technically difficult. Thickened parts of the septum are always flattened with a cylindric drill.

32.6.1 Correction of the ANS

Before replantation of the neoseptum, the ANS must be positioned in the midline. A side-to-side fixation of the replanted septum is only possible in cases of minor dislocation. Then the ANS is perforated with a drill to allow a transosseous fixation of the neoseptum placed next to the dislocated spine.

In most cases, we cut the displaced ANS with a Lindemann fraise, put it in the midline, and fix it there by an angulated four-hole microplate that is secured by microscrews.[6] The septum itself is sutured after replantation (see below) directly to the microplate.

32.6.2 Correction of the Bony Pyramid

Before the septum is put back, the deviated and asymmetric bony pyramid has to be straightened.

Parasagittal medial osteotomies are necessary for explanting the septum. The lateral as well as the transverse osteotomies are performed percutaneously. We do not respect Webster's triangle, because in more than 10,000 rhinoplasties we have not seen problems with medialization of the lower turbinate's head. After marking the low-to-low lateral osteotomy line, we make a stab incision, push away the vessels by scratching on the bone, and make a continuous transsection of the maxillary process with a 3 mm osteotome. The transverse osteotomy is performed analogously in the intercanthal line.

32.7 Septal Correction, Part 2

After bringing the fragments in the right position, replantation of the neoseptum starts. Safe fixation of the replant is essential for success.

After smoothing the dorsal line by trimming the nasal bones with a drill and the ULC with a scissor, the neoseptum is put back. To avoid the need of a columella strut, the neoseptum is put in a more caudal position to allow a tongue-and-groove technique for tip correction.

First, the cartilaginous dorsum is reconstructed by fixing the neoseptum to the ULC with horizontal mattress sutures, followed by reconstruction of the keystone area. This is a most important step. The best and easiest way to fix the neoseptum to the nasal bones is a criss-cross technique: After drilling a hole into the cranial-caudal part of the right nasal bone, a 4-0 PDS suture is placed downward and penetrates the upper edge of the LLC of the opposite left side. Then the nasal bone on the left side is perforated and the same thread is placed analogous through the right ULC—so that, in the end, the thread can get knotted on the outer side at the junction from the nasal bone to the ULC on the right side.

In the end, the neoseptum is fixed to the ANS, respectively, to the microplate (see above). The length of the caudal border can be adapted by trimming the septum at its base. Then the anterior septum is fixed with three passes of a nonresorbable suture either through a drill hole in the ANS or directly to the microplate in case a transposition and osteosynthesis of the ANS is necessary.

32.7.1 Tip Correction

A strong and straight caudal border of the septum is also essential for the tip correction. The goal is a symmetric cartilaginous framework of the LLCs. If trimming of the cephalic portion on the noncleft side seems appropriate, we do not resect this part, but dissect off the vestibular skin from the alar cartilage and turn the excess under it so that it gets stronger. Furthermore, this procedure helps to flatten the lateral crus. On the cleft side, we prefer to dissect out the lateral crus completely and form symmetric domes by a lateral-steal technique. The complete dissection of the lateral crus enables us to give it a symmetric orientation to the noncleft side. By transferring the cartilage medially, a lateral deficiency may result, which can be corrected by a lateral crural strut graft or a batten graft taken from residual septum parts, straight parts from the concha, or from rib cartilage.

For stabilizing the nasolabial angle and preventing postoperative drooping, we like a tongue-and-groove technique and fix the medial crura to the caudal border of the replanted septum. If it is not possible to follow this principle, we use a septal extension graft for the same purpose. If this does not work, a columella strut from a double-layered conchal graft is our favorite technique.

The tip itself is contoured as usual with transdomal sutures and sometimes with additional intradomal sutures. The strong lateral crura can be molded by ala spanning sutures, which are combined with a tip suspension suture, fixing the tip complex to the dorsal septum (tip suspension with posterior sling technique). In case stronger lateral crura are needed to apply spanning sutures without any risk of creating an iatrogenic deformity, we prefer to use horizontal mattress sutures as suggested by Gruber[7] for flattening and strengthening the alar cartilages.

The soft tissue does not always follow the changes of the framework, and an asymmetry may persist. In such cases we perform a triple flap repair.[5,8] The principle of this technique is to lengthen the short columella on the cleft side by a flap, based on the columella, and swing it inward 90 degrees after incising the vestibular skin for lengthening. The typically hanging ala on the cleft side is elevated into normal position by raising a second flap, based on the ala, and swinging inward accordingly. By transposing these two flaps, a gap results at the apex of the nostril. To achieve roundness, a third flap is created from the excessive vestibular skin, which remains after transposing the skin flaps.

32.7.2 Correction of the Alar Base

The position and the shape of the alar base on the cleft side depend a lot on the primary cleft closure and the effect of bone grafting. If there is a maxillary deficiency, we compensate it with diced cartilage fascia (DCF), made from allogenic fascia lata and autogenous diced ear or rib cartilage. We prefer rib cartilage because of its unlimited quantity. In minor asymmetries, we use fine diced cartilage as free graft.

In most cases, the ala on the cleft side is displaced laterally and/or superolaterally.

If the alae are positioned at the same horizontal level, a lateral displacement can be corrected by an island flap from inside to outside, based on the small nasal muscles. This technique works inversely too and has the great advantage that, by the pull of the muscle pedicle, the effect of narrowing or widening is increased. Additionally, this lineament creates a nice crease and therefore gives a more natural appearance.

If there is simultaneously a vertical asymmetry, we use transposition flaps for correction. If the ala base is positioned too cranially, we harvest a flap based on the upper lip mediocaudally to the ala. The lower incision has to be placed at the same level like the ala position on the healthy side. The vestibular skin is incised, the gap is filled with this transposition flap, and by closing the donor side the ala is brought into a symmetric position. In case the ala base is placed too caudally, the same principle is used vice versa.

Case 50

An 18-year-old woman with left-sided CLP deformity presented for revision surgery after previous cleft nose correction (operation by Wolfgang Gubisch).

The axis was deflected typically to the noncleft side, and the columella was oblique with consecutive asymmetric nostrils. The anterior nasal spine was dislocated to the noncleft side and the caudal border of the septum was subluxated to the same side. The central septum was bowed to the left; on the right side, the lower turbinate was hypertrophic. The ala on the cleft side was pinched—the ala base was displaced superolaterally. In the profile, the maxilla was hypoplastic (the nasal tip was hanging) because the support to it was insufficient (**Fig. 32.1a–f**).

After exposing the typical deformity using an external approach via an inverted V transsection, we found the ANS dislocated 9 mm from the midline (**Fig. 32.1g, h**) to the noncleft side. The caudal border of the septum was displaced in the same way.

After dissection of the deflected anterior septum (**Fig. 32.1i**) from the dislocated ANS, we cut the spine with the Lindemann fraise (**Fig. 32.1j**), put it in the midline, and fixed it there with an angulated four-hole microplate and micro screws (**Fig. 32.1k, l**). Before fixing the ANS, we augmented the hypoplastic maxilla with a DCF (**Fig. 32.1m**) from autogenous rib graft and allogenic

fascia lata (Tutoplast). On top of the DCF we placed a septal extension graft (**Fig. 32.1n**), harvested from the central septum. We fixed it to the anterior septum and then directly to the microplate (**Fig. 32.1o**), which secured the ANS in the midline. This septal extension graft kept the deformed septum straight.

The hypertrophic turbinate bone on the right side was removed by a submucous resection.

Tip asymmetry was balanced by suturing the medial crura to the septal extension graft using a tongue-and-groove technique (**Fig. 32.1p**) combined with a lateral crural steal technique (**Fig. 32.1q**). After trimming the asymmetric cephalic portions (**Fig. 32.1r**), the domes were contoured by intradomal sutures and then the tip was shaped by a transdomal suture (**Fig. 32.1s**). A very thin, extended shield graft was fabricated from the rib sutured in position and turned backward to cover the whole tip (**Fig. 32.1t**) to increase the projection. To avoid any irregularities this construction was covered with a single layer of allogenic fascia lata (Tutoplast) (**Fig. 32.1u**). Before putting the skin flap back, an underbatten graft was placed to the right ala (**Fig. 32.1v**), fixed with transcutaneous sutures (**Fig. 32.1w**), and a rim graft was placed to the right side. After closing the columella, before closing the infracartilagenous incision, the final contouring was performed with a finely diced, pastelike cartilage (**Fig. 32.1x**), using it as a free graft injected through a tuberculin syringe (**Fig. 32.1y**).

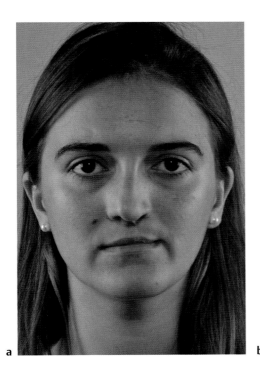
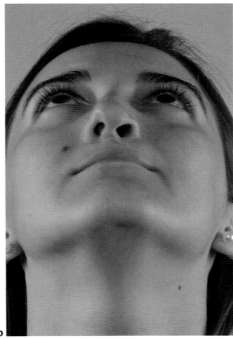
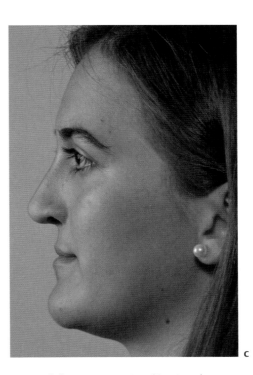

a   b   c

Fig. 32.1 An 18-year-old woman with left-sided CLP deformity presented for revision surgery after previous cleft nose correction. *(Continued on next page)*

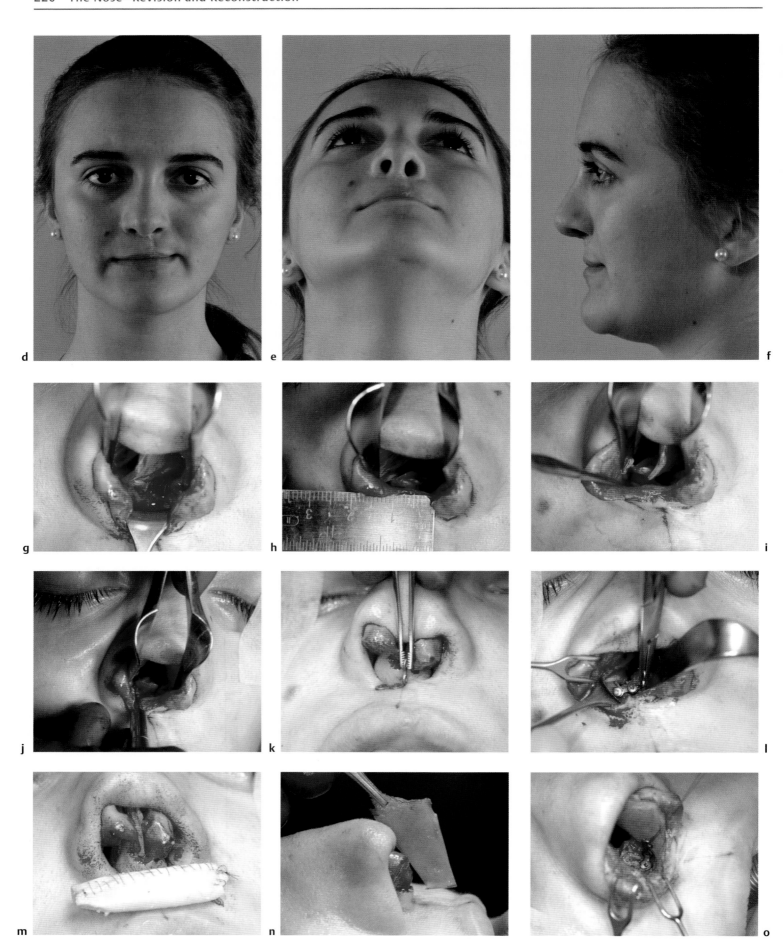

Fig. 32.1 (*Continued*)

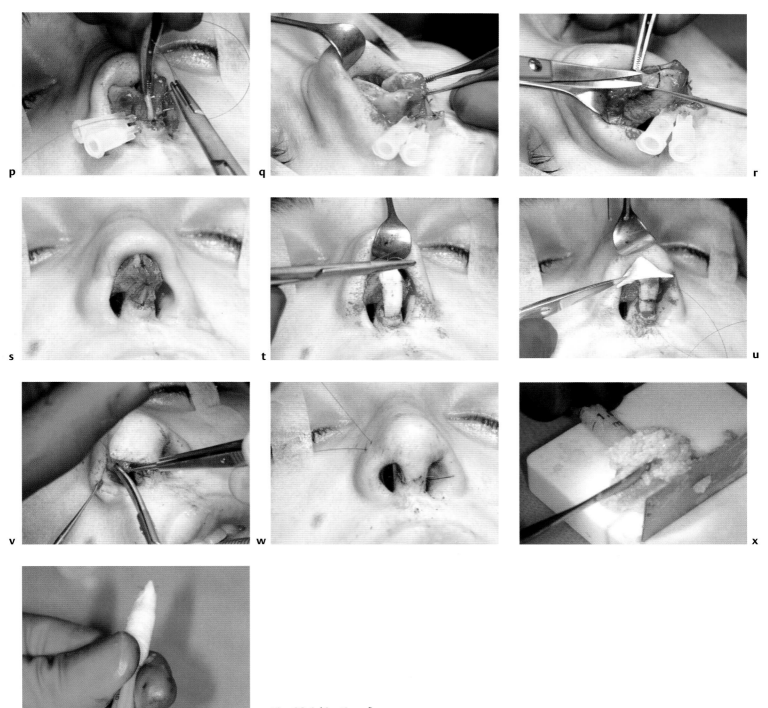

Fig. 32.1 (*Continued*)

Case 51

Introduction

The patient presented for an aesthetic rhinoplasty at 55 years of age. She had undergone six previous operations for cleft lip and palate repair. She now sought an improvement of middle-third and alar symmetry and improved nasal tip projection.

Findings

Fig. 32.2a, Fig. 32.2b, and **Fig. 32.2c** show the patient as she appeared at presentation after six previous operations both to repair her cleft lip and palate and to improve the function and appearance of her nose.

Surgical Procedures

A total of three revision rhinoplasties were performed by Hans Behrbohm:

1. In 2006: Tragal cartilage was harvested, and the nasal septum was medialized through a hemitransfixion incision. The nasal sidewall and middle vault were augmented on the left side. The alar base was transposed and repositioned on the left side.

2. In 2007: The nose was refined by reaugmenting the same region with retroauricular connective tissue.

3. In 2009: Very firm, stable tragal cartilage was harvested from the opposite side to make a columellar strut, which was inserted through an open approach and fixed with 5–0 Prolene sutures. The left nasal sidewall was again camouflaged with conchal cartilage (**Fig. 32.2g**).

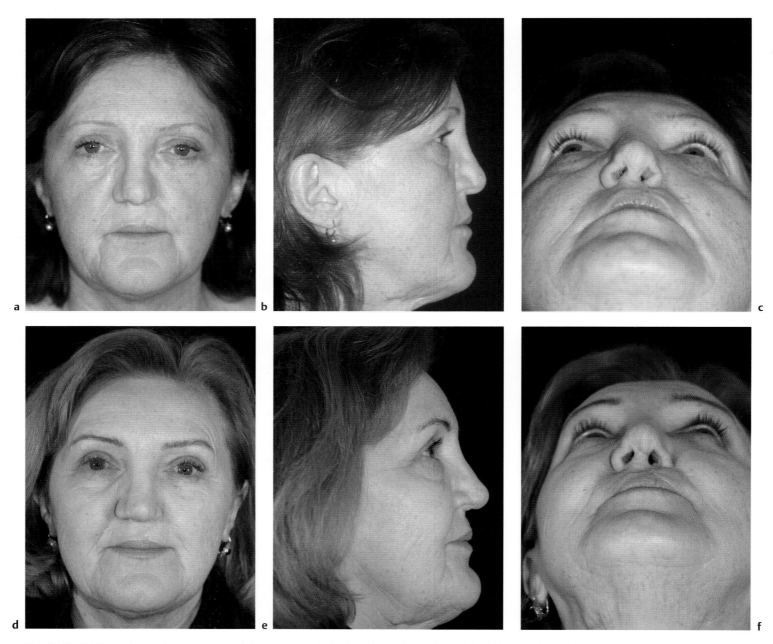

Fig. 32.2 (**a**) Frontal view shows asymmetric brow-tip aesthetic lines due to hypoplasia of the left upper lateral cartilage, depression of the left nasal sidewall, and upward retraction and medialization of the left ala due to scarring. (**b**) Profile view shows an underprojected nasal tip with an acute nasofrontal angle and typical flat profile associated with a cleft lip and palate. (**c**) Basal view shows severe vestibular stenosis and medial alar retraction due to scarring. (**d–f**) Findings 2 years after the revisions.

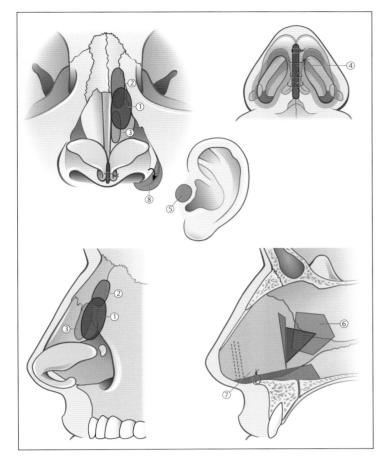

Fig. 32.2 (**g**) Intraoperative details: blue = cartilage implants (dorsal onlay grafts, columellar strut), red = resections. 1, 2, 3, conchal cartilage onlay grafts; 4, columellar strut; 5, tragus cartilage removal; 6, reconstruction of the cartilaginous and bony septum; 7, fixation of the straightened septal cartilage; 8, new positioning of the alar wing.

Psychology, Motivation, Personal Background

Cleft lip and palate is not just a surgical problem; it affects the whole individual. Rehabilitation of the deformity proceeds in a series of steps that culminate in rhinosurgery. A successful operation can help to heal a psychological wound that has existed for years.

Discussion

Rhinoplasty is the last step in the reconstructive rehabilitation of patients with cleft lip deformities. It is important to establish a closed nasal sill, as it will create a foundation for constructing symmetrical columellar and alar anatomy. Previous cleft repairs leave scars that will direct the rhinosurgical procedure. In the case described, the patient's desire for further improvements developed gradually, starting with a very minor improvement in symmetry and proceeding to increased nasal tip projection. Cleft lip produces typical anatomic changes depending on whether the deformity is unilateral or bilateral. Cleft lip repairs leave behind firm scars that tend to contract and distort the surrounding tissues. These factors must be taken into account when planning the placement of stable, tension-free implants in cleft lip rhinoplasties.

The term "cleft lip and palate" is somewhat incomplete, as it fails to express the significant functional and aesthetic nasal prob- lems that always coexist with a cleft lip. The primary treatment goals are centered on the cleft repair, while secondary treatment options are directed toward optimizing the form and function of the nose.[9] The goals of a secondary rhinoplasty are determined by the congenital anomaly itself and by the results of the primary repairs. Unilateral and bilateral cleft deformities present differ- ent starting conditions for septorhinoplasty. Patients with a bi- lateral cleft have a short columella. The nasal tip is broad and flat, and the nostrils have a transverse oval shape. The nasal sill is frequently absent, and the alar base is displaced laterally and cephalad. The alar cartilages show an S-shaped deformity.

Unilateral clefts are usually associated with nasal deviation to the opposite side and significant septal deviation. Typically the anterior septum is dislocated toward the affected side, with the anterior septum deviated to the noncleft side and the posterior septum deviated to the cleft side. The nasal spine is displaced to the noncleft side.[9,10]

Given this initial situation, septorhinoplasty is a highly complex operation that has a different scope and time frame than other rhinoplasties. Complete symmetry often cannot be achieved, and many cases require a staged approach to surgical treatment. Optimum symmetry of the nasal tip and nostrils can be achieved only by repositioning the cartilages and reshaping the soft-tissue envelope.[11,12]

The following specific issues need to be addressed: the septal deformity, turbinate hyperplasia, the deformed bony nasal pyramid, the deformed nasal tip, the alar displacement on the cleft side, and the short columella.

1. The septum: It is important to approximate the septum to the palatal shelves. The septum is the central structural element. Good exposure is obtained with a U-shaped incision over the columella that extends into the alar cartilages on both sides. An extracorporeal septoplasty is often advised.[13]

2. It is often essential to perform a moderate, structure-conserving reduction of a hyperplastic inferior turbinate on the side opposite the deviation.

3. The axial deviation usually affects both the cartilaginous and bony portions of the nose. Tailored osteotomies are often required.[14]

4. Contrary to the usual sequence of steps, the nasal tip should be addressed after correction of the septum and bony nasal pyramid. It is important to relax and lengthen the columella through a U-shaped approach.

5. The alar base, which is usually displaced laterally or laterally upward on the cleft side, is repositioned by an elliptical skin excision and sutured into place.

6. The columella can be lengthened by a V-Y skin flap advancement from the nasal floor. The alar base is transposed medially.

References

1. Anderl H. Simultaneous repair of lip and nose in unilateral cleft (a long term report). In: Jackson IT, Sommerlad BC, eds. Recent Advances in Plastic Surgery. Vol 3. Edinburgh: Churchill Livingston; 1985

2. Salyer KE. Primary correction of the unilateral cleft nose: a 15-year experience. Plast Reconstr Surg 1986;77:558–566

3. McComb H. Primary correction of unilateral cleft lip nasal deformity: a 10 year review. Plast Reconstr Surg 1985;75:791–797

4. Huffmann WC, Lierle DM. Studies on the pathological anatomy of the unilateral harelip nose. Plastic Reconstr Surg 1949;4(3):225–234

5. Gubisch W. In: Naumann HH, ed. Head and Neck Surgery. Vol. 1. Face, Nose and Facial Skull, Part 1. New York: Thieme; 1995: 286–301

6. Gubisch W. Treatment of the scoliotic nose with extracorporeal septoplasty. Facial Plast Surg Clin N Am 2015;23(1):11–22

7. Gruber RP, Nahai F, Bogdan MA, et al. Changing the convexity and concavity of nasal cartilages and cartilage grafts with horizontal mattress sutures. Part II: clinical results. Plast Reconstr Surg 2005;115:595–606

8. Gubisch W. How to obtain symmetry in a unilateral cleft nose. A new technique. Eur J Plast Surg 1990;13:241–246

9. Grzonka M, Koch H, Koch J. Die Lippen-Kiefer-Gaumen-Spalte: Ausprägung, Auswirkungen, Korrektur der Nasenfehlbildung. Forum HNO 2005;7:192–198

10. Pausch N, Hemprich A. Möglichkeiten und Grenzen, Komplikationen und Fehler der chirurgischen Korrektur spaltbedingter Nasendysplasie. Journal DGPW Chir 2009;21(40):32–39 http://www.dgpw.org/fileadmin/dgpw.org/PDF-Dateien/Journal_Ausgabe_Nr.40.pdf

11. Stellmach R. (1973) Operative Korrektur und Nachbehandlung der spaltbedingten Schiefnase. In: Schuchardt K, Steinhardt G, Schwenzer N, eds. Lippen-Kiefer-Gaumenspalten: Primär- und Sekundärbehandlungen. Fortschritte der Kiefer- und Gesichtschirurgie 16. Stuttgart, West Germany: Thieme; 1973:261–265

12. Tolhurst DE. Secondary correction of the cleft nasal deformity. Br J Plast Surg 1983;36:449–454

13. Gubisch W. Principles of cleft nose correction [in German]. Laryngorhi- nootologie 1997;76(11):682–685

14. Nolst Trenité GJ. Secondary rhinoplasty in the cleft lip patient. B-ENT 2006;2(Suppl 4):102–108

33 Iatrogenic Overresection of the Nasal Framework

In cooperation with Wolfgang Gubisch

Case 52

This case involves a severe deformity of the nasal tip with loss of support to the anterior septum (operation by Wolfgang Gubisch).

Introduction

After undergoing two previous operations elsewhere as a child, the patient suffered from an unusual aesthetic deformity of the nasal tip and a severe impairment of nasal breathing.

Findings

Inspection revealed a conspicuous deformity of the nasal tip with loss of tip support and projection (**Fig. 33.1a–c**). The tip defining points were spaced far apart, and the tip appeared completely undefined (**Fig. 33.1a, b**). On palpation, the anterior part of the septum and anterior nasal spine were found to be missing. Internal examination revealed a severely deviated septum.

Surgical Procedure

An open approach was done through a standard inverted-V midcolumellar incision. Analysis showed massive scar formation at the nasal tip (**Fig. 33.1g**). After dissecting the tip, we found that the lower cartilages had been overresected and the remaining cartilages were deformed. The anterior nasal spine was missing. The anterior part of the septal cartilage was absent and the rest was deviated. When the scars at the nasal base were dissected, the septal cartilage became straight. Conchal cartilage was harvested on one side, and a double-layer conchal sandwich graft was placed as a septal extension graft (**Fig. 33.1h**). The sandwich graft was fixed to the premaxilla through a V-shaped drill hole in the area of the missing anterior nasal spine and also to the anterior border of the septal cartilage. We used the bending technique for reconstruction of the lower cartilages (**Fig. 33.1i, j**).[1,2] Costal cartilage was harvested because there was not enough

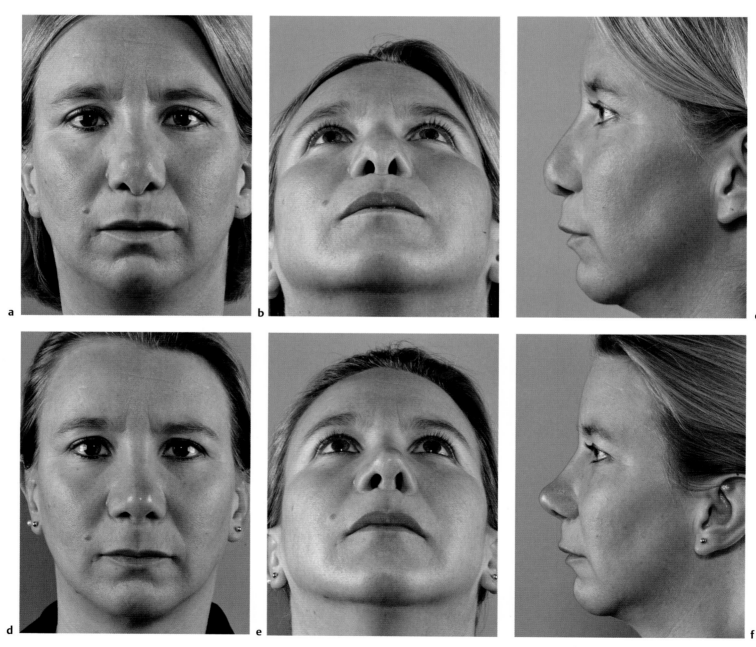

Fig. 33.1 Pre- and postoperative views. (**a**) Preoperative frontal view shows a severe deformity of the nasal tip and a short nose. The tip defining points are too far apart. The nose is disharmonious with the rest of the face. (**b**) Lack of tip definition is appreciated in the basal view. (**c**) Profile view shows the loss of projection. There is a conspicuous loss of tip support and definition. (**d**) Frontal view one year after revision rhinoplasty. The tip is corrected, and nasal length is in harmony with the rest of the face. (**e**) Basal view after the revision. (**f**) Profile view one year after revision rhinoplasty documents the correction of tip projection and tip support.

material in the septum and not even enough conchal cartilage for a cartilaginous reconstruction. Two strips of costal cartilage were sculpted with a bur to create a defined arch in the new dome area. The new alar cartilages were sutured medially to the stumps of the medial crura and also to the septal extension graft. Laterally they were affixed to the vestibular mucosa. The tip was reshaped with inter- and transdomal sutures and a spanning suture.

Psychology, Motivation, Personal Background

After two previous operations during childhood, the patient had a severe residual septal deviation that was causing significant breathing issues. The nasal tip was grossly deformed and had caused the patient significant emotional distress over the years.

She was strongly motivated to have another revision rhinoplasty to improve both the function and appearance of her nose. One year later she is very pleased with the functional and aesthetic outcome of her surgery (**Fig. 33.1d–f**).

Discussion

Lengthening can also be achieved with a columellar strut held in place by extended spreader grafts. But this procedure would create an unnatural and unpleasant fullness in the vestibule, which the patient would find objectionable. Auricular cartilage can be used instead of rib cartilage, as described by Pedroza,[3] but rib cartilage seemed to be more predictable in this case owing to the absence of a predefined cartilage shape.

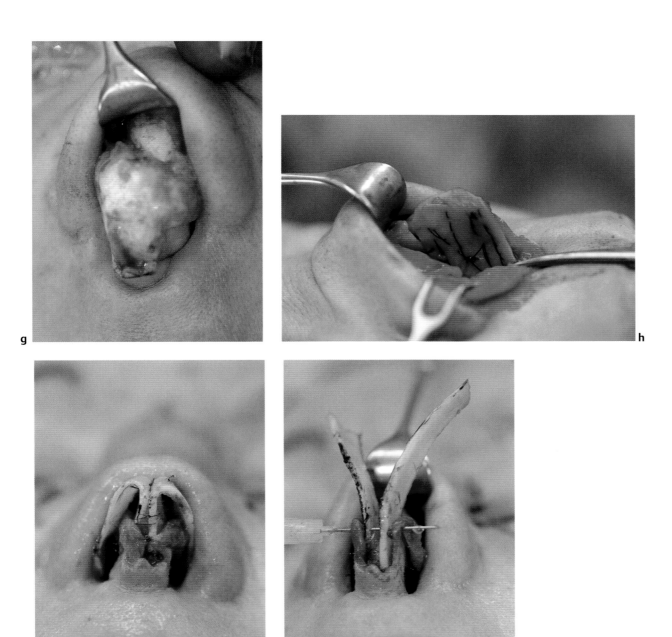

Fig. 33.1 (**g–j**) Intraoperative views. (**g**) Intraoperative view of scarring at the nasal tip. (**h**) View after fixation of the septal extension graft (double-layer conchal cartilage graft). (**i, j**) Reconstruction of the lower cartilages by the bending technique. (**i**) The strips of costal cartilage are fixed medially to the stumps of the medial crura. (**j**) The new alar cartilages are sutured laterally to the vestibular mucosa and are joined together medially with an intercrural suture.

Case 53

Introduction

A 36-year-old woman presented 1 year after undergoing a septo-rhinoplasty elsewhere. She sought improvement in the appearance of her nose and the quality of nasal breathing, especially on the left side.

Findings

On examination, it was found that both the bony and cartilaginous portions of the nasal skeleton were severely destabilized. Treatment consisted of a combination of revision surgery and refinement (**Fig. 33.2a–f**).

Surgical Procedures

1. Conchal cartilage was harvested on the right side. An open approach and swinging double-door technique were used to perform the septoplasty and place a columellar strut, alar button grafts, a dorsal onlay graft, and a tip graft. Medial and lateral curved osteotomies were performed on both sides.

2. Reosteotomy was performed on the right side to revise the nasal dorsum and eliminate its tendency for lateral deflection. Bilateral spreader grafts were placed to widen the stenotic left nasal valve (**Fig. 33.2g**).

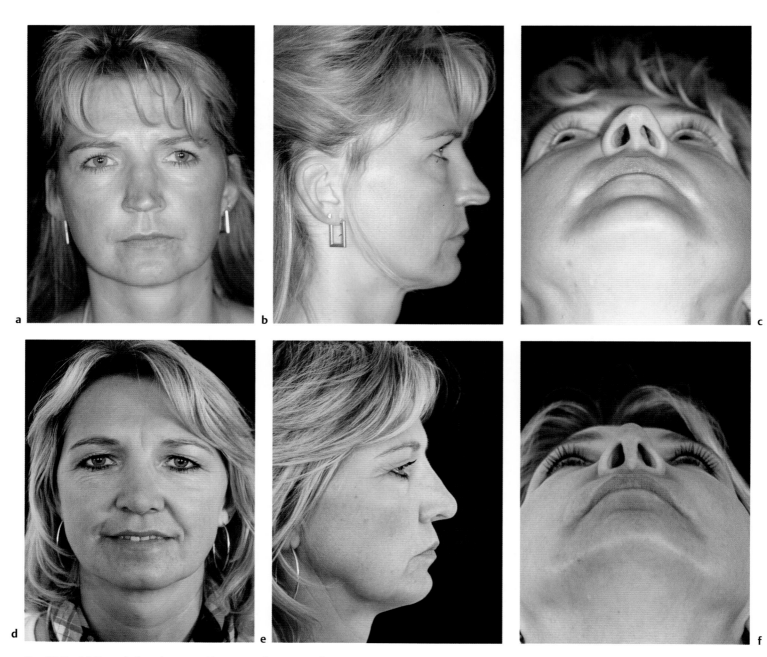

Fig. 33.2 (**a**) Frontal view shows a wide nose with an amorphous tip, an open roof, and paradoxical alar cartilages due to previous overresection. (**b**) Profile view: pseudohump, saddle nose, ptotic tip. (**c**) Basal view: The septum is deflected to the right. Endonasal inspection showed vestibular stenosis on the right side. (**d**) Frontal view 10 years after the revisions. (**e**) Profile view 10 years after the revisions. (**f**) Basal view 10 years after the revisions.

Psychology, Motivation, Personal Background

The primary rhinoplasty was considered a failure. The patient, who was deeply disappointed, traveled a considerable distance to seek treatment at our clinic. She was strongly motivated to undergo a revision rhinoplasty that would improve both the function and appearance of her nose.

Discussion

This case illustrates a complex reconstruction involving all structural components of the nose. The revision resulted in significant functional and aesthetic improvement. Other techniques would also have been an option, as illustrated in the case below.

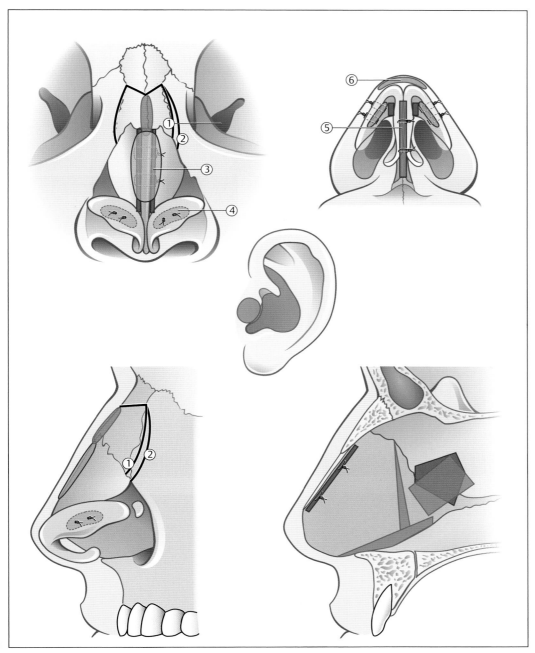

g

Fig. 33.2   (**g**) Intraoperative details. 1,2, lateral osteotomies; 3, dorsal onlay graft; 4, alar strut graft; 5, columellar strut; 6, camouflage with fascia; red, resections.

Case 54

Introduction
A 51-year-old woman had wanted a "new nose" since her early youth. She had undergone surgery of the nasal tip and septum at 29 years of age, but that was followed by the development of a severe nasal deformity with breathing problems.

Findings
Examination revealed a severe cartilaginous deformity of the nose with significant breathing difficulties relating to bilateral inspiratory alar collapse (**Fig. 33.3a–f**).

Surgical Procedure
Conchal cartilage was harvested, and an extracorporeal septoplasty was performed through an open approach. Cartilage grafts consisted of a columellar strut, alar button grafts, and tip and shield grafts. Perichondrium was used for camouflage. Medial and lateral curved osteotomies were performed on both sides (**Fig. 33.3g**).

Psychology, Motivation, Personal Background
As an author, the patient writes about her life in gripping autobiographical novels. Her desire for a "new" nose was deeply rooted in both aesthetic and functional concerns. I met the patient years after her operation in New York, where a long personal search had led her. She describes her quest in a novel. She was happy with her new nose.

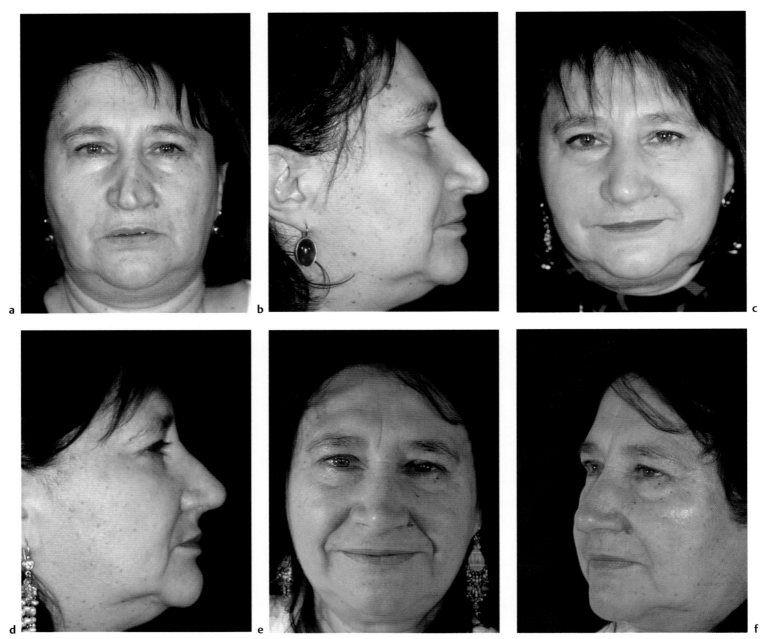

Fig. 33.3 (**a**) Frontal view shows a cartilaginous crooked nose with an inverted-V deformity, overresected alar cartilages with paradoxical curvature, and a pinched nasal tip that is more prominent on the right side. (**b**) Profile view shows a long nose with a bony and cartilaginous hump and a ptotic tip. Endonasal inspection showed septal deviation to the right and nasal valve stenosis. (**c–f**) Postoperative views at 4 and 10 years after revision rhinoplasty.

Discussion

The complex reconstruction of all unstable or overresected structural components required an extracorporeal septoplasty and the construction of a straight, symmetrical nasal shape through an open approach.

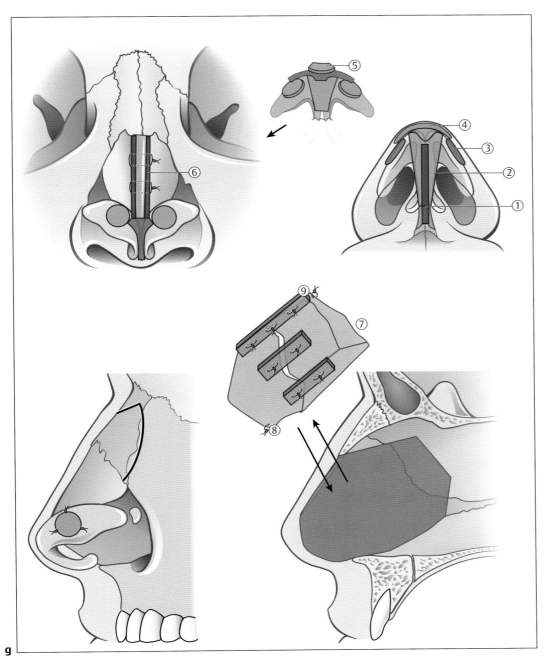

g

Fig. 33.3 **(g)** Intraoperative details. Red = resections, blue = grafts, purple = camouflage with perichondrium. 1, columellar strut; 2, shield graft; 3, alar button graft; 4, camouflage with fascia; 5, tip graft; 6, spreader grafts; 7, extracorporeal septoplasty with spreader grafts and fixation with sutures on the anterior nasal spine (8) and keystone areas (9).

References

1. Gubisch W, Eichhorn-Sens J. Overresection of the lower lateral cartilages: a common conceptual mistake with functional and aesthetic consequences. Aesthetic Plast Surg 2009;33(1):6–13

2. Eichhorn-Sens J, Gubisch W. Ausgedehnte Resektion der Flügelknorpel—ein falsches Konzept zur Verschmälerung der Nase. HNO 2009;57(11):113–120

3. Pedroza F, Anjos GC, Patrocinio LG, Barreto JM, Cortes J, Quessep SH. Seagull wing graft: a technique for the replacement of lower lateral cartilages. Arch Facial Plast Surg 2006;8(6):396–403

34 Reconstructive Surgery

The didactic goal of this book is to provide a practical guide to the large field of revision rhinoplasty and reconstructive nasal surgery. The surgical spectrum ranges from minimally invasive procedures in patients who seek the aesthetic refinement of one or more features to partial or complete reconstructions of the nose.

We have tried consistently to begin each case presentation with an analysis of the morphologic, aesthetic, or functional problems relevant to the case. This enables us to work from general principles to more concrete problem situations and from the simple to the complex. On the other hand, this approach is not applicable to all nasal problems since every nose is attached to a human being who often views the problem differently from the surgeon.

Whether to use an open or closed approach is a "matter of faith" that we have not addressed. It does not matter. Every approach has its advantages and disadvantages. In one case I prefer a closed approach based on a particular situation, while in another case I favor an open approach. The important thing is for the surgeon to develop a repertoire of as many surgical techniques as possible rather than use the same procedure over and over again.

The psychological aspects of revisions and reconstructive surgery play an important role. Jacques Joseph repeatedly alluded to them in his work:

> It is not vanity which is the driving motivation, but the feeling of being disfigured and, conversely, the aversion to disfigurement and its psychological consequences. Rhinoplasty seeks to cure psychological depression by restoring a normal shape to the nose. Its social importance is beyond question, and it represents a significant branch of surgical psychotherapy.

The following chapter gives the reader practical tips for analyzing defects in the nose and formulating a "surgical plan" for reconstructing small, large, and complex tissue defects. It concludes with the surgical replacement of a nose that has been lost as a result of trauma or malignancy.

Case 1: Extrusion of a Nasal Implant after 51 Years

Introduction

This 68-year-old woman presented with extrusion of a nasal implant. When she was 17 years old, the L-shaped plastic splint had been inserted for dorsal augmentation. Forty years later a slowly progressing atrophy of the surrounding tissue and formation of spider veins affected the appearance. The visible extrusion in the tip area developed within 4 weeks, painless and without other symptoms (**Fig. 34.1a–c**) (operation by Joachim Quetz).

Diagnosis

Inspection showed a prominent contour of the implant tightly encased by atrophic skin with conspicuous spider nevi. The defect at the tip had a diameter of 4 mm (bottom) extending to 6 mm (outside edges) with the exposed implant in the center. The wound edges were epithelialized and showed hardly any signs of inflammation. Palpation of the nose revealed a highly atrophic and inelastic skin around the surface of the implant, while the glabella region showed a dilatable skin. Aim of the upcoming operation was removal and replacement of the implant by rib cartilage grafts,[1] reinforcement of the skin, and, preferably primary closure of the defect.

Surgical Procedure

Rib cartilage was harvested first to gain time for carving, observation, and refinement of the grafts. The first layers were taken off the surfaces right away to prepare two balanced blocks. Special feature: The No. 10 blade had to be exchanged for a micro circular saw and a cutting burr because of advanced calcification. Fascia lata was harvested afterward. The defect was symmetrically enlarged as a transverse-oval excision, bilaterally prolonged by short incisions running parallel to the edges of the soft triangles (**Fig. 34.1d**). To minimize tension for later closure, the nasal skin was widely undermined up to the glabella region. Explantation of the graft was easy and the enlarged scarry pocket suitable as a recipient bed for the grafts. A typical columella strut and a meticulously tailored dorsal strut were fitted into the final position and fixed with permanent sutures. The columella strut, length 25 mm, was tightly fixed to the remnant of the septum and the spine area (5–0 monofil) to prevent upward rotation of the tip and shortening of the nasal dorsum. The alar cartilages, so far depressed by the implant, were augmented and fixed to the strut. The dorsal graft, 45 × 11 × 5 mm, concave undersurface and very thin edge on the nasal bone (**Fig. 34.1e, f**), was fixed with multiple fine sutures (7–0 monofil) to the underlay and a strong suture to the columella strut. Dead spaces were obliterated by perichondrium and fascia. The atrophic skin was reinforced by a single layer of fascia lata and a double layer above the new tip (**Fig. 34.1g**). The former defect could be closed with some additional excision and little tension. The spider veins were obliterated by cauterization.

Healing was disturbed by a small necrosis at the tip, progressing to the diameter of the old defect within 10 days (**Fig. 34.1h, i**). Formation of delicate granulation tissue on the edges could not prevent central necrosis of the two-layered fascia and exposure of rib cartilage after 5 weeks. At the end of 6 weeks, tissue had recovered and the defect slightly contracted. Decision was taken against a forehead flap and in favor of a composite ear graft.

Six weeks postoperatively the edges were freshened and the defect, 5 mm in diameter on the bottom, was closed with a composite ear graft, diameter of the skin when harvested 7 mm (**Fig. 34.1j–l**). Healing process went well; the early and late result was good (**Fig. 34.1m, n**).

Psychology, Motivations, Personal Background

An open nasal trauma of the 4-year-old girl could not be treated adequately shortly before the end of the Second World War. The adolescent girl suffered from a severely underprojected profile and a groove in the midline. Being 17 years old, she was offered a modern plastic implant at a university clinic—a "method with no alternative," as she was told. The result was much appreciated by the patient, family, and friends. The actual shape with the rib grafts is viewed as being more harmonic, more natural, and less "pinched" compared with the shape as it appeared for decades with the implant.

Discussion

In most of our cases, replacement of implants by rib cartilage with reinforcement of the skin and primary closure is possible. In this case, a slight elongation of the dorsum may have been too ambitious even though tension of the skin was low during primary closure. A skin graft for secondary repair might have been sufficient some weeks earlier with the fascia still intact. Such a graft (e.g., taken from the glabella region) would have led to a better color match and probably to a better contour.

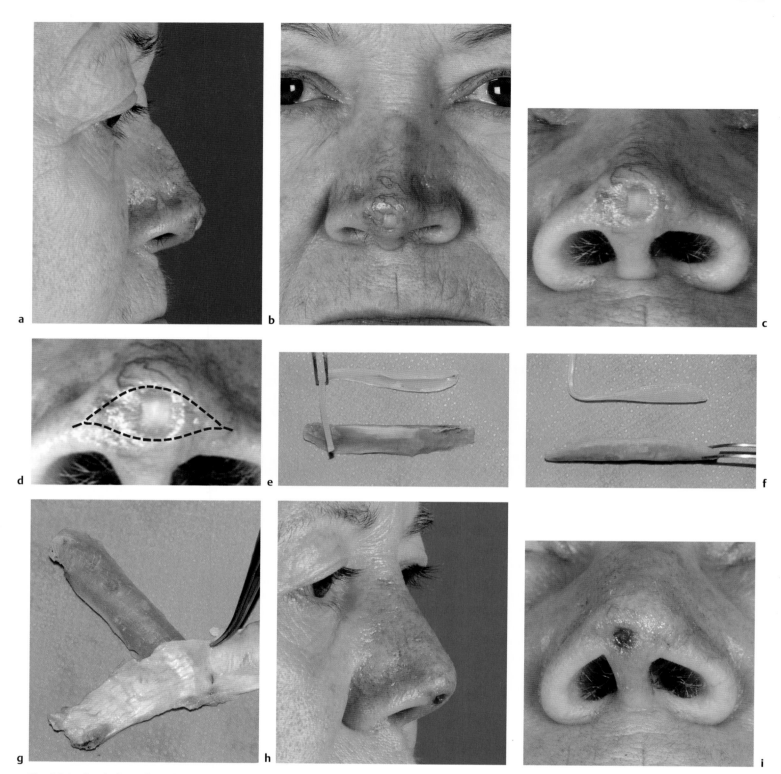

Fig. 34.1 (**a–c**) The L-shaped plastic splint is penetrating the skin at the most typical point. (**d**) Fusiform resection of some of the atrophic skin provides a modified open approach and will allow primary closure if skin can be mobilized sufficiently. (**e, f**) The dorsal graft from rib cartilage while being carved, 45 × 11 × 5 mm, compared with the former implant. Note the thin outer ends that will rest on the nasal bone and columella strut. (**g**) Fascia lata for protection and reinforcement of the atrophic skin. (**h, i**) Small necrosis below the tip in spite of good and relaxed condition of the surrounding skin. *Later:* Minor signs of secondary healing, loss of fascia and exposure of rib graft without protrusion.

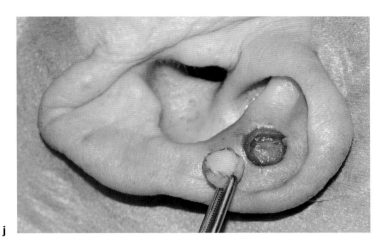

j

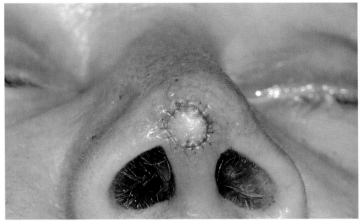

k

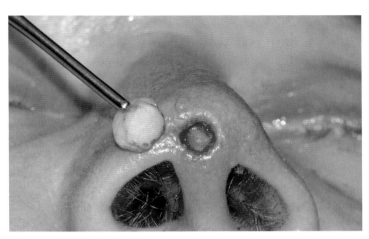

l

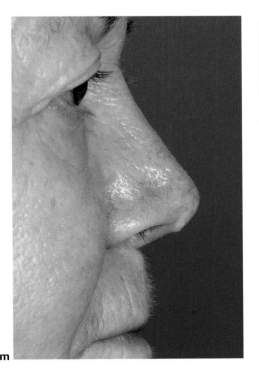

m

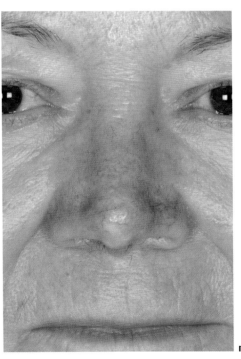

n

Fig. 34.1 (**j–l**) A skin cartilage composite ear graft is harvested for repair of the full thickness skin defect. Note the beveled edges of the cartilage and the smaller diameter of the skin component. This design ensures a stepless incorporation of the graft and survival of the skin. (**m, n**) Side and front view after 1 year showing improvement of shape and skin quality. A slight color mismatch and an irregularity of the composite graft are conspicuous.

Case 2: Severe Saddle Nose Deformity by Granulomatosis with Polyangiitis (Wegener)

Introduction

This 27-year-old woman presented with severe saddle nose deformity. Granulomatosis with polyangiitis (GPA; Wegener granulomatosis) had been verified only 2 years ago even though typical symptoms had occurred already at the age of 17: severe inflammations of the left middle ear and the nasal septum. Slow formation of a saddle nose soon became noticeable while three tympanoplasties were performed in rapid succession. Augmentation of the nasal dorsum with bank cartilage by closed approach had been tried elsewhere at the age of 24. A revision 1 year later by the same surgeon did not improve the result (**Fig. 34.2a, b**). We had to wait 5 years for complete remission and yet another year for stable remission and performed the reconstructive rhinoplasty at the age of 33 (operation by Joachim Quetz).

Diagnosis

Inspection and palpation showed a severe saddle nose deformity with a prominent contour of the inappropriate rib transplant tightly encased by scarred and shrunk skin. Destruction of the nasal spine area and the nasal bone was conspicuous by loss of projection of the midface in the lateral view. Endonasal endoscopy revealed a total loss of septal cartilage manifesting as a subtotal septal perforation. Protection of the deprojected tip felt almost normal. Diagnostic investigation was completed by a lateral cephalographic X-ray (**Fig. 34.2c**), providing good information about soft-tissue relation to the bony midface and a basis for the traditional planning with transparent paper and pencil on a scale of 1:1 (**Fig. 34.2d**).

Surgical Procedure

As in most cases, rib cartilage was harvested first to gain time for carving, observation, reshaping, and refinement of the grafts (**Fig. 34.2h**). The first layers were taken off the surfaces right away for later preparation of two balanced blocks. According to the destroyed spine area and preoperative planning, an unusually long columella strut of ~ 4 cm and a dorsal graft of 5 cm was prepared (**Fig. 34.2i, j**). Perioperative antibiotic prophylaxis and repeated accurate disinfection—basic precautions in patients with increased risks—were performed. An endonasal approach by hemitransfixion incision was used to partly uncover the remnants of the septal cartilage, a narrow falx; to elevate the dorsal skin, strictly avoiding damage to the atrophic inner lining; and to remove the old graft (**Fig. 34.2e**). The columella strut was tentatively inserted into a dissected pocket and caused an extreme saddle of the dorsum and overrotation of the tip by lack of elastic skin (**Fig. 34.2k**). Large-scale undermining of the surrounding facial skin could provide just about a sufficient amount to achieve the aspired profile and projection (**Fig. 34.2l**). A stable gearing between columella strut and spine area and between the grafts was essential to keep up the profile while withstanding significant tension of the skin. The dorsal graft was fixed with a long titanium screw in the area of the former nasal bone for the same reason (**Fig. 34.2f, g**). Closure of the incision was tight and ended up in a small necrosis at the hemitransfixion incision some days later with an exposure of the grafts. Secondary healing under permanent antiseptic occlusive dressing did not work. The defect was finally closed with a vestibulum oris mucosal flap 4 weeks later without further problems. One year later the patient was—unsuccessfully—offered a correction of an alar rim retraction on the right side. This retraction was preexisting but had become more noticeable by the augmentation. The plan was—and still is—to push down the alar rim by a skin cartilage composite ear graft. The graft would be placed into a created vestibular pocket, the cutaneous component facing the nasal vestibule.

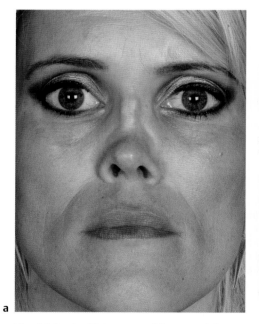
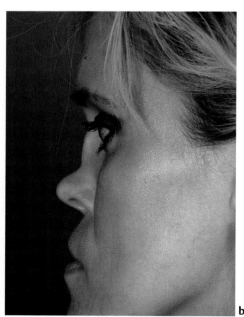

a
b

Fig. 34.2 (**a, b**) Severe saddle nose deformity with additional loss of projection by destruction of nasal spine and bone. Two operations for augmentation with rib cartilage have been performed elsewhere.

Psychology, Motivations, Personal Background

GPA started at the age of 14 years as a limited disease (ear and nose) and progressed some years later, undetected and untreated, to a systemic vasculitis with multi-organ involvement (lymph nodes, kidney, lung, and brain with slight stroke). Her caring family, a sympathetic boss (the patient worked in a barbershop), and a happy marriage helped her to stay mentally stable while experiencing the stigmatizing change in her midface and suffering the long and serious illness. After two rhinoplasties with very limited improvement she was not pushing for the reconstruction. Postoperatively she was pleased but not enthusiastic about the result. The positive reaction of her family, friends, and her clients in the barbershop helped her to fully accept and appreciate her new nose (**Fig. 34.2m, n**). Special feature: Putting on heavy makeup had been her way to cope with formation of the saddle.

Discussion

Complete remission for at least 1 year seems to be an adequate period before repair of a GPA nose. A closed approach was chosen because no work on the tip had to be done and at that time a closed approach seemed to us to be safer in GPA patients with big septal perforation.[2] In the meantime, open approaches have proved to be just as safe. Even in patients with steroid medication combined with anti-rheumatic drug therapy we have seen perfect healing processes in most cases. Fixation of the dorsal graft with a Kirschner wire (K-wire) is a good alternative to a titanium screw. Three major issues had to be and were successfully resolved in this case: Mobilization of the surrounding skin, creation of a very strong scaffold, and a semi-rigid fixation by gearing and screwing the scaffold to the damaged bony anatomy to prevent disintegration and dislocation.

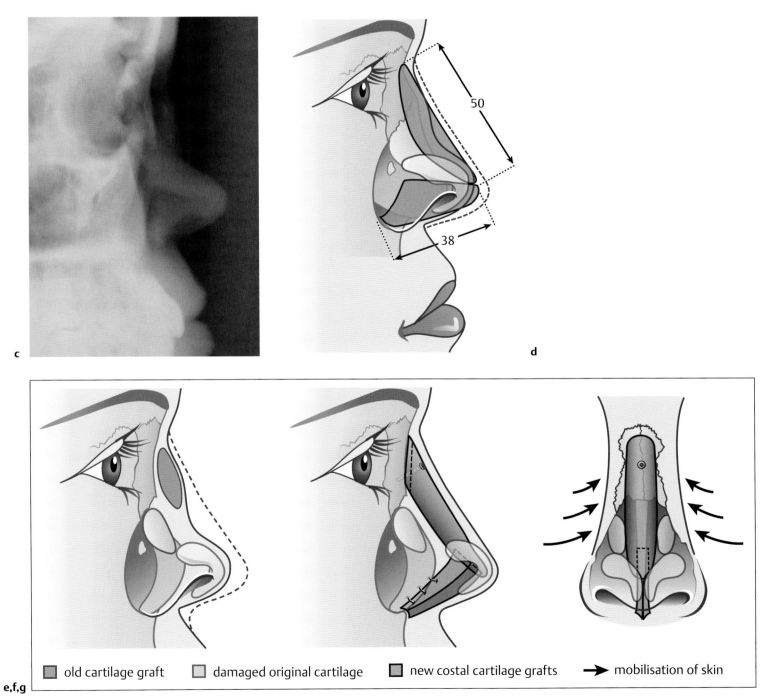

old cartilage graft   damaged original cartilage   new costal cartilage grafts   → mobilisation of skin

Fig. 34.2 (**c, d**) A lateral cephalographic X-ray provides good information about soft-tissue relation to the bony midface and a basis for traditional planning with transparent paper and pencil on a scale of 1:1. Nasal scaffold at the beginning (**e**) and end (**f, g**) of the operation. Note the interlocking of columella strut and former nasal spine, supported by permanent sutures to the remnant of the septum (**f**) and the anchorage of the dorsal beam to the remnant of the nasal bone by a long titanium screw (**f, g**). (*Continued on next page*)

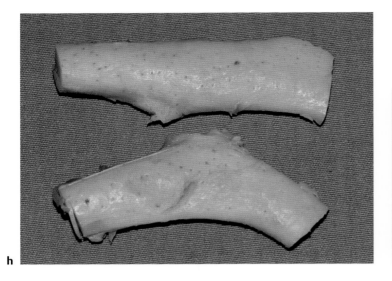

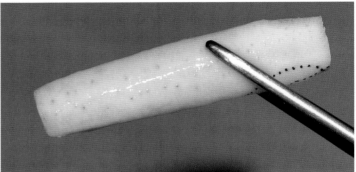

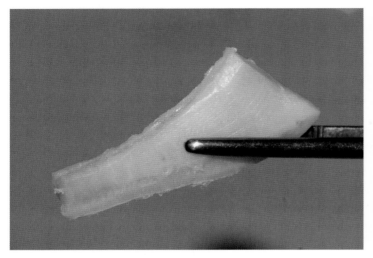

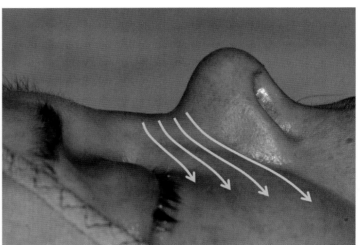

Fig. 34.2 (*Continued*)   (**h–j**) Costal cartilage grafts after being harvested and while being carved, dorsal beam 5 cm and columella strut 4 cm long. (**i**) Note narrowing of the tip (*dotted blue line*) that will be placed under the domes and (**j**) the groove along the short curve of the strut where the edge of the septal remnant will be inserted. (**k**) Tentative insertion of the columella strut into a dissected pocket causes an extreme saddle and overrotation of the tip by lack of elastic skin. *Blue arrows:* Direction of extensive undermining of surrounding skin.

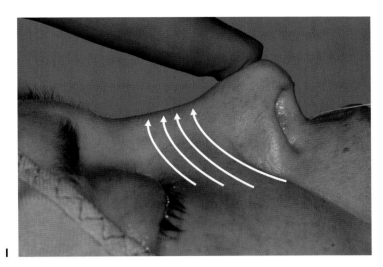

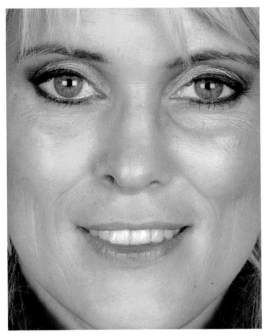

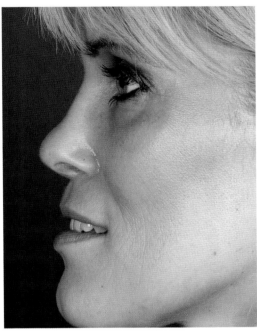

Fig. 34.2 (**l**) Undermining of the skin is in progress and the required amount for augmentation partly mobilized (*white arrows*): Attempt to push the tip in the final position. (**m, n**) Front and side view after 1 year: Saddle, underprojection, and overrotation of the nose as well as retrusion of the lip are corrected as far as possible via closed approach. Lowering of the right ala rim by a composite ear graft is planned.

Case 3: Subtotal Loss of Cartilaginous Scaffold

Introduction

Initially, this patient had had his paranasal sinuses operated on, followed by four septorhinoplasties elsewhere: removal of a big hump, revision rhinoplasty, second revision for extracorporeal septal reconstruction with polydioxanone foil, and a fourth operation some weeks later following abscess formation—foil and cartilage had to be removed. One year after this last revision and 9 years after the initial sinus surgery the patient, then 37 years old, returned with impaired nasal breathing and deformation of the nose by loss of cartilaginous scaffold to a large extent (operation by Joachim Quetz).

Diagnosis

Inspection showed a deformed nose with an uneven surface, deviation, and loss of projection (**Fig. 34.3a, l**). A contracted scar of the soft triangle on the right side was particularly conspicuous. Palpation revealed a severe lack of protection, whereas rigidity of the thickened skin seemed to contribute significantly to the stability of the whole nose. Endoscopy showed septal deviation to the left and hyperplasia of the lower turbinates. The aim of the upcoming operation was complex restoration of form and function. Reconstruction of the scaffold had to be strong enough to mount and straighten the rigid skin and to withstand later scar contraction.

Surgical Procedure

Building of a new thin septal plate from rib cartilage needs some hours' time for observation and reshaping to overcome the tendency to warping. For this reason rib cartilage was harvested first and work on the grafts started prior to work on the nose. Curved chips were created by removing the superficial layers off the surfaces with a No. 10 blade (**Fig. 34.3e**). They are carefully preserved and thus provide a useful collection of differently shaped chips for later replacement of the subsurface framework. An open approach was employed for excellent insight and anatomically correct reconstruction of the destroyed and deformed components. Exposure of the remnants of the nasal skeleton and troublesome separation of the septal mucosal sheets were per-formed with an operating microscope. Only the lateral segments of the upper lateral and the right lower lateral cartilage could be identified (**Fig. 34.3c**). Reconstruction started with replacement of the septum, assembled by two plates, width less than 3 mm (**Fig. 34.3d, f, g**). The bigger plate was tailored to match the dorsal end of the septal defect and to be dovetailed with the spine area (**Fig. 34.3i**). It was fixed to the spine by a drill hole and permanent suture. The upper plate was fitted in the remaining gap; minor deviation of both components was balanced by assembling them directly opposed. They were interconnected by simple interrupted and 8-shaped stitches alternately (**Fig. 34.3d**). Final shape of the new septum was designed and trimmed in situ, dimension of the lower edge resembling an integrated extension graft (**Fig. 34.3c, d, i**). The two plates were bridged by spreader grafts on both sides and thus firmly locked in the desired straight position.[3] The grafts, size ~ 20 × 3 × 2 mm, were tentatively fixed with a fine injection needle and joined with the upper lateral cartilages: four horizontal mattress sutures, following the direction of the injection needle, allowed later shaping of the dorsum without cutting the threads (**Fig. 34.3j**). Finally the whole left and medial part of the right alar cartilage was replaced by choosing suitable elements from the collection of curved chips (**Fig. 34.3k**). The medial crura were fixed to the caudal extension of the neoseptum by permanent mattress sutures and the new tip shaped by modified inter- and transdomal sutures.

Psychology, Motivations, Personal Background

The patient didn't like to talk about his motivation for the preceding rhinoplasties and his approach to the severe complications. His desire for repair of function and form was easy to follow. In contrast to the evaluation of the surgeon and the good outcome (**Fig. 34.3b, m**), the patient was not entirely pleased with the result.

Discussion

When inner lining and soft-tissue envelope are intact, the anatomically correct reconstruction of the framework with rib cartilage may be the best technique for a superior outcome and a predictable long-term stability. The warping forces of shaped rib grafts can be sufficiently harnessed by the described technique.

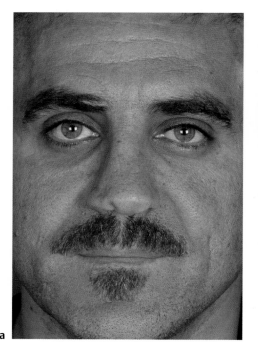
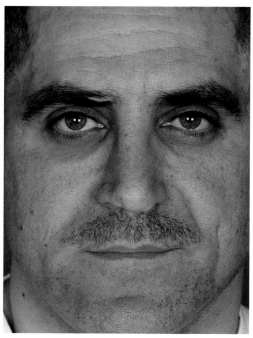

a   b

Fig. 34.3 Frontal view (**a**) before and (**b**) 1 year after reconstruction of the framework shows only limited changes: The nasal base is narrowed and definition of tip and alar lobule slightly improved.

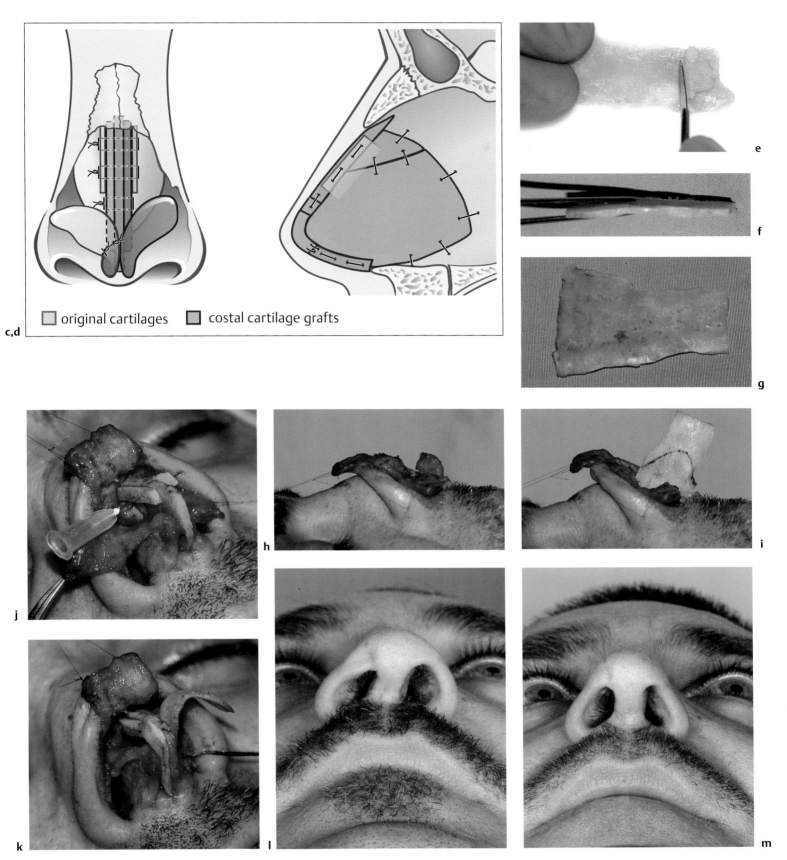

Fig. 34.3 (**c, d**) See-through frontal view and paramedian sagittal section shows shape, position, and attachment of the cartilage grafts. Note the spreader grafts bridging and firmly locking the two septal plates in a straight position. (**e–g**) Carving of two well-balanced plates for reconstruction of the septum, width less than 3 mm. Minor deviation will be equalized by assembling them in an opposite sense. (**h**) After troublesome separation of the septal mucosal sheets with a surgical microscope: Exposure of the remnants of the nasal skeleton. (**i**) The final shape of the new septum is trimmed in situ, dimension of the lower edge is designed as an integrated extension graft. (**j**) The spreader grafts are fixed with a fine injection needle and joined with neo-septum and upper lateral cartilages by horizontal mattress sutures that allow shaping of the dorsum without cutting them. (**k**) The whole left and medial part of the right alar cartilage are replaced by suitable elements from the collection of curved chips. (**l, m**) Pre- and postoperative view after 1 year from below showing restoration of projection, definition, and symmetry.

Case 4: Conspicuous Skin Graft

Introduction

Five years ago, when the patient was 59 years old, a basal cell carcinoma of the nasal tip and dorsum had been excised and the defect closed by a free skin graft. The patient asked for revision of the poor result (operation by Joachim Quetz).

Diagnosis

Color match was the only positive detail about the skin graft, whereas all other aspects were unsatisfying: Position of the graft was asymmetrical, the subunit principle had been neglected, the shiny atrophic texture did not match the surrounding sebaceous skin, the graft was not in level with the surface, and the contour looked unnatural. Most eye-catching were the resultant misplaced highlights (**Fig. 34.4a, b, j, k**). Aim of the revision was to correct all of these aspects by reshaping the defect by bringing it close to the tip subunit (**Fig. 34.4c**), rearranging the alar cartilages, and replacing the skin with a two-stage forehead flap.

Surgical Procedure

The skin graft was excised and the defect symmetrically enlarged, bringing it as close as possible to the shape of the tip subunit (**Fig. 34.4e**). Skin of the nasal dorsum was completely undermined and gently pulled down to make the defect smaller, thus bringing it closer to the desired shape (**Fig. 34.4c, d**). The skin was fixed in the new position, taking care not to rotate the tip upward. The intermediate and lateral portions of the alar cartilages were found on a level with the top edge of the septum. They were repositioned and reshaped by inter- and transdomal sutures. A foil of a suture pack was used to accurately cut and mold a template representing a three-dimensional copy of the defect (**Fig. 34.4f**). The foil was flattened to two dimensions and transferred to the forehead, turning it upside down. Length and size of the pedicle were defined and marked with ink along with the outline of the template. Base of the pedicle measured 13 mm and was positioned on the right side. The flap was elevated and transposed to resurface the defect. The last steps were performed with a surgical microscope. Excess subcutaneous fat was excised within the distal half of the flap, preserving axial dermal vessels as far as possible. It was inserted in its final position with 5–0 subcutaneous sutures and the skin closed with 7–0 nylon simple interrupted and running sutures (**Fig. 34.4g–i**). For closure of the donor site, the adjacent forehead and scalp tissue was widely elevated and fixed under moderate tension with subcutaneous sutures and a running suture of the skin by 7–0 nylon. The area that would have required more than moderate tension was only approached with resorbable threads and the dog ear excised at the upper end. Granulation tissue filled up the missing volume in the following weeks under permanent semi-occlusive dressing. Three weeks later the pedicle was transacted, the proximal end reduced to a small triangle and reintegrated resembling the "frown lines" of the opposite side. The distal end was meticulously thinned, trimmed, integrated into the defect, and fixed with 7–0 nylon simple interrupted sutures. Waste skin from the middle portion of the pedicle was thinned and used as a free transplant to close off the remaining defect of the forehead now in line with the adjacent skin.

Psychology, Motivations, Personal Background

The patient had never been satisfied with the result, and the surgeon had not been either. As a private person and a tourist guide she always had replied with wisecracks when people commented on her nose. She had been determined to live with this defect. But one day her grandson refused to be collected from school by his grandmother because his classmates had been joking about the "fingernail" on his granny's nose. That was the moment when she changed her mind and desperately wanted a revision. She was happy with the result and repeatedly remarked that "a new nose is like a new life" (**Fig. 34.4j–m**).

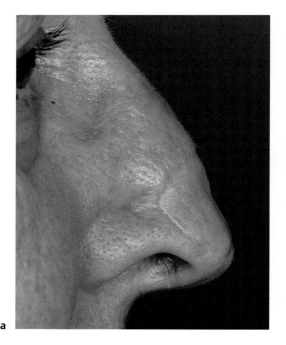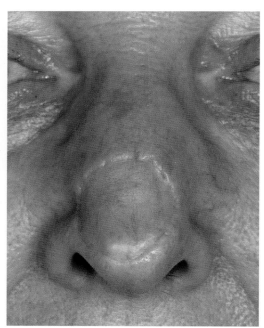

a   b

Fig. 34.4 (**a, b**) Asymmetric skin graft, not in line with the subunit and below level of the surrounding surface, texture shiny and atrophic, highlights misplaced.

Discussion

Repair of "small surface defects" can be more challenging than a full thickness defect of a whole subunit. The level of difficulty is frequently underestimated by both patients and surgeons. Such a defect of less than 15 mm with an intact underlying framework might have sufficiently been repaired by a skin graft in the thin-skinned area of dorsum and sidewalls. This case demonstrates the problem of a mature shiny skin graft within the area of thick sebaceous skin of the tip.[4] The outcome is worsened by asymmetry and incongruity with the subunit. Decision was in favor of a forehead flap and against, e.g., a Rieger's flap, because of the size of the defect and the sun-damaged skin of the upper dorsum.

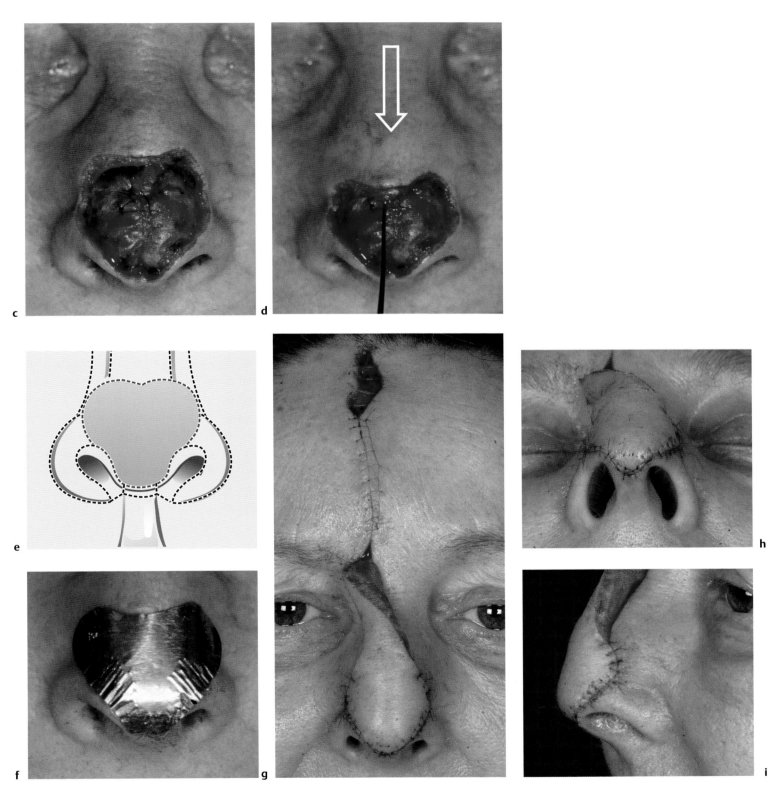

Fig. 34.4 (**c–e**) Defect after resection of the graft, symmetrical enlargement and mobilization of the cranial skin, which is gently pulled down (**d**) to make the defect smaller, thus getting it closer to the shape of the subunit (**e**). (**f**) A foil of a suture pack is used to create a template representing a three-dimensional copy of the defect. (**g–i**) The flap has been elevated and transposed, the distal half thinned and inserted to resurface the defect. Half of the donor site was closed primarily. The area that would have required more than moderate tension was only approached with resorbable threads and the dog ear excised at the upper end. (*Continued on next page*)

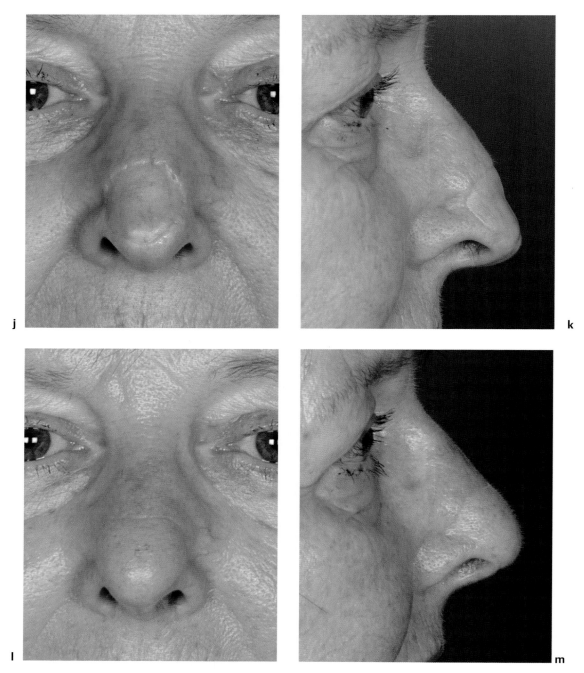

j

k

l

m

Fig. 34.4 (*Continued*)   (**j–m**) Frontal and lateral views before and 1 year after the revision.

Case 5: Full-Thickness Defect of the Right Alar and Tip Subunit

Introduction

This 32-year-old woman presented with a full-thickness defect of the right ala and tip after resection of a basal cell carcinoma. She was mainly suffering from a metastatic breast cancer. The reconstruction was expected to take little time and the result to be excellent (operation by Joachim Quetz).

Diagnosis

The ventral half of the alar and the lateral quarter of the tip subunit had been excised (**Fig. 34.5a, b**). For a superior result, a paramedian forehead flap was planned, braced by a septal cartilage transplant. The decision was in favor of a two-stage procedure (see discussion below). Enlargement of the defect to apply the subunit principle was considered for both ala and tip. Residual skin at the alar base would normally be discarded and replaced by a one-piece skin envelope of the whole ala. This would have moved the posterior scar away from the visible to the shadowed area—the alar–facial groove. The idea was abandoned because sacrifice of intact skin would have been relatively large and a slight dimple within the subunit seemed to be able to conceal the scar. Enlargement of the tip subunit exactly to the midline, thus creating a sagittal straight edge, might have led to

symmetry and natural-looking appearance.[5] But the right tip defining point was just intact and the amount of visible scar would have increased significantly—two further reasons to neglect the subunit principle in this case (**Fig. 34.5b**). Standardized photos were—as always—of utmost importance for successful planning. Rotation, inversion, bilateral comparison, for example, should be possible, and tools for measurements and drawings should be at hand.

Surgical Procedure

The procedure started by freshening and slightly modifying the edges for precise alignment of the flap later on. Ink marking of all subunits and a template from the opposite side were dispensable in this case because of the relatively small dimension and stable margins of the defect. An exact template of the lining and cover was cut out of aluminum foil, bent and crimped with a sufficient distance between both surfaces for easy folding of the flap (**Fig. 34.5c, d**). The foil was flattened to two dimensions, transferred to the forehead, turned upside down, and twisted 180 degrees. It was positioned vertically above the right supratrochlear vessels and provided with an extra-long pedicle for easy primary positioning of the cartilage graft (**Fig. 34.5e**). Width of the base of the pedicle: 14 mm. The full-thickness forehead flap was harvested with the segment for inner lining extending into the hairline. The distal 2 cm were carefully thinned by removing muscle and fat with short scissors progressing close to the hair-

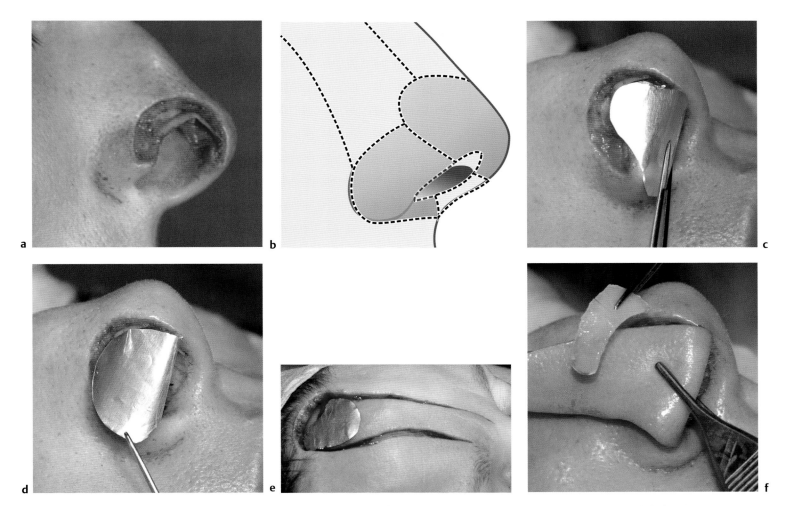

Fig. 34.5 (**a, b**) The full-thickness defect comprises the ventral half of the alar and the lateral quarter of the tip subunit. (**c, d**) A template for lining (**c**) and cover is cut out of aluminum foil, bent and crimped with a sufficient distance between both surfaces for easy folding of the flap. (**e**) The foil is flattened and transferred to the forehead, turned upside down, and flipped 180 degrees. The flap is positioned vertically above the right su-

pratrochlear vessels and provided with a long pedicle for easy primary positioning of the cartilage graft (two-stage procedure in this case). (**f**) The shaped septal graft will be firmly fixed to the stumps of the lower lateral cartilage and covered on the in- and outside by the carefully thinned distal flap. (*Continued on next page*)

bulbs at the distal end. Fine distal arteries were visualized with a surgical microscope and avoided as much as possible. The shaped septal graft was firmly fixed by small pockets and multiple 6–0 and 7–0 permanent sutures to the stumps and the surrounding tissue (**Fig. 34.5f**). The graft was coated by the thinned flap for internal lining and external cover. The distal edge was sutured to the residual mucosal lining with 6–0 absorbable sutures. Symmetry of the alar margins was checked and adjusted several times and then the cover sutured to the external skin (**Fig. 34.5g**). Both layers with the cartilage in between were gently linked with some 7–0 quilting sutures for several days to protect the position and prevent formation of hematoma.

For closure of the donor site, the adjacent forehead and scalp tissue was widely elevated and fixed under moderate tension with subcutaneous sutures and a running suture of the skin by 7–0 nylon. The area that would have required more than moderate tension was only approached with absorbable threads and a small dog ear excised at the upper end beyond the extension. Granulation tissue filled up the missing volume in the following weeks under permanent semi-occlusive dressing. Three weeks later, the pedicle was transected, the proximal end reduced to a small triangle, and reintegrated resembling the "frown lines" of the opposite side. The distal end was meticulously thinned, trimmed, integrated into the defect, and fixed with 7–0 nylon simple interrupted sutures. Waste skin from the middle portion of the pedicle was thinned and used as a free transplant to close off the remaining defect of the forehead now in line with the adjacent skin (**Fig. 34.5i**).

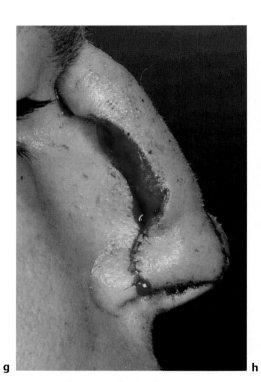

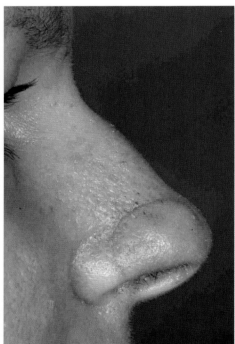

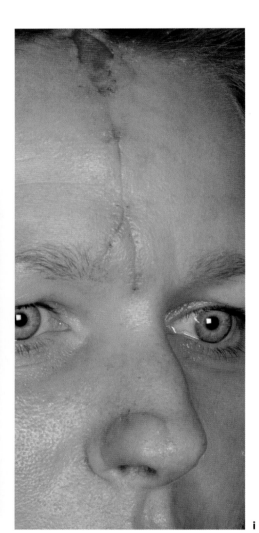

g   **h**   **i**

Fig. 34.5 (*Continued*) (**g, h**) Lateral view 1 week after the first and 1 week after the second step (division of the pedicle). (**i**) One week after division of the pedicle—sutures and bolster dressing of the skin graft have just been removed: The graft is vital, a revision zone of the frontal scar reddened, triangular base of the former pedicle in the desired position, swelling of the flap moderate.

Psychology, Motivations, Personal Background

Carcinoma and defect of the nose in addition to the underlying malignant disease weighed upon the young patient's mind. Physically, she was slightly handicapped by the effects of a metastasis followed by a stabilizing operation of the cervical spine. The reconstruction was expected to be done in one or two operations at the most and the result to be, for psycho-oncologic reasons, very good.

Discussion

All technical alternatives, such as composite graft or adjacent local flaps, were considered as too venturous and the conceivable result not good enough. A two-stage forehead technique was chosen in this case for a fast procedure and a predictable good outcome. Thinning and grafting was done during the first step;

thus the reconstruction could be accomplished after three weeks by division of the pedicle with a good result (**Fig. 34.5h, j, k**). In many other cases, however, the tissue would have been too thick and stiff for sufficient primary thinning, and positioning of a cartilage graft simply impossible. In all such cases, a three-stage procedure is the adequate solution.[6] In the first operation, the full-thickness forehead flap is thinned only as much as necessary to be folded onto itself and no primary cartilage graft is placed. After 3 to 4 weeks a second stage is performed: The outside part of the flap is divided from the inner part completely, re-elevated, and thinned. The inner portion has become part of the surrounding normal lining and is no longer dependent on the pedicle for blood supply. The cartilage grafts are placed in this intermediate second stage. The third stage, division of the pedicle and minor revisions, is performed 6 to 8 weeks after the first.

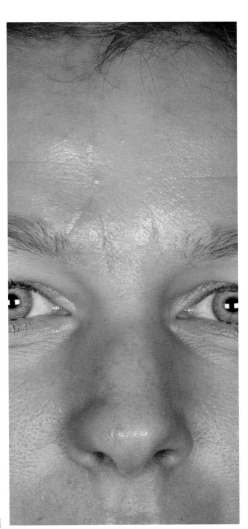

j

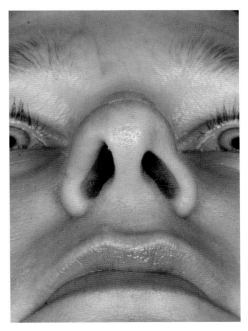

k

Fig. 34.5 (**j, k**) Ten months after last operation: The skin graft is re-epithelized, frontal scar almost invisible, and the triangle resembles the "frown lines" of the left side; thus the donor site is inconspicuous. The most important aspect of the reconstructed ala came out well: Symmet-ric borderline between nostril (dark) and adjacent alar rim (bright) compared with the opposite side. Due to the two-stage procedure the upper part of the nostril is a bit bulky.

Case 6: Full-Thickness Defect Overlapping Three Subunits: Tip, Ala, and Columella

Introduction

This 74-year-old woman presented with a recurrence of a basal cell carcinoma in the area of the soft triangle. A full-thickness defect of the tip and the right ala had to be repaired after resection with clear additional marginal excisions (**Fig. 34.6a**; operation by Joachim Quetz).

Diagnosis

Nearly half of the right tip and ventral third of the right alar subunit had been excised. Half of the columella with the right middle crus, domes of both sides, and a segment of the right lateral crus of the lower lateral cartilage were missing. An unwanted delay of 4 weeks led to secondary healing and shrinkage, but the lateral view still showed the real dimension of the defect by significant loss of tip projection. In this case, decision was taken in favor of enlargement of the defect, thus applying the subunit principle for inconspicuous reconstruction of almost the whole tip unit (**Fig. 34.6b**).[4–6] A paramedian forehead flap in two or three stages was planned, braced by septal cartilage transplants for repair of the scaffold and especially the tip defining points.

Surgical Procedure

First, the scarred defect had to be reconstructed and the edges freshened and brought back to their original position. A small version of the tip subunit was designed and marked around the defect, carefully controlled and modified several times (**Fig. 34.6c**). The residual skin within the unit was excised and septal cartilage grafts shaped, superficially scored, and bent for replacement of the domes and the adjacent missing structures. They were firmly fixed by small pockets and multiple 6–0 and 7–0 permanent sutures to the stumps and the surrounding

tissue (**Fig. 34.6d, e**). The defect with its final dimension was then transferred to an exact template for lining and cover in one piece. It was cut out of aluminum foil, bent and crimped with a sufficient distance between both surfaces for easy folding of the flap. The foil was flattened to two dimensions and transferred to the forehead, turned upside down, and twisted 180 degrees (**Fig. 34.6f**). It was positioned vertically above the right supratrochlear vessels with the segment for inner lining extending into the hairline. The flap was provided with an extra-long pedicle to reach the columella and for primary positioning of the cartilage graft if considered possible. Width of the base of the pedicle: 13 mm. The full-thickness forehead flap was harvested, the blood supply proved to be excellent, and the tissue was subtle, ready to be thinned in the first stage. Thus, decision for a two-stage procedure was taken, the distal 2 cm were carefully thinned by removing muscle and fat progressing close to the hairbulbs at the distal end. Fine distal arteries were visualized with a surgical microscope and avoided as much as possible. The grafts were coated by the thinned flap for internal lining and external cover. The distal edge was sutured to the residual mucosal lining with 6–0 absorbable sutures. Symmetry of the domes was checked and adjusted several times and then the cover sutured to the external skin. Both layers with the cartilage in between were gently linked with some 7–0 quilting sutures for some days to protect the position and prevent formation of hematoma.

For closure of the donor site, the adjacent forehead and scalp tissue was elevated and fixed without tension with subcutaneous sutures and a running suture of the skin by 7–0 nylon. The area that would have required more than moderate tension was only approached with absorbable threads and a small dog ear excised at the upper end beyond the extension. Granulation tissue filled up the missing volume in the following weeks under permanent semi-occlusive dressing (**Fig. 34.6g, h**). Four weeks later, the pedicle was transected, the proximal end reduced to a small triangle and reintegrated resembling the "frown lines"

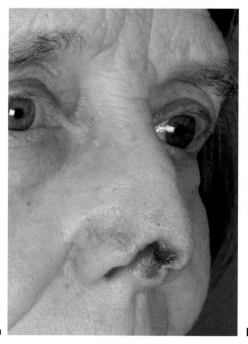
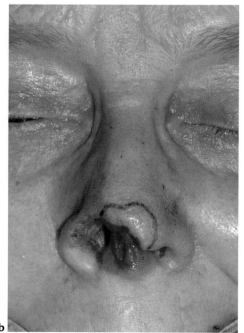
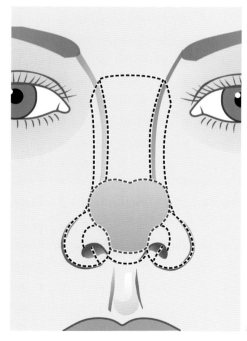

Fig. 34.6 (**a–c**) Defect per subunit: Almost half of the right tip, ventral third of the right ala, half of the columella with right middle crus, domes of both sides, and a segment of the right lateral crus of the lower lateral cartilage are missing. Minimum size of enlargement of the defect (**b**) for applying the subunit principle (**c**).

of the opposite side. The distal end was meticulously thinned, trimmed, integrated into the defect, and fixed with 7–0 nylon simple interrupted sutures. Waste skin from the middle portion of the pedicle was thinned and used as a free transplant to close off the remaining defect of the forehead now almost in line with the adjacent skin.

Psychology, Motivations, Personal Background

The lively and relaxed former teacher was ready for any sort of surgery necessary. But she didn't care too much about her looks and preferred a two-stage procedure with less perfection to a three-stage repair. She had always had a rather pointed nose and was very satisfied with the result (**Fig. 34.6i–k**).

Discussion

Contraction of the pedicle, temporarily distorting the tip in this case, can be prevented by an envelope of split skin graft. Refinement of minor deficits after 12 months, e.g., leveling of the slightly faulted neo-columella, was not desired by the patient. Thinning and grafting could be done during the first step, thus performing a two-stage forehead procedure. In many other cases, however, the tissue would have been too thick and stiff for sufficient primary thinning and positioning of grafts. In those cases, a three-stage procedure is the adequate solution with re-elevation of the outside part of the flap, thinning and placing the grafts as an intermediate second stage after 3 to 4 weeks.[7] The third stage, division of the pedicle and minor revisions, is performed 6 to 8 weeks after the first in such cases.

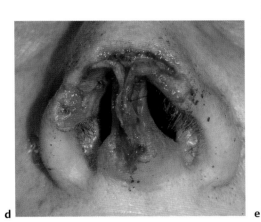
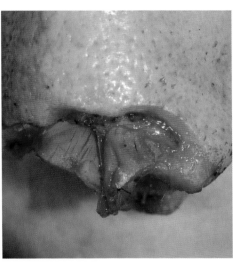
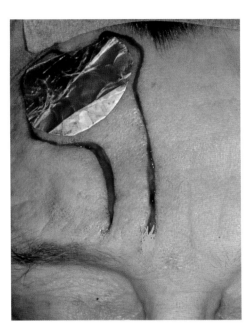

d   e   f

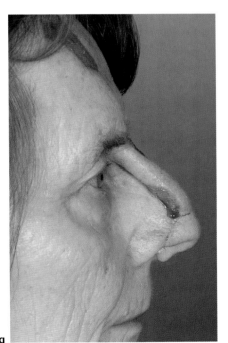
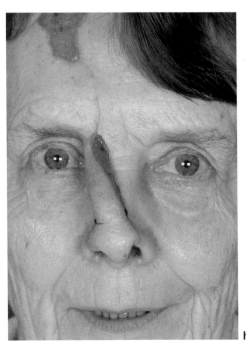

g   h

Fig. 34.6 (**d, e**) Septal cartilage grafts are shaped, superficially scored, and bent for replacement of the domes and the adjacent missing framework. They are firmly fixed by small pockets and multiple 6–0 and 7–0 permanent sutures to the stumps and the surrounding tissue. (**f**) Enlarged defect with repaired framework is represented by an exact template for lining and cover in one piece. The aluminum foil is transferred to the forehead, flattened, turned upside down, and flipped 180 degrees. Its position lies vertical above the right supratrochlear vessels, segment for inner lining reaching the hairline. (**g, h**) Four weeks after the first and a day before the second and last step. The relatively short pedicle will be divided and release the slightly distorted left side of the tip. Granulation tissue has partly filled up the missing volume under permanent semi-occlusive dressing. It will be covered by a skin graft taken from the pedicle. (*Continued on next page*)

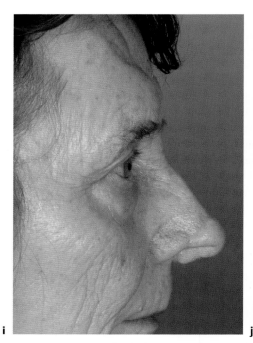
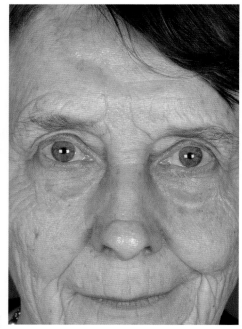
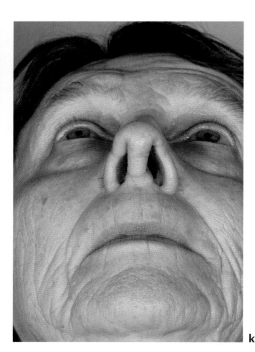

i j k

Fig. 34.6 (*Continued*)   (**i–k**) 11 months after last operation. Note the particularly important symmetry of the tip defining highlights, symmetry of the nostrils (*front view:* very eye-catching black-and-white contrast between dark nostrils and bright alar rims) and symmetry of the newly defined top of the tip subunit. Refinement of minor deficits was not desired by the patient.

Case 7: Subtotal Nasal Defect

Introduction

Recurrence of a squamous cell carcinoma of the nasal vestibule (Wang classification: T2) had been treated surgically without radiotherapy. Result was a subtotal loss of the inner structures and a vast open defect on the outside (operation by Joachim Quetz).

Diagnosis

Most of the cartilaginous septum and the complete nasal dorsum had been excised. About 50% of the outside skin was preserved but hollowed out with subtotal loss of subsurface framework and inner lining. Remnants of tip and columella had descended because of lack of support (**Fig. 34.7a, b**). Decision was taken in favor of a primary reconstruction and it was planned as a total replacement of the skin envelope within the borders of the nasal unit. A delay of 6 weeks between resection and reconstruction was observed to provide the opportunity to use the skin as turnover flaps for partial repair of inner lining. Otherwise, the skin within the nasal unit would have had to be discarded completely.

Surgical Procedure

A typical three-stage procedure was planned.[7,8] *First Stage:* Reconstruction of the septum with a bi-pedicled composite septal pivot flap[4,8] of the inner lining and cover with a full-thickness paramedian forehead flap. *Second Stage,* after 3 to 4 weeks: Reelevation of the forehead flap, thinning of its layers, and reconstruction of the nasal framework using autogenous rib cartilage. *Third Stage,* after 4 to 8 weeks: Minor corrections and division of the pedicle.

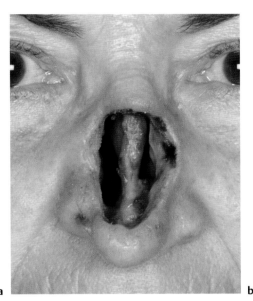
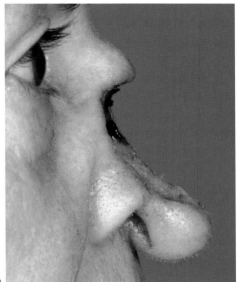
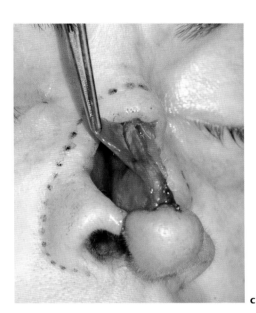

a   b   c

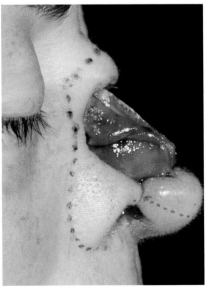
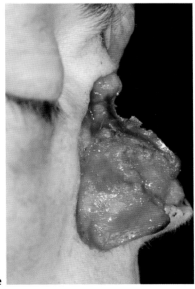
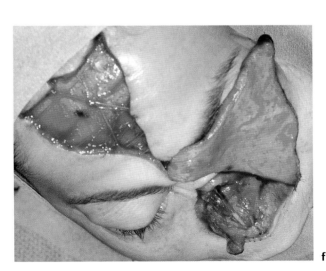

d   e   f

Fig. 34.7 (**a, b**) Subtotal nasal defect: Most of the cartilaginous septum and subsurface framework are resected. Complete nasal dorsum is missing. About 50% of the outside skin is preserved but hollowed out with subtotal loss of inner lining. (**c, d**) The septal pivot flap has been rotated out of the piriform aperture, excess bone and cartilage removed from between the bilateral mucosal flaps to achieve the desired nasal profile. The flaps are turned laterally to contribute some lining to the nasal domes. The drooped remnant of tip and columella are lifted and fixed to the neo-septum, thus establishing the former projection. Border of the nasal unit is marked (*dotted blue line*). (**e**) The defect is significantly enlarged according to the (aesthetic) unit of the nose: The residual skin was incised all along the nasal unit, elevated, and discarded in the upper half, converted into turnover flaps for inner lining in the lower half. Small remaining gaps are bridged with full-skin grafts. (**f**) A full-thickness paramedian forehead flap is elevated with all layers above the periosteum. Subcutaneous fat and frontalis muscle is partially removed only along the distal edges. An extension for repair of the columella is not needed in this case. The adjacent forehead and scalp tissue was widely elevated and fixed under slight tension with subcutaneous sutures. The area that would have required more than moderate tension is only approached with absorbable threads and three small dog ears were excised at the most distal edges of the donor site in the hair-bearing scalp. (*Continued on next page*)

First Stage: The inner part of the septum had been preserved and could be used for reconstruction of the septum as a *pivot flap.* The septal branches of the superior labial artery allow almost the entire septum to be elevated and rotated forward. The upper edge of the flap was separated from the anterior base of the skull with straight scissors, the dorsal edge then perforated with a 60-degree angle blade and a curved chisel to be freed completely. Finally, the lower edge was ventrally severed using a scalpel and chisel by maintaining an at least 12-mm-wide mucosal bridge. After harvest of a bony-cartilaginous wedge from between the mucosal bridges, the whole septal composite flap could be rotated out of the piriform aperture anteriorly (**Fig. 34.7g**). The base of the flap was—as in most cases—sufficiently interlocked with the spine area and additionally fixed by the gently twisted pedicles. The upper part was wedged by the inner structures of the nasal bone and additionally fixed to it by drill holes and a permanent suture. There was now enough protection for support of the lining and for the upcoming forehead flap (**Fig. 34.7h**). The drooped remnant of tip and columella was lifted and fixed to the neo-septum, thus establishing the former projection. Excess bone and cartilage was removed from between the bilateral mucosal flaps to achieve the desired nasal profile. The mucosal flaps, when turned laterally, could contribute some *lining* to the nasal domes (**Fig. 34.7c, d, i**). The shape of the defect was then modified according to the aesthetic unit of the nose: The residual skin was incised all along the nasal unit and thereby the defect significantly enlarged. In the upper half of the nose, the skin was elevated and discarded. In the lower half, it was converted into turnover flaps for inner lining and connected to mucosal flaps and upper edge of the neo-septum. Small remaining gaps were bridged with full-skin grafts (**Fig. 34.7e**). During reconstruction the new lining was supported by bent aluminum foils and gauze swabs. A three-dimensional model of the new nose according to the defect was prepared by cutting and bending aluminum foil (superfluous suture package). An ideal pattern as illustrated by Burget and Menick[4] is helpful, slightly oversized then modified and thus reduced according to the defect. Flattened into two dimensions, it served as a template on the forehead. Its position was chosen as vertically as possible, reaching into the hair-bearing scalp, the base of the pedicle narrowed to ~ 1.2 cm. A full-thickness *paramedian forehead flap* was elevated with all the layers above the periosteum. Subcutaneous fat and frontalis muscle were partially removed only along the distal edges. An extension for the columella was not needed in this case. The flap was flipped over 180 degrees and hinged down another 180 degrees for cover of neo-septum and lining (**Fig. 34.7f**). For closure of the donor site, the adjacent forehead and scalp tissue was widely elevated and fixed under slight tension with subcutaneous sutures. The short segment that could be closed primarily was stitched up with 7–0 nylon simple interrupted sutures. The area that would have required more than moderate tension was only approached with absorbable threads, and three small dog ears were excised at the most distal edges of the donor site in the hair-bearing scalp. Granulation tissue was expected to fill up the surface area that remained open in the following 8 weeks under permanent semi-occlusive dressing. The forehead flap was carefully brought into line and fixed to the surrounding wound edges with subcutaneous sutures and 6–0 as well as 7–0 nylon simple interrupted and running sutures. The lining was fixed to the flap by 7–0 quilting sutures for several days to protect the position and prevent formation of hematoma: skin grafts with slight tension and vascularized flaps loosely. Furthermore, the neo-cavity was packed with dry cotton wool for at least two days.

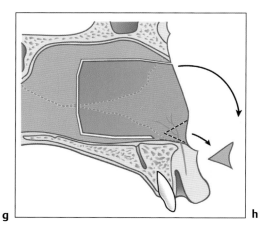 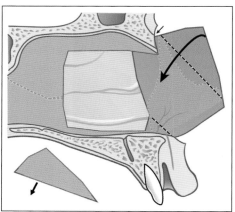 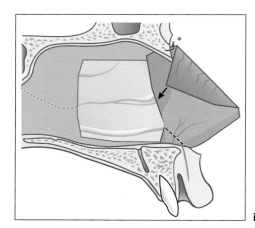

g   h   i

Fig. 34.7 (*Continued*)   (**g**) The flap is supplied by branches of the superior labial artery within a 15-mm-wide mucosal bridge. The other edges are severed totally. A bony-cartilaginous wedge is removed (*small arrow*) from between the mucosal bridges to allow rotation of the flap. (**h**) Rotation is done by bending the flap, pulling it out of the nasal cavity, and in this case, chiseling a groove into the nasal bone (*small arrow*). After the mucosa is separated as far as necessary for the trimming (*large arrow*), the profile is created by removing a bony-cartilaginous segment (*medium-sized arrow*). (**i**) The excess mucosa is turned laterally to contribute to the repair of inner lining. A suture through the nasal bone (*asterisk*) may secure the position of the rotation flap.

Blood supply of the forehead flap was carefully controlled. The inner lining was regularly checked with an ear microscope, patient in a supine position. Only this sort of overview, magnification, and illumination guarantees a reliable control of the inner surfaces: Mucosal and turnover flaps showed sufficient perfusion, the skin grafts had positively healed after 8 days. Otherwise, an intermediate operation would have been performed immediately, i.e., re-grafting full skin to a necrotic area of the lining or mending a bigger defect with a local or regional flap. The regular second step would have to be postponed as long as septum and lining are not in perfect condition. When all layers have healed properly, the second stage can be performed. The new nose now has about its final dimension, but looks bulky and uneven. Typical shape and attractive details are still missing (**Fig. 34.7j, k**).

Second Stage, after 4 weeks: *Rib cartilage* was harvested in the beginning of the operation to have all the time needed for further processing, shaping, and observation of this material. Some fascia and perichondrium were taken at the same time. Immediately after being harvested, the two 5-cm long pieces of rib cartilage were split into curved chips and straight struts of various dimensions. Stored in saline solution, they were observed, carved, and observed again until being fixed to the recipient bed, thus minimizing the risk of warping and getting deformed later on. At the same time, the entire delayed forehead flap was easily and safely *re-elevated* in an unscarred subcutaneous plane and extensively thinned (**Fig. 34.7l**). Thinning was done under a surgical microscope and short scissors to avoid damage to the axial vessels. The pedicle area and the distal wings of the flap were thinned conservatively to not endanger the blood supply. The patchwork of skin grafts, mucosal flaps, and turnover flaps were thus completely separated from the overly-ing skin cover, forming a soft and homogeneous surface, coated by the fat of the forehead flap (**Fig. 34.7l**). This surface was also carefully thinned, trimmed, and sculptured to a symmetric, well-proportioned, and reliably vascularized recipient site for the cartilage grafts. Again a microscope was used and the lower edge of the rims permanently controlled for sufficient blood supply. The *subsurface framework* was now replaced by extensive and more than anatomically correct cartilage grafting. In multiple steps, the straight and curved cartilaginous pieces had been carved parallel to the thinning until the desired shapes were achieved. The dorsal strut was fixed to the dorsal edge of the neo-septum with a series of 7–0 permanent sutures. This element is statically and optically the most important piece of the new framework. It had a concave underside precisely matching the convex base. A columella strut—in this case made from two pieces—provided reinforcement of the lower edge of the new septum and gave additional support to the dorsal strut. It replaces the medial genua of the alar cartilages and defines the columella show. Alar battens are next in importance. They were made from elastic strips of rib cartilage approximated to the shape of typical alar lobules. Additional elements extended into the soft triangle region to give support to the nostril margins. The battens and elements were sutured to the caudal end of the lining, again with 7–0 monofil threads. Replacement of the alar cartilages was and can be incomplete: They have to reinforce the cover and shape of the hard nasal tip and the supratip area. Conchal cartilage is best suited to this end; alternatively, thin elements of rib cartilage can be carved and assembled. However, the latter have to be covered by a perichondrial layer at the end. The remaining unprotected surfaces of the sidewalls were splinted with thinly sliced pieces of rib cartilage. All the small gaps and cavities were filled with adequate pieces of cartilage and perichondrium (**Fig. 34.7m–o**).

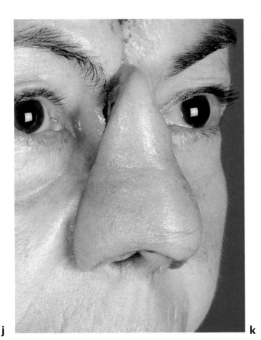
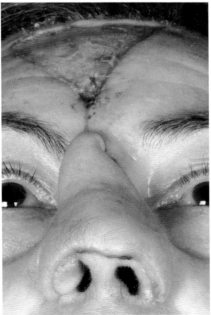
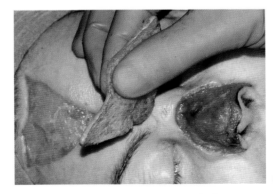

j   k   l

Fig. 34.7   (**j, k**) Three days before second stage: All layers have healed properly. The new nose now has about its final dimension, but looks bulky and uneven; attractive details are still missing. (**l**) Second stage: The delayed forehead flap was easily and safely re-elevated in an unscarred subcutaneous plane and extensively thinned. The pedicle area and the distal wings of the flap were thinned conservatively for not endangering the blood supply. The patchwork of skin grafts, mucosal flaps, and turnover flaps is thus completely separated from the overlying skin cover, forming a soft and homogeneous surface, coated by the fat of the forehead flap. (*Continued on next page*)

The nasal tip especially sometimes needs an extra cover of fascia or perichondrium. All grafts were dipped into disinfectant before being finally fixed. The forehead flap was now repositioned and fixed onto the recipient bed by lightly tied mattress quilting sutures (7–0 and 6–0) to close the dead spaces. These sutures have to be removed some days later to avoid marks in the skin. The cavity was packed with dry cotton wool for at least two days.

Blood supply of forehead flap and inner lining was carefully controlled. To make sure no seroma or hematoma stays below the flap, a "rolling out" procedure in the direction of the pedicle was performed at least twice every day. Antibiotics were given for 10 days.

When transplants and cover have healed and symmetry and shape meet the expectations, the third stage can be done. Otherwise, an intermediate operation is necessary, e.g., for modifying and repositioning the grafts or for repair. Division of the pedicle is postponed as long as major revision is within the realms of possibility. Three weeks after the second stage, when the swelling had gone down sufficiently and the last step was considered, some unsatisfying details had become obvious: The nasal dorsum was slightly tilted to the right side, the tip was too narrow, the alar lobules too broad, and definition of both needed improvement (**Fig. 34.7p–r**). A revision of the second step was agreed upon.

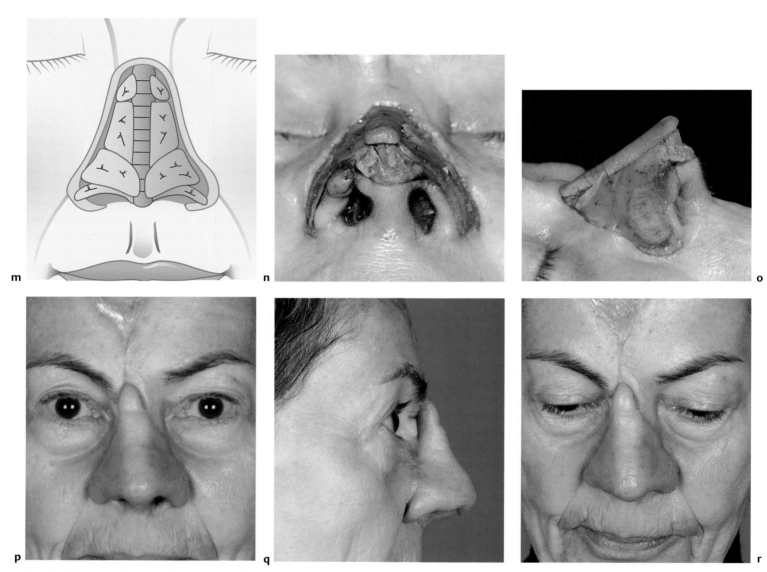

Fig. 34.7 (*Continued*)   (**m–o**) Ideal pattern of a reconstructed subsurface framework by extensive and more than anatomically correct cartilage grafting (**m**). Dorsal strut on the way to be fixed to the dorsal edge of the neo-septum with a series of 7–0 permanent sutures. It has a concave underside precisely matching the convex base. A columella strut—in this case made from two pieces—provides reinforcement of the lower edge of the new septum, gives additional support to the dorsal strut, and defines the columella show. Additional elements extend into the soft triangle region to give support to the nostril margins. The remaining unprotected surfaces of the sidewalls are splinted with thinly sliced pieces of rib cartilage. All small gaps and cavities are filled with adequate pieces of cartilage and perichondrium. (**p–r**) Three weeks after the second stage, swelling has gone down sufficiently. The shape has improved, but some unsatisfying details are obvious: Nasal dorsum is slightly tilted to the right side, the tip is too narrow, the alar base too broad, and definition of both needs improvement.

Revision of the second stage, 6 weeks after the regular second stage: The forehead flap was re-elevated a second time without problems, again carefully thinned, the framework explored and analyzed, and sufficiently big pieces of conchal cartilage were harvested from both ears. The dorsal strut was repositioned, grafts of the alar lobules reduced, and definition of the tip improved by a modified shield graft, extended by elements for shape and support of the soft triangles (**Fig. 34.7s, t**). Again all the small gaps and cavities were filled with adequate pieces of cartilage and fat and the tip additionally covered with perichondrium (**Fig. 34.7u, v**). All grafts were—as always—dipped into disinfectant before being put into place. Repositioning of the forehead flap went the same way as in the second stage, but the skin was slightly trimmed around the area of the alar lobules. Postoperative control was like after the second stage. The improvement developed satisfyingly while the swelling decreased.

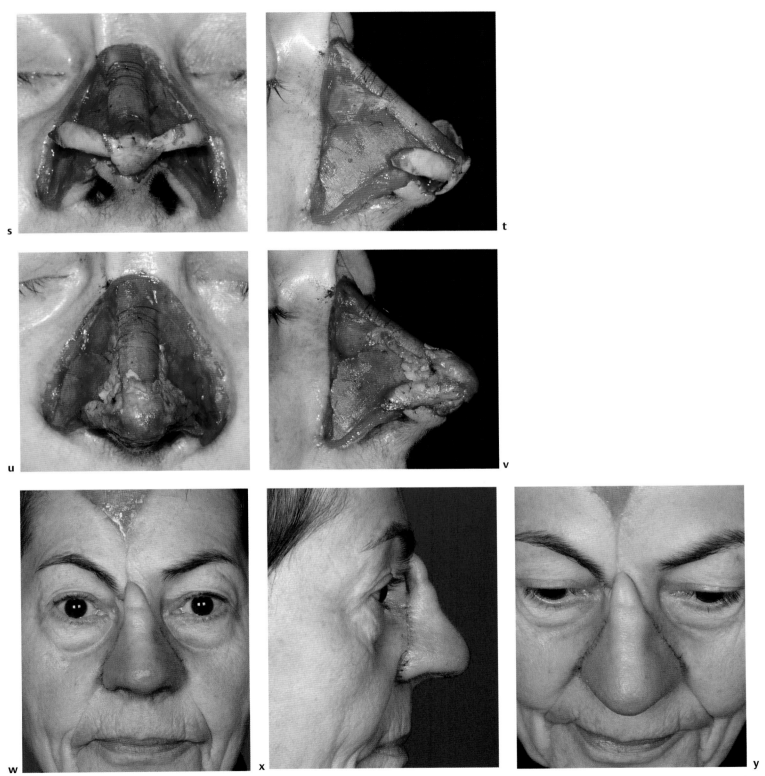

Fig. 34.7 (**s, t**) Revision 6 weeks after the regular second stage: Second re-elevation of the flap, framework explored and analyzed. Some grafts are reduced, volume and definition of the tip improved by a modified shield graft, extended by elements for shape and support of the soft triangles by conchal cartilage. (**u, v**) All small gaps and cavities are filled with adequate pieces of cartilage and fat, and the tip is additionally covered with perichondrium. All grafts are dipped into disinfectant before being put into place. Skin of the forehead flap was slightly trimmed around the area of the alar lobules. (**w–y**) One week after the revision: Improvement starts being noticeable (see **Fig. 34.7p–r**). (*Continued on next page*)

Third Stage, 10 weeks after the unscheduled revision: The pedicle was transected, the proximal end reduced to a small triangle and reintegrated resembling the "frown lines" of the opposite side. The distal end was meticulously thinned, trimmed, integrated into the defect, and fixed with 7–0 nylon simple interrupted sutures. Waste skin from the middle portion of the pedicle was thinned and used as a free transplant to close the lower third of the remaining defect of the forehead now almost in line with the adjacent skin (**Fig. 34.7z**).

Four weeks later, the granulation tissue of the harvesting defect was completely epithelialized, inconspicuously in line with the skin graft. The aesthetic result was good, nasal breathing and an uncompromised sense of smell (**Fig. 34.7aa**).

Psychology, Motivations, Personal Background

The patient was—as a matter of routine—made familiar with the extent of surgery she would have to face, compared with modern implant-supported prostheses mostly ensuring good camouflage, predictable results, fast rehabilitation, and the absence of donor site morbidity.[9] Both methods were demonstrated by pictures showing intermediate stages and average results. The kind, modest, and nonsmoking patient decided without question for direct reconstruction. She was—as are all patients—informed

about the fact that the new nose will look like a "potato sack" after the first stage and that she should not be worried. After the second stage, the patient was rather pleased with the result and at first not sure about revision and refinement. When the deficits became more obvious, she finally agreed to our suggestion, and told us afterward that it had been worthwhile.

Discussion

Many advantages are coming along with the total nasal repair as a regular three-stage procedure. The option of using skin grafts in the first stage is one of them. Re-elevation of the—then delayed—forehead flap allows thinning to be pushed to the limits and the cartilage grafts can be fixed to a reliable and shaped surface without putting them at risk. The second operation offers the opportunity of repositioning the flap, using surplus tissue where needed or resecting it where it is overlapping. At the same time, the second stage allows the total length of the nose to be slightly extended or shortened. Late division of the pedicle always allows—as in the case of this patient—an unscheduled revision for functional or aesthetical improvement. So the three-stage procedure to reconstruct a nose layer by layer offers great security. Thus, the rate of complications and revisions may drop and results should improve.[7]

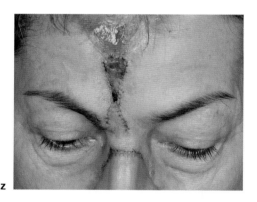

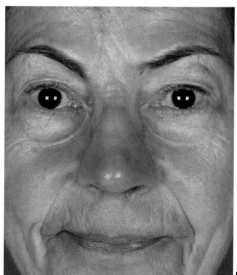
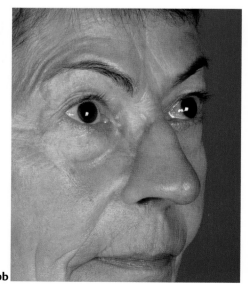
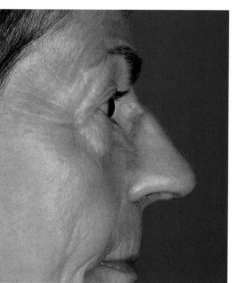

Fig. 34.7 (*Continued*) (**z**) Third Stage: Pedicle transected, proximal end reduced to a small triangle and reintegrated, distal end meticulously thinned, trimmed, integrated into the defect, and fixed with 7–0 nylon suture. Waste skin from the pedicle is thinned and used as a free transplant to close the lower third of the remaining defect of the forehead now almost in line with the adjacent skin. (**aa–cc**) Eleven months after the last operation: Well-balanced result of the unscheduled revision is fully visible (see **Fig. 34.7s–v**).

Case 8: Supratotal Nasal Defect

Introduction

This 79-year-old woman presented with the second relapse of a basal cell carcinoma that had totally distorted the small pre-operated nose. After total ablation, including and going beyond the nasal bone and extending into the right cheek, only the left nostril was left over. In spite of her age the healthy older woman decided against an implant-supported prosthesis and for total repair (operation by Joachim Quetz).[9]

Diagnosis

The whole nose but the left nostril had been resected, including nasal bone and right sidewall, extending into the right cheek and reaching the right upper lip including nasal spine and bone of the right piriform aperture. The inner part of the septum was in good condition, but soft tissue of the upper lip had been resected down to the bone, thus destroying the vessels between the septal mucosa and the supralabial artery on the right side (**Fig. 34.8a, d**).

Surgical Procedure

A typical three-stage procedure was planned.[7,8,10] *First Stage:* Reconstruction of the septum with a bi-pedicled composite septal pivot flap, of the inner lining and cover with a full-thickness paramedian forehead flap. *Second Stage,* after 3 to 4 weeks: Re-elevation of the forehead flap, thinning of its layers and reconstruction of the nasal framework using autogenous rib cartilage. *Third Stage,* after 4 to 8 weeks: Minor corrections and division of the pedicle.

First Stage: The inner part of the septum had been preserved and could be used for reconstruction of the septum as a *pivot flap*. The septal branches of the superior labial artery allow almost the entire septum to be elevated and rotated forward. But in this case the right side had been completely destroyed—a severe handicap for the pivot flap. Rotation was tried anyway: The upper edge of the flap was separated from the anterior base of the skull with straight scissors, the dorsal edge then perforated with a 60-degree angle blade and a curved chisel to be freed completely. Finally, the lower edge was ventrally severed using a scalpel and chisel by maintaining an at least 12-mm-wide

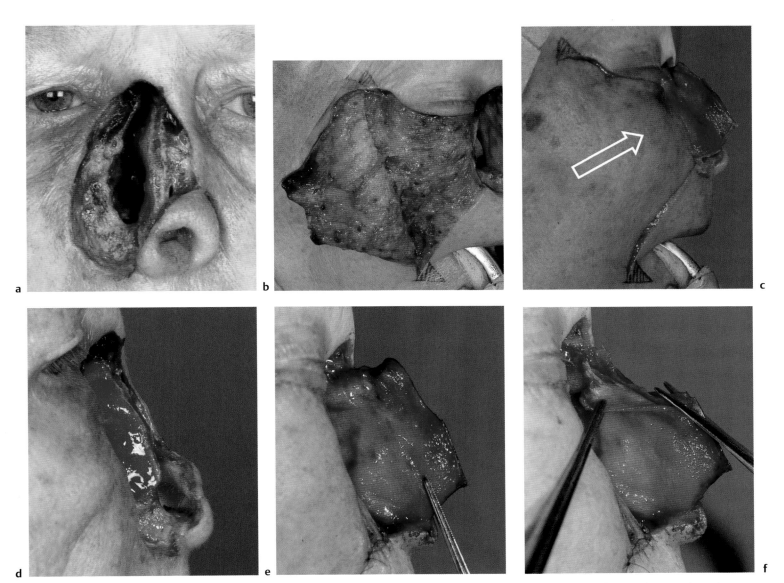

a b c

d e f

Fig. 34.8   (**a, b**) The whole nose but the left nostril is destroyed, including nasal bone, medial cheek, nasal spine, and piriform aperture reaching the upper lip on the right side. The inner part of the septum is in good condition, but the vessels between the septal mucosa and the supralabial artery on the right side are resected. A septal rotation is planned even so. (**c, d**) The septal pivot flap has been rotated out of the piriform ap- erture, blood supply is unexpectedly good. Excess bone and cartilage are removed from between the bilateral mucosal flaps to achieve the desired nasal profile. The flaps are turned laterally to contribute some lining to the nasal domes. (**e, f**) The defect is scaled down according to the (aesthetic) unit of the nose by a cheek advancement flap. (*Continued on next page*)

mucosal bridge. After harvesting of a bony-cartilaginous wedge from between the mucosal bridges, the whole septal composite flap could be rotated out of the piriform aperture anteriorly (**Fig. 34.8e, g**). Blood supply of the right septal mucosa was better than expected and decision was taken to go on with the normal procedure after an hour of recovery.[10] This hour was used to modify the shape of the defect according to the aesthetic unit of the nose: Size of the defect was diminished and a basis provided for the upcoming new alar lobule on the right side by a cheek advancement flap (**Fig. 34.8b, c, g**). The base of the pivot flap was sufficiently interlocked with the spine area and additionally fixed by the gently twisted pedicles. The upper part was wedged by remnants of the nasal bone and additionally fixed to it by drill holes and a permanent suture. There was now enough protection for support of the lining and for the upcoming forehead flap.

Excess bone and cartilage were removed from between the bilateral mucosal flaps to achieve the desired nasal profile (**Fig. 34.8f**). The mucosal flaps were turned laterally and contributed some *lining* to the nasal domes (**Fig. 34.8f, h**). Most of the lining was restored by full-skin grafts that were fixed to the mucosal flaps, the upper edge of the neo-septum, and all along the lateral aspects of the piriform aperture on both sides. For reconstruction of the nasal bone, a calvarial bone graft was harvested, divided, and fixed with small titanium screws and plates (**Fig. 34.8n**). During reconstruction the new lining was supported by bent aluminum foil and gauze swabs. A three-dimensional model of the new nose according to the defect was prepared by cutting and bending aluminum foil (superfluous suture package, **Fig. 34.8l**). An ideal pattern as illustrated by Burget and Menick[4] is helpful, slightly oversized and then modified, and thus reduced according to the

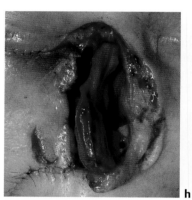 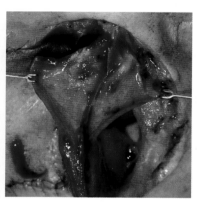

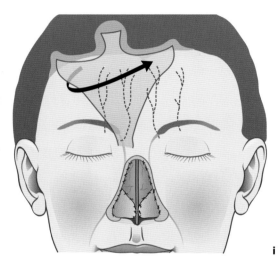

Fig. 34.8 (*Continued*)   (**g**) Frontal view on the septal pivot flap. The "blue edge" of the check advancement flap will later be partly resected. Note the incision for the new alar base. (**h**) Excess mucosa of the pivot flap is turned laterally to contribute some lining to the nasal domes. (**i, j**) First stage of total reconstruction with septal pivot flap if available, repair of intranasal lining and repair of the cover by a full-thickness paramedian forehead flap. Lining is partly restored by excess mucosa (*red*) of the pivot flap (*blue*), partly with full-skin grafts (*gray*). If available, turnover flaps built from remnants of the old nose can be integrated into the patchwork. A three-dimensional model of the new nose is prepared with aluminum foil, flattened out on the forehead as a template, positioned as vertical as possible, base of the pedicle narrowed to less than 1.5 cm. A full-thickness paramedian forehead flap is elevated with all layers above the periosteum, flipped, and turned down 180 degrees. Distal edges of the flap are thinned to be able to form columella and nostril rims. The flap is sutured to its final position. Lining is fixed to the forehead flap by quilting sutures: skin grafts tightly and vascularized flaps loosely, supported by dry cotton wool tamponade. The mobilized wound edges of the donor site are approximated (*short arrows*) by strong resorbable sutures and dog ears excised at the most distal edges of the donor site (*long arrow*). The remaining defect will heal secondarily under permanent semi-occlusive dressing. (**k**) Second stage, after ~ 4 weeks: Re-elevation and thinning of the forehead flap, thinning and shaping of intranasal lining, and reconstruction of nasal framework using autogenous rib cartilage. The entire delayed forehead flap is re-elevated in the unscarred subcutaneous plane and thinned, lining thus completely separated from the overlying skin, coated by the fat of the forehead flap. Lining is also carefully thinned and trimmed to a symmetric, well-proportioned, and reliably vascularized recipient site for the cartilage grafts. The subsurface framework is built by extensive cartilage grafting: A dorsal strut is the most dominant element, a separate strut defines the exposition of the columella (not visible in the frontal view), and alar battens shape and stabilize the nostrils. The unprotected surfaces of the sidewalls have also to be splinted with thinly sliced pieces of cartilage. The nasal tip mostly needs an extra cover of fascia or perichondrium. Lining is again carefully fixed to the forehead flap with thin quilting sutures running in between and through the grafts. A tight dry cotton wool tamponade helps obliterate the dead spaces.

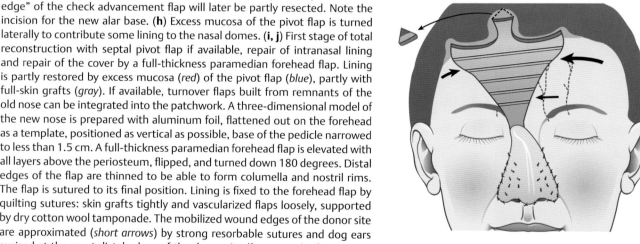

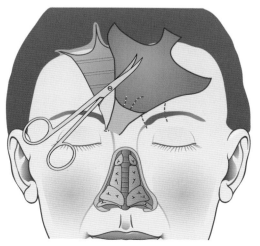

defect (e.g., typical distances from nasion to base of columella and between alar-facial grooves about 8 cm each). Flattened into two dimensions, it served as a template on the forehead (**Fig. 34.8m**). Its position was chosen as vertically as possible, reaching into the hair-bearing scalp, the base of the pedicle narrowed to ~ 1.2 cm after the supratrochlear artery had been identified with a Doppler. A full-thickness *paramedian forehead flap* was elevated with all the layers above the periosteum (**Fig. 34.8i**). Subcutaneous fat and frontalis muscle were removed only along the distal edges to be able to form columella and nostril rims. The flap was flipped over 180 degrees and hinged down another 180 degrees for cover of neo-septum and lining (**Fig. 34.8j, n**). For closure of the donor site, the adjacent forehead and scalp tissue was widely elevated and fixed under slight tension with subcutaneous sutures. The short segment that could be closed primarily was stitched up with 7–0 nylon simple interrupted sutures. The area that would have required more than moderate tension was only approached with absorbable threads and two small dog ears were excised at the most distal edges of the donor site in the hair-bearing scalp (**Fig. 34.8j**). Granulation tissue was expected to fill up the surface area that remained open in the following 10 weeks under permanent semi-occlusive dressing. The forehead flap was carefully brought into line and fixed to the surrounding wound edges with subcutaneous sutures and 6–0 as well as 7–0 nylon simple interrupted and running sutures. The lining was fixed to the flap by 7–0 quilting sutures for some days to protect the position and prevent formation of hematoma (**Fig. 34.8j**). Furthermore, the neo-cavity was packed with dry cotton wool for at least two days.

Blood supply of the forehead flap was carefully controlled. The inner lining was checked with an ear microscope, patient in a supine position. Only this sort of overview, magnification, and illumination guarantees a reliable control of the inner surfaces: Mucosa of the pivot flap did survive completely and most of the skin grafts had visibly healed after 7 days. The new nose now had about its final dimension, but looked bulky and uneven. The typical shape and any sort of attractive details were still missing (**Fig. 34.8o, p**). A small necrosis of the lining with significant loss of volume in the most distal area, the left neo-ala, was replaced by a nasolabial flap (**Fig. 34.8q, r**). The regular second step had to be postponed for two weeks for this reason. When all layers had healed properly, the second stage was performed.

Second Stage, after 5 weeks: *Rib cartilage* was harvested in the beginning of the operation to have all the time needed for further processing, shaping, and observation of this material. Immediately after being harvested, the two 5-cm-long pieces of

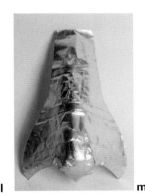
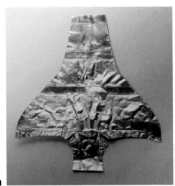
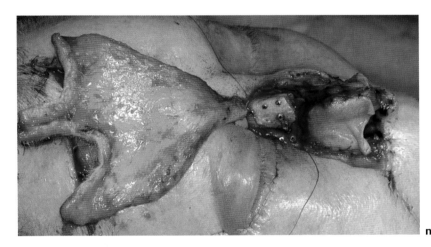
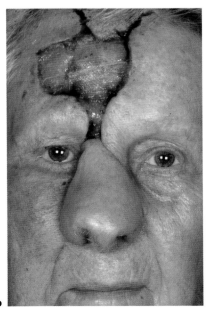
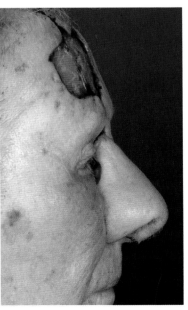

Fig. 34.8 (**l, m**) A three-dimensional model of the new nose according to the defect is prepared by cutting and bending aluminum foil (0.06–0.09 mm, e.g., suture package). Flattened into two dimensions, it serves as a template on the forehead. (**n**) The full-thickness paramedian forehead flap is elevated, flipped 180 degrees, distal edges are thinned and formed to columella and nostril rims. The nasal bone is repaired by calvarial bone grafts, fixed with small titanium screws and plates. Lining is partly restored by excess mucosa of the pivot flap and mainly with full-skin grafts. (**o, p**) The new nose now has about its final dimension, but looks bulky and the typical shape and any sort of attractive details are still missing. (*Continued on next page*)

rib cartilage were split into curved chips and straight struts of various dimensions. Stored in saline solution, they were observed, carved, and observed again until being fixed to the recipient bed, thus minimizing the risk of warping and getting deformed later on. At the same time, the entire delayed forehead flap was easily and safely *re-elevated* in an unscarred subcutaneous plane and extensively thinned (**Fig. 34.8s**). Thinning was done under a surgical microscope and short scissors to avoid damage to the axial vessels. The pedicle area and the distal wings of the flap were thinned conservatively in order not to endanger the blood supply. Lining was thus completely separated from the overlying skin cover, forming a soft and homogeneous surface, coated by the fat of the forehead flap. This surface was also carefully thinned, trimmed, and sculptured to a symmetric, well-proportioned, and reliably vascularized recipient site for the cartilage grafts (**Fig. 34.8t**). Again a microscope was used and the lower edge of the rims permanently controlled for sufficient blood supply. The *subsurface framework* was now restored by extensive and more than anatomically correct cartilage grafting. In multiple steps the straight and curved cartilaginous pieces had been carved parallel to the thinning until the desired shapes were achieved (**Fig. 34.8u**). The dorsal strut was fixed to the dorsal edge of the neo-septum with a series of 7–0 permanent sutures. This element was statically and optically the most important piece of the new framework. It had a concave underside precisely matching the convex base. No columella strut was needed in this case. Alar battens were next in importance. They were made

from elastic strips of rib cartilage approximated to the shape of typical alar lobules and rims. They extended into the soft triangle region to give support to the nostril margins. The battens and elements were sutured to the caudal end of the lining, again with 7–0 monofil and some fine resorbable threads. Replacement of the alar cartilages can be incomplete: They have to reinforce the nose and to cover and shape the hard nasal tip and the supratip area. Conchal cartilage is best suited to this end, but as an alternative thin elements of rib cartilage can be carved and assembled (**Fig. 34.8v, w**). However, the latter should be covered by a perichondrial layer at the end. The remaining unprotected surfaces of the sidewalls were splinted with thinly sliced pieces of rib cartilage. All grafts were dipped into disinfectant before being finally fixed. The forehead flap was now repositioned and fixed onto the recipient bed by lightly tied mattress quilting sutures (7–0 and 6–0) to close the dead spaces. These sutures have to be removed some days later to avoid marks in the skin.

When transplants and cover have healed and symmetry and shape meet the expectations (**Fig. 34.8x, y**), the third stage can be performed. Otherwise, an intermediate operation is necessary, e.g., for modifying and repositioning the grafts or for repair. Division of the pedicle is postponed as long as major revision is within the realms of possibility.

Third Stage, after 8 weeks: The pedicle was transected, the proximal end reduced to a small triangle and reintegrated resembling the "frown lines" of the opposite side. The distal end was meticulously thinned, trimmed, integrated into the defect,

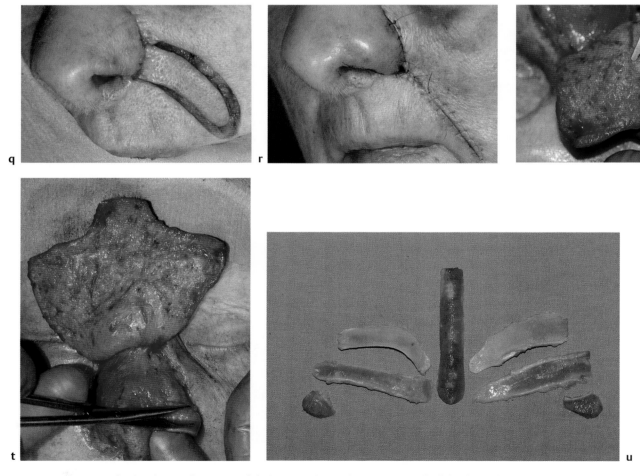

Fig. 34.8 (*Continued*)   (**q, r**) A small necrosis of the lining with significant loss of volume in the most distal area, the left neo-ala, was replaced by a nasolabial flap. Note: It is important not to use those local flaps primarily for reconstruction! (**s, t**) Thinning of forehead flap and lining with a surgical microscope to avoid damage to the axial vessels and for permanent control of blood supply along the most distal edges. The pedicle area and the distal wings of the flap are thinned very conservatively. (**u**) Main components of new subsurface framework from rib cartilage that have been carved parallel to the re-elevation and thinning.

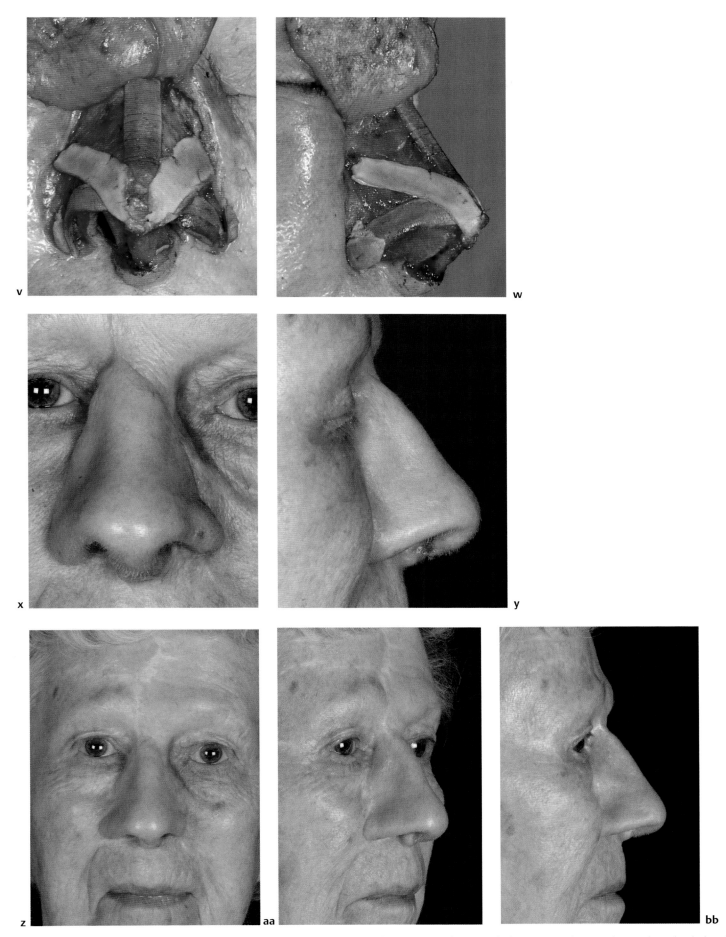

Fig. 34.8 (**v, w**) Main components of the new framework fixed to the lining. (**x, y**) Three weeks later: Transplants and cover have healed and symmetry and shape meet the expectations. (**z–bb**) Result 3 years after reconstruction. (*Continued on next page*)

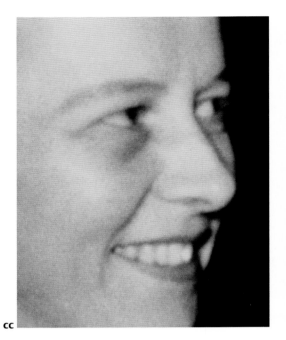
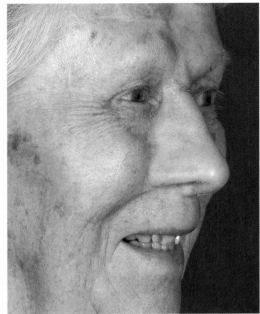

cc   dd

Fig. 34.8 (*Continued*)   (**cc, dd**) Reconstructed nose compared with a 50-year-old photograph.

and fixed with 7–0 nylon simple interrupted sutures. The granulation tissue on the forehead was covered with a skin graft from the preauricular region.

Psychology, Motivations, Personal Background

The patient was explicitly informed—as a matter of routine—about two ways of repair: reconstruction or implant-supported prostheses. Both methods were demonstrated by pictures showing intermediate stages and average results. The relaxed older woman, always accompanied by her caring husband, was not worried by the extent of surgery she would have to face and decided in favor of a total reconstruction. She was very happy with the aesthetic result and even discovered similarities with the original shape of her nose that she had lost years before (**Fig. 34.8z–dd**).

Discussion

The three-stage total reconstruction went basically as planned with a good result at the end. Nasal breathing and the sense of smell were unimpaired. A delay of some weeks before division of the pedicle was caused by a minor healing problem at the left alar lobule. The septal rotation flap proved very robust in this case with no vascular support from the labial artery on the right side. Reconstruction of the nasal bone with calvarial grafts is time consuming and makes things more complicated, e.g., bringing the dorsal strut in line with the bone during the second stage—in this case the reason for the little hump. A combination graft of cartilage attached to bone would have been a better choice in this case, providing a longer strut, preventing formation of a step, and even reducing the risk of warping.

References

1. Sherris DA, Kern EB. The versatile autogenous rib graft in septorhinoplasty. Am J Rhinol 1998;12(3):221–227

2. Quetz J. Sattelnase bei M. Wegener: Rekonstruktive Rhinoplastik mit autologen Rippenknorpetransplantaten durch geschlossene Technik. Presented at the 79th Annual Meeting of the German Society of Oto-Rhino-Laryngology, Head and Neck Surgery, April 30–May 5, 2008, Bonn, Germany. http://www.egms.de/static/en/meetings/hnod2008/08hnod540.shtml

3. Sheen JH. Spreader graft: a method of reconstructing the roof of the middle nasal vault following rhinoplasty. Plast Reconstr Surg 1984;73(2): 230–239

4. Burget GC, Menick FJ. Aesthetic Reconstruction of the Nose. St. Louis, MO: Mosby; 1994:117–156

5. Burget GC, Menick FJ. The subunit principle in nasal reconstruction. Plast Reconstr Surg 1985;76(2):239–247

6. Burget GC, Menick FJ. Nasal support and lining: the marriage of beauty and blood supply. Plast Reconstr Surg 1989;84(2):189–202

7. Menick FJ. A 10-year experience in nasal reconstruction with the three-stage forehead flap. Plast Reconstr Surg 2002;109(6):1839–1855, discussion 1856–1861

8. Quetz J, Ambrosch P. Total nasal reconstruction: a 6-year experience with the three-stage forehead flap combined with the septal pivot flap. Facial Plast Surg 2011;27(3):266–275

9. Fischer H, Gubisch W. Nasal reconstruction: a challenge for plastic surgery. Dtsch Arztebl Int 2008;105(43):741–746

10. Quetz J. Update on the Septal Pivot Flap. Facial Plast Surg 2014;30(3):300–305

Appendix

Jacques Joseph—My Personal Tribute

In cooperation with Walter Briedigkeit†

Each morning on my way to work, I pass by the grave of Jacques Joseph. Through a large gate in the side wall of the Jewish Cemetery in Berlin-Weissensee, not far from the Park-Klinik Weissensee hospital, I bid good morning to the founder and father of modern rhinoplasty. His grave was thought to have been destroyed by a bombing raid on Berlin during the Second World War and was believed to be lost.[1] Today, however, a large stone made of black granite bears large golden letters that commemorate his life and passing (**Fig. A.1**).

It was not always so. But although his grave was believed to be lost, in 2003, a few days before our "Essentials of Septorhinoplasty" international conference, Prof. Walter Briedigkeit informed me that, after years of persistent research, he was sure that he had located the grave and tombstone of Jacques Joseph (**Fig. A.2**).

The Jewish Cemetery in Berlin-Weissensee is the largest Jewish cemetery in Europe. Its long and tragic history was detailed in the recent film and book *Himmel auf Erden* (*Heaven on Earth*) by Britta Wauer and Amelie Losier.[2]

On just the second day of the conference, Prof. Briedigkeit called upon the participants from over 30 nations to launch a fund-raising effort for the restoration of Jacques Joseph's grave. The initiative and support of M. E. Tardy, Jr., were instrumental in finding numerous donors throughout the world.

On October 17, 2004, the grave was consecrated by the eminent Rabbi Andreas Nachama (**Fig. A.3**). During the international conference on "The Nose and Face" held in 2005, several attendees visited the restored grave site of Joseph (**Fig. A.4**).

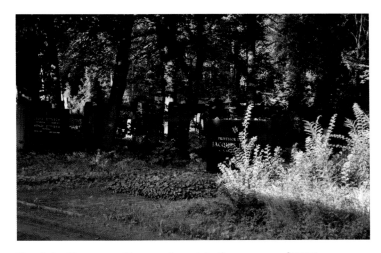

Fig. A.1 The grave of Jacques Joseph in the summer of 2012.

The biography of Jacques Joseph stayed with Prof. Briedigkeit and me, prompting us to follow several vague leads to documents dating from the period of Joseph's work in Berlin. One clue led us to Mrs. E. Stellmach, the widow of Prof. Rudolf Stellmach. We knew from the documentary film *Don't Call it Heimweh* by Thomas Halaschinski that a collection of original Jacques Joseph instruments did exist. Throughout his lifetime, Joseph developed

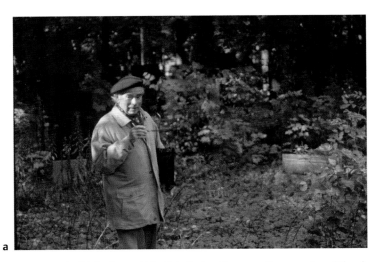

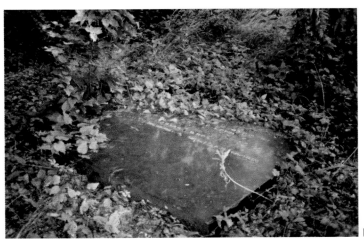

Fig. A.2 (**a, b**) Professor Briedigkeit standing near the remains of the damaged and partially buried tombstone of Jacques Joseph.

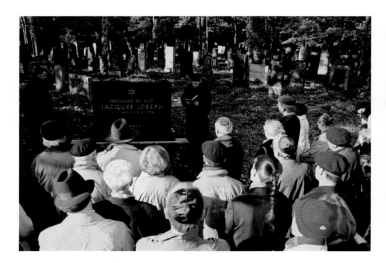

Fig. A.3 Consecration of the restored grave site.

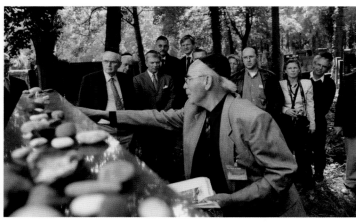

Fig. A.4 A visit to Jacques Joseph's grave during the international conference "Nose and Face" held in Berlin in 2005. The visitors included M. E. Tardy Jr., Regan Thomas, and Richard Goode.

special instruments for his own operations. He had each of his instruments engraved with the words "Prof. Joseph." Many of his students and close comrades-in-arms emigrated from Germany during the Nazi era. His original instruments were scattered all over the globe and were closely guarded like religious relics by renowned plastic surgeons. In 1969, Prof. Rudolf Stellmach (1924–2003) received several of Joseph's original instruments from Dr. Pabst, a plastic surgeon from Berlin-Grunewald. Stellmach, himself a respected plastic surgeon and a specialist in the field of facial malformation surgery, gathered together many more instruments from Joseph's star pupils including Gustave Aufricht, Joseph Safian, Samuel Fomon, Jacques Maliniac, and John Maurice Converse.[3,4]

We visited Mrs. Stellmach in her home and learned many details about the unique collection of the master's instruments. And then, she laid before us the collection of original instruments that had belonged to Jacques Joseph. At the end of our visit, Mrs. Stellmach made us a remarkable offer: "Why don't you just take the instruments with you! They'll be safer with you than with me." And so we finally did. Since 2007, the instruments have been on display at the Berlin Medical History Museum of the Charité as part of its permanent collection, *Dem Leben auf der Spur* (*On Life's Trail*) (**Fig. A.5**).

The exhibit includes an "historical infirmary" that traces the fates of eight illustrative patients. Visitors can experience how medicine affected people's lives in different periods of history. The patients' stories include that of an educator, Dr. Karl Hasbach,[5] who was conscripted as a lieutenant in the German Army in November, 1914. While Hasbach was serving on the French front in February of 1915, his nose and upper jaw were shattered by exploding shell fragments. In 1915 and 1916 he underwent 19 operations, apparently with poor results as he found it necessary to wear an artificial nose. Then, from 1916 to 1918, definitive reconstruction of his facial defects was performed by Jacques Joseph in Berlin.

Joseph had a private practice until June 2, 1916, when the Prussian Ministry of Education and Cultural Affairs appointed him the head of the newly formed Department of Facial Plastic Surgery at Berlin Charité Hospital. His department in the Ear and Nose Clinic was active from 1916 to 1922. Wounded soldiers were transported in railroad cars directly from the battlefield to the Friedrichstrasse train station and from there to Joseph's eight-bed unit (**Figs. A.6, A.7**).

Aided by the use of regional or forehead and upper-arm flaps as well as free cartilage and bone grafts, Joseph was able to accomplish masterful reconstructions of the face, like that achieved

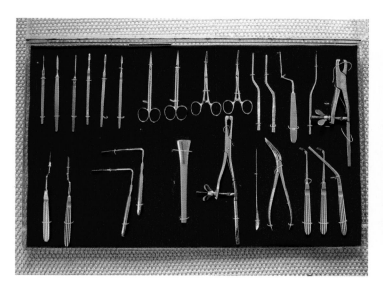

Fig. A.5 Original instruments that belonged to Jacques Joseph.

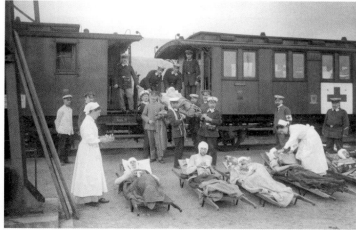

Fig. A.6 Wounded German soldiers arriving from the front. Combatants in World War I were sustaining craniofacial injuries on a previously unknown scale.

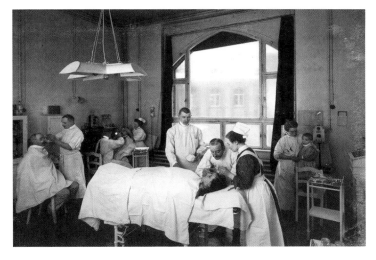

Fig. A.7 Admission ward at the Ear and Nose Clinic of Berlin Charité during Joseph's time.

for Karl Hasbach. He even fashioned implants out of ivory from the Bechstein piano factory in Berlin. Panels **a–f** in **Fig. A.8** show some examples of his surgical art during that time.

But who was Jacques Joseph really? The Hall of Fame of German surgeons contains only scant references to a man who today is credited with monumental advances in facial plastic surgery and especially in rhinosurgery. Joseph's career began in the Germany of Kaiser Wilhelm, earned him the highest professional acclaim and social reputation during the years of the Weimar Republic, and ended under the National Socialists with humiliation and blacklisting during the systematic persecution of the Jews. Joseph worked in Berlin all his life and refused to leave, although his wife Leonore and daughter Bella later emigrated to the United States.

Even during his lifetime, Joseph was a Berlin legend and was known as *Nasen-Joseph* ("Nose Joseph") or "Noseph" by Berliners. When the Army stopped financing the Department of Facial Plastic Surgery in 1922, Joseph returned to his private practice

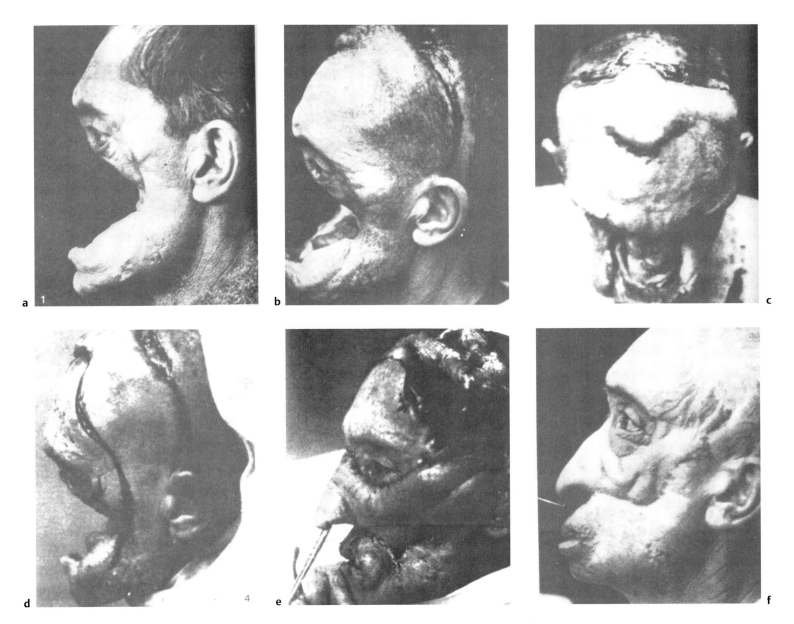

Fig. A.8 (**a–f**) Reconstructions of severe war injuries by Jacques Joseph during his time at the Berlin Charité.

at 63 Kurfurstendamm and devoted himself increasingly to corrective and aesthetic surgery (**Fig. A.9**).[6] Most of his work now involved plastic surgery on the nose and "sagging cheeks" as well as mammoplasties. Joseph gave surgical courses at a local hospital on Bulow Street and taught dissection classes at the Department of Anatomy at Charité Hospital.

An article published by the "roving reporter" Egon Erwin Kisch in 1922 gives us a glimpse of how Joseph ran his surgical practice from a waiting-room perspective. (Incidentally, Joseph's office was located in the same building as my current satellite clinic and office at 61 Kurfurstendamm in Berlin.)

> In his office on the Kurfurstendamm, Professor Joseph received people who were sick with vanity. He asked each one what he was, whether he was rich, and from which neighborhood he came. Then and only then did he ask about their character... and he needs to know their character, for he shapes their nose accordingly. "Would you like a saucy nose or an intelligent one, a flirty one or an energetic one?" .... The Professor hands his patients an album filled with hundreds of photographs of former patients, before and after the operation. They flip through the album pages and choose the nose that they would like to have. "Fine," says the Professor, and grabs them by the nose. He twists it with his hand and fingers to show them what they will look like after the surgery. "Come to my private clinic at Bülowstrasse 22 at ten o'clock tomorrow morning."

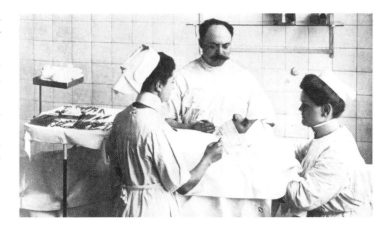

Fig. A.9 Jacques Joseph in his private clinic.

References

1. Natvig P. Jacques Joseph: Surgical Sculptor. Philadelphia, PA: WB Saunders; 1982

2. Wauer B, Losier A. The Weissensee Jewish Cemetery—Moments in History, 2010, be.bra verlag, 176 pp

3. Behrbohm H, Briedigkeit W, Kaschke O. Jacques Joseph: father of modern facial plastic surgery. Arch Facial Plast Surg 2008;10(5):300–303

4. Behrbohm H. Dem Leben auf der Spur—Jacques Joseph, ein Wegbereiter der plastischen Gesichts- und Nasenchirugie. ebook, Nasenkorrekturen, Oemus-media, 2011, www.zwp-online.de

5. Weerda H, Pirsig W. Jacques Joseph und der Patient Dr. Karl Hasbach. HNO aktuell 2006;14(7–8):274–278

6. Natvig P. Some aspects of the character and personality of Jacques Joseph. Plast Reconstr Surg 1971;47(5):452–453

7. Briedigkeit W, Behrbohm H. Jacques Joseph—ein Pionier der plastischen Gesichtschirurgie. Jüdische Miniaturen. Hentrich-Verlag; 2006, 61 pp

8. Briedigkeit W, Behrbohm H. Die Büste des Jacques Joseph Face. Oemus-Media 2012;3:56–58

Index

Note: Page numbers followed by f indicate figures.